Radiographic Imaging for the Dental Team

Sally M. Mauriello, RDH, MEd
Associate Professor
The University of North Carolina at Chapel Hill
School of Dentistry

Vickie P. Overman, RDH, MEd
Clinical Assistant Professor
The University of North Carolina at Chapel Hill
School of Dentistry

Enrique (Rick) Platin, RT, MS, EdD
Clinical Assistant Professor
The University of North Carolina at Chapel Hill
School of Dentistry

J.B. Lippincott Company
Philadelphia

Acquisitions Editor: Andrew Allen
Coordinating Editorial Assistant: Laura Dover
Production Service: Chernow Editorial Services, Inc.
Cover Designer: Larry Pezzato
Production Manager: Janet Greenwood
Editor Production: Mary Kinsella
Printer/Binder: Quebecor/Kingsport

6   5   4   3   2   1

Library of Congress Cataloging-in-Publication Data

Mauriello, Sally M.
    Radiographic imaging for the dental team / Sally M. Mauriello,
  Vickie P. Overman, Enrique Platin.
        p.   cm.
    Includes bibliographical references and index.
    ISBN 0-397-55020-0 (acid-free paper)
    1. Teeth—Radiography.   2. Dental auxilliary personnel.
  I. Overman, Vickie P.   II. Platin, Enrique.   III. Title.
  RK309.M384   1995
  617.6'07572—dc20   94-47615

♾ This Paper Meets the Requirements of ANSI/NISO Z39.48-1992 (Permanence of Paper).

To my family and friends who made the writing of this book possible. My husband Michael, for his patience, support, and understanding; my children Steven, Joseph, and Megan for their inspiration; my mother Thelma W. Murr for her unwavering love; and in memory of my father, George L. Murr, Jr.

Sally M. Mauriello

To my wonderful family with whom I have been blessed. A great deal of love and gratitude to my children, Emily and Zachary; my husband Gary for providing love and support; and my parents, Mr. and Mrs. J.E. McGuire, Sr., for their never ending support of my endeavors throughout my life.

Vickie P. Overman

To my family for always believing in me, especially my wife, Mary Ann, and my son, Ryan, who are a constant source of strength and inspiration.

Enrique (Rick) Platin

The authors also dedicate this book to Dr. Stephen R. Matteson for his mentoring and friendship during our educational and professional careers.

Preface

Dental radiology is one of the most important diagnostic components of dentistry. In the last few years, it has undergone dramatic changes. The use of computers and the integration of high-level technology requires that practitioners be better educated. Thus, the ability to provide radiologic services that are appropriate and safe to the patient and clinician can not be overemphasized. This premise is used for the foundation for this book. As such, it was written to reflect changes brought about by research, regulations, and the technological revolution. The authors hope that the information presented will fill this void.

This book is written by dental radiography professionals for dental team members. Therefore, readers will find the material presented in a logical sequence with extensive information, practical applications, and "know-how" techniques that will be useful in the clinical setting. Many examples, illustrations, and photographs complement the text. There are in-depth chapters on infection control, alternative radiographic procedures, supplemental radiographic procedures, patient management, quality assurance, pitfalls, radiology administration, and other relevant subjects.

In essence, our goal is to provide both the instruction and the rationale for the safe use of ionizing radiation and to maximize the practice of the ALARA (as low as reasonably achievable) principle. The book is divided into three main areas. The first provides information on x-ray production, biological effects of radiation, image receptors, and darkroom management. The second discusses topics dealing with patient care, such as infection control, projection geometry, radiographic techniques, patient management, radiographic anatomy, and interpretation. The third deals with radiographic administrative issues, such as quality assurance, pitfalls, and administrative policies.

Each chapter provides a set of objectives to guide the reader on expected outcomes, review questions for self-assessment, and suggested readings for the curious learner. The chapters are self-contained, designed to complement one another, and can be presented in any order. They are written in an easy to understand manner, with several examples provided to explain difficult concepts. The technique chapters were written in a step-by-step format to assist both the beginning learner and the experienced clinician. They describe the proper psychomotor skills needed for exposing radiographs, discuss problems that can occur with individual components, and offer appropriate problem-solving strategies. The content and radiographic techniques presented in this book are in compliance with the recommendations from the American Association of Dental Schools curricular guidelines, the American Academy of Oral and Maxillofacial Radiology, and the Commission on Dental Accreditation.

The authors hope that the content and format of this book will provide the reader with the necessary tools needed to become a competent dental radiographer and to provide a high level of patient care.

ACKNOWLEDGMENTS

The authors wish to express their appreciation and gratitude to the artist and photographers of the Learning Resources Center of the University of North Carolina School of Dentistry. Their contributions and talents complemented the text by bringing our ideas into visual concepts. In addition, we appreciate the patience and support of our colleagues and staff during the writing of this text, especially Donald A. Tyndall who provided valuable assistance in the preparation of the interpretation chapter. Ms. Overman extends her appreciation to Mary George, who has served as a mentor, colleague, and friend for many years, and to Dr. John Ludlow for his assistance with the anatomy chapter. Dr. Platin wishes to acknowledge Donald Tyndall, DDS, MPH, PhD, and Mark Kutcher, DDS, MS, for their time, efforts, and feedback in the writing of his chapters, and Ms. Angie Harper for providing her professional clerical skills. Appreciation is extended to our students, past and present, for their suggestions and encouragement, and for demonstrating that our educational techniques are effective. We thank the editor and staff of the J.B. Lippincott for their patience and guidance.

We are also grateful to those who reviewed the book: Su-Yan L. Barrow, RDH, RDA, BS, MA, of New York University; Barbara A. Brabandt, CDA, of Phoenix College; Bunny L. Byle, CDA, RDA, RDH, MS, of Grand Rapids Community College; Sharon Golightly, BS(N), MS(N), of Pierce College; Kathleen J. Hinshaw, CDA, EFDA, LDH, MSEd, of Indiana University Northwest; Florence Hockhauser, CDA, Guest Dental Assisting Lecturer; Frances Holbrook, CDA, Med, of Morton College; Mel L. Kantor, DDS, of UMDNJ Dental School New Jersey; Sandra L. Kolsom, CDA, RDA, of City College of San Francisco and Santa Rosa Junior College; and Stephanie Schmidt, CDA, RDA, CDT, of Simi Valley Adult School and Pasadena City College.

Sally M. Mauriello
Vickie P. Overman
Enrique Platin

Contents

Radiographic Imaging for the Dental Team,
by Sally Mauriello. J.B. Lippincott Company,
Philadelphia © 1995.

1

Development of Dental Radiology

Upon the completion of this chapter, the student should be able to:

1. Discuss the major events in the development of dental radiology.

2. Identify major contributors and researchers in radiation development and technology.

3. Discuss the public and governmental agencies that regulate the use of ionizing radiation.

HISTORY OF DENTAL RADIOLOGY

To fully understand the evolution of dental radiography, it is important to know the developments that led to the discovery of x-rays. The first step occurred in 1870, when Wilhelm Hittorf determined that the rays emitted by a partially evacuated discharge tube produced heat and had a greenish-yellow glow where they struck the glass. A scientist named Varley then determined that these rays were negatively charged particles by placing a magnet nearby and changing the path of the rays. These emissions were called "**cathode rays**" by Goldstein of Germany.

To experiment with these cathode rays, Sir William Crookes developed a tube that was subsequently named the Hittorf–Crookes tube. J.J. Thompson identified these particles as electrons after he compared their speed and the relationship between their mass and charge. Then in 1894 Philip Lenard developed a tube with an aluminum window that enabled him to study the cathode rays' behavior. By placing screens containing fluorescent salts outside the aluminum window, Lenard discovered that enough of the rays were able to penetrate the window to cause the fluorescent screens to glow. If he moved the screens further away, the amount of light emitted decreased. This revealed that cathode rays could be detected as far away as 6 to 8 cm.

As a result of these investigations, the following conclusions were made about the nature of cathode rays: 1) they were negatively charged particles; 2) they could be absorbed by 5 cm or less of air; 3) they caused fluorescence; and 4) they had mass.

On November 8, 1895, after repeating all of Lenard's known experiments, Dr. Wilhelm Conrad Roentgen, a professor of physics at the University of Wurzberg in Germany, studied the rays emitted from the Hittorf–Crookes tube in a darkened laboratory. He noticed that a faint glow was being produced on a fluorescent screen some distance away from the tube. As he applied power to the tube, which he had covered in black cardboard, he realized the source causing the screen to glow was well beyond the distance that known cathode rays could be detected. Dr. Roentgen deemed this unknown type of energy "x-radiation." By accident, he also discovered that if he placed his hand in the line of the beam, the bones of his hand could be seen on the screen. This was the beginning of radiology.

Roentgen continued to experiment with the rays by placing different objects in their path. He determined that the beam could be diminished by varying degrees depending on what was placed in its path. The only material that completely absorbed the beam was lead. Following these discoveries, he learned that images of the body could be produced on photographic plates. He placed his wife's hand on a photographic plate and exposed it to the rays for 15 minutes. When the plate was developed, it showed the outlines of the bones of her hand and the shadows of the surrounding flesh. This was the first radiograph taken of the human body. After many experiments, he defined the following properties of x-rays:

1. they exhibited differential attenuation (distinguished between various thicknesses of materials);

2. they caused a screen to fluoresce and affected photographic plates;

3. they were made of pure energy (had no mass);

4. they traveled in straight lines; and

5. they had no charge.

For this work, Roentgen was awarded the first Nobel Prize in Physics in 1901.

Just 14 days after Roentgen's discovery, Otto Walkhoff of Germany took the first dental radiograph. This exposure took approximately 25 minutes. But it was Dr. W.J. Morton, a physician who promoted the use of x-rays in dentistry, who took the first whole body radiograph. Although it is difficult to determine who took the first dental radiograph in the United States, Dr. C. Edmund Kells, a New Orleans dentist, made many significant contributions to dental radiography. In 1896, he took the first *intraoral* radiograph on a patient using his own equipment and a technique he had devised. In July 1896, he presented the first clinical demonstration of dental x-rays in Asheville, North Carolina, at the Southern Dental Association meeting.

Unfortunately, Dr. Kells also demonstrated the potentially harmful effects of x-rays with his practice of "setting the tube." He used this procedure to adjust the quality of the beam. He placed his hand in front of the beam and adjusted the tube until the image of his hand was seen clearly. As a result of this exposure, he experienced increasing erythema (redness of the skin) and pain. Subsequently, his fingers, hand, and ultimately his arm had to be amputated. After numerous operations, he committed suicide on May 7, 1928, at the age of 72.

In addition to Kells, other early pioneers in dental radiography include William H. Rollins, who developed the first dental x-ray unit in 1896, as well as intraoral film holders, and W.D. Coolidge, who developed the hot cathode tube, a forerunner of today's x-ray tubes. In addition, Rollins proposed several innovative ideas concerning radiation protection that have served as forerunners for today's safe use of radiation. They included the use of filters to remove the dangerous parts of the x-ray beam, the use of collimation to reduce the beam size, and draping the patient with a material that the x-rays could not penetrate. He also urged that the use of a long target-to-film distance would increase the quality of the image. He suggested that, with the exception of the port, the tube should be shielded. Rollins also introduced the concept of placing film between two intensifying screens to reduce patient exposure. Twenty-two years before the establishment of the maximum permissible dose, Rollins indicated that both safe and harmful dose limits should be set. Around 1918, Coolidge and the General Electric (G.E.) Corporation introduced the Victor CDX dental x-ray machine, which placed the x-ray tube in an oil-filled, grounded compartment. This eliminated the patient's accidental exposure to high voltage shock, while also insulating and cooling the machine. Current x-ray units employ a similar design.

Further developments and improvements in x-ray imaging include variable kVp machines, introduced by G.E. in 1957, electrical timers, constant potential generators, filtration, and improvements in film speed. In addition, imaging techniques were enhanced. Weston Price of Cleveland devised the bisecting the angle technique. Kells recommended the paralleling technique, which McCormack pioneered for use in dentistry.

Dr. H. Numatat of Japan first proposed the concept of rotational panoramics in 1933. He placed a curved film in the patient's mouth and used a narrow x-ray beam (or slit) that rotated around the patient's jaw to expose the film. Then in 1946, Dr. Yrjo Paatero, of the University of Helsinki, experimented with this method. First he used a curved intraoral film and a stationary narrow x-ray beam. The patient rotated by means of a moving chair. Later he continued to have a stationary x-ray beam, but placed the film external and had both the patient and film moving.

In the early 1950s, Dr. Robert J. Nelson, of the University of Washington, and Mr. John Kumpula also experimented with the development of an automatic panographic machine that would allow the selection of a variety of movements according to the patient's size and shape. But it was Dr. Paatero who in 1959 created the first orthopantomograph unit that would take acceptable radiographs. In 1961, the first commercially manufactured Orthopantomograph became available.

In a later advance, Dr. Donald Hudson and John Kumpula designed a system in which the film and radiation source moved in opposite directions while the patient remained stationary. This was the beginning of the panoramic x-ray machine (later called the Panorex). In 1980, Dr. Charles Morris developed the Panorex II, which allowed either a split or continuous image to be made.

Since the early 1970s many types of panoramic x-ray machines have become available. These offer a variety of imaging features and focal trough shapes to accommodate the needs of the patient and the dentist.

X-ray film also changed from the original glass photographic plates. In 1913 Eastman Kodak introduced the first hand-wrapped dental x-ray film packets. Then in 1924, Dr. Howard R. Raper designed the first bitewing film packet. As a result, film packets now offer high-speed, double-emulsion films that produce excellent quality images with minimal exposure to the patient.

OVERVIEW OF RADIATION EFFECTS

Scientific journals, government agencies, and the public media have frequently discussed the hazardous effects of **ionizing radiation** from both natural and artificial sources. With the growing concern about sources of radiation, the public has exhibited an increased awareness of the effects of low-level radiation exposure. It is not unusual for a patient to refuse essential diagnostic radiographic examinations. As health professionals, we need to be aware of the public concern and be informed about the hazards, as well as the benefits, of radiographs. Only then, can we give accurate information in a meaningful manner to our patients about the risks versus the benefits of diagnostic radiographic examinations. We can no longer simply inform a patient that radiation exposure during dental x-rays is so small that it is nothing to worry about. As allied dental professionals, we need to be able to explain the biological effects of radiation, dose equivalents, and the risks versus benefits of radiographic examinations used in the dental profession.

Certainly, we are not using a risk-free medium to record this diagnostic information. The largest man-made source of radiation exposure for humans is through medical and dental examinations (about 15 percent of the average annual dose for the U.S. population). Yet, we are all exposed to other sources and types of radiation (Table 1-1). These include man-made sources, such as building materials and luminous goods (i.e., television), as well as natural sources (i.e., cosmic rays, rock, soil, and minerals) (Table 1-2).

To regulate radiation exposure for the general public as well as for professional personnel, the use of radiation and radiation-producing equipment is governed by state, national, and international agencies. The International Commission on Radiologic Protection (ICRP) is a nongovernmental organization that strongly influences the regulations enacted by many national and international agencies. This commission regularly publishes recommendations on dose limits that serve as the basis for legislative action. The **National Council on Radiation Protection and Measurements (NCRP)** is a nonprofit agency that makes many recommendations on occupational radiation exposure.

TABLE 1-1
Average annual effective dose equivalent of ionizing radiations
for a member of the U.S. population

	mSv	*%*
Natural		
Radon	2.0	55.0
Cosmic	0.27	8.0
Terrestial	0.28	8.0
Internal	0.39	11.0
Artificial		
Medical		
X-ray diagnosis	0.39	11.0
Nuclear medicine	0.14	4.0
Consumer products	0.10	3.0
Other		
Occupational	<0.01	<0.3
Nuclear fuel cycle	<0.01	<0.03
Fallout	<0.01	<0.03
Total	3.6	100

Reprinted with permission from HEALTH EFFECTS OF EXPOSURE TO LOWER
LEVELS OF IONIZING RADIATION. Copyright 1990 by the National Academy of Sciences. Courtesy of the National Academy Press, Washington, D.C.

This agency defines the occupational radiation exposure an individual
can receive during a specified period of time without any significant radiation side effects. Although this agency has significant impact on
radiation practices, it has no force of law with which to enforce its
recommendations. The International Commission on Radiation Units
and Measurements (ICRU) is an agency that makes recommendations on radiological units of measurement. The organization that
establishes radiation protection regulations is the **Nuclear Regulatory**

TABLE 1-2
Sources of natural and man-made radiation

Type	*Natural Source*	*Man-Made Source*
alpha	Soil, rock, minerals	Self-illuminating materials
beta	Soil, rock, minerals, po-tassium 40 (internally)	Television
gamma	Cosmic radiation	Dental and medical x-rays
neutron	None	Nuclear power plants, nuclear waste, nuclear weapons

Commission (NRC), formally known as the Atomic Energy Commission. Its regulations apply to the nuclear reactors, reactor fuel, and radioactive materials produced by reactor operation. The **Environmental Protection Agency (EPA)** is responsible for setting environmental radiation standards which are generally acceptable. The **Occupational Safety and Health Administration (OSHA)** is responsible for all occupational radiation protection regulations that are not regulated by the NRC. OSHA can choose to transfer its responsibility to the states. The **Bureau of Radiological Health (BRH),** now called the National Center for Devices and Radiological Health, regulates the manufacture of radiation-producing equipment, such as x-ray machines and microwave ovens. In addition, the **Bureau of Mines and Mining Safety and Health Administration** is responsible for occupational radiation protection regulation for uranium mines. Each state also has its own bureau of radiation safety, which governs practices within that state. These state bureaus are responsible for upholding the state practice acts governing radiation practices.

In addition to these agencies and bureaus, an important program has provided us with valuable information concerning radiation exposure practices. Entitled the **National Evaluation of X-ray Trends (NEXT),** it is carried out jointly by the state and federal governments in order to compile nationwide data on radiation exposure in dental offices. This data is collected yearly and analyzed to provide the most recent dose comparisons depending on technique and examination type.

SUMMARY

This chapter has reviewed the major events in the development of dental radiology. It has also identified the significant people in the history of radiation technology. The agencies, both private and public, that regulate the use of radiation have also been discussed.

BIBLIOGRAPHY

BENNETT J. Oral Care of Cancer Patients Undergoing Head and Neck Irradiation. *Dental Hygiene* 1979; 53(5): 209–212.

BOMBERGER A, DANNENFELSER BA. *Radiation and Health Principles and Practice in Therapy and Disaster Preparedness.* Rockville, MD: Aspen, 1984.

BUSHONG SC. *Radiologic Science for Technologists: Physics, Biology and Protection,* 3d ed. St. Louis: CV Mosby, 1984.

COUNCIL ON DENTAL MATERIALS, INSTRUMENTS, AND EQUIPMENT. Recommendations in Radiographic Practices. *JADA* 1984; 109(5): 764–765.

COUNCIL ON DENTAL MATERIALS, INSTRUMENTS, AND EQUIPMENT. Biological Effects of Radiation from Dental Radiography. *JADA* 1982; 105 (Aug.): 275–281.

COUNCIL ON DENTAL MATERIALS, INSTRUMENTS, AND EQUIPMENT. Recommendations in Radiographic Practices: An Update, 1988. *JADA* 1989; 118(1): 115–117.

CURRY III TS, DOWDY JE, MURRY JR RC. *Christensen's Physics of Diagnostic Radiology,* 4th ed. Philadelphia: Lea & Febiger, 1990.

FROMMER H. *Radiology for Dental Auxiliaries,* 5th ed. St. Louis: Mosby Year Book, 1992.

GIBBS SJ, ET AL. Patient Risk from Rotational Panoramic Radiography. *Dentomaxillofac Radiol* 1988; 17(1): 25–32.

GIBBS SJ ET AL. Radiation Doses to Sensitive Organs from Intra-oral Dental Radiography. *Dentomaxillofac Radiol* 1987; 16(2): 67–77.

GIBBS SJ, PUJOL JR A, CHEN TS, JAMES JR A. Patient Risk from Intraoral Dental Radiography. *Dentomaxillofac Radiol* 1988; 17(1): 15–23.

GOAZ PW, WHITE SC. *Oral Radiology Principles and Interpretation,* 2d ed. Philadelphia: CV Mosby, 1987.

GRANIER R, GAMBINI DJ. *Applied Radiation Biology and Protection.* New York: Ellis Horwood, 1990.

HENDEE WR. *Health Effects of Low-Level Radiation.* Norwalk, CT: Appleton-Century-Crofts, 1984.

HORIOT JC, BONE MC, IBRAHIM E, CASTRO JR. Systematic Dental Management in Head and Neck Irradiation. *Radiation Oncology– Biology Physics* 1981; 7(8): 1025–1029.

KEIFER, JURGEN. *Biological Radiation Effects.* New York: Springer-Verlag, 1990.

LANGLAND OE ET AL. *Panoramic Radiology.* 2d ed, Philadelphia: Lea and Febiger, 1989.

LANGLAND OE, SIPPY FH, LANGLAIS RP. *Textbook of Dental Radiology,* 2d ed. Springfield, IL: Charles C. Thomas, 1984.

MATTESON SR, WHALEY C, SECRIST VC. *Dental Radiology,* 4th ed. Chapel Hill, NC: University of North Carolina Press, 1988.

MILES DA, VANDIS ML, JENSEN CW, FERRETTI A. *Radiographic Imaging for Dental Auxiliaries.* Philadelphia: WB Saunders, 1989.

NATIONAL COUNCIL ON RADIATION PROTECTION AND MEASUREMENTS. *Exposure of the U.S. Population from Diagnostic Medical Radiation.* NCRP Report No. 100, Bethesda, MD, 1989.

NATIONAL COUNCIL ON RADIATION PROTECTION AND MEASUREMENTS. *Exposure of the U.S. Population from Occupational Radiation.* NCRP Report No. 101, Bethesda, MD, 1989.

NATIONAL RESEARCH COUNCIL. *BEIR V: Health Effects of Exposure to Low Levels of Ionizing Radiation.* Washington, DC: National Academy Press, 1990.

NORTH CAROLINA DEPARTMENT OF ENVIRONMENT, HEALTH, AND NATURAL RESOURCES, DIVISION OF RADIATION PROTECTION. *North Carolina Regulations for Protection Against Radiation.* Raleigh, NC, 1991.

SULLIVAN DM, FLEMING TJ. Oral Care for the Radiotherapy-Treated Head and Neck Cancer Patient. *Dental Hygiene* 1986; 60(3): 112–114.

WHITE SC. An Update on the Effects of Low-Dose Radiation. *AAOMR Newsletter* 1990; 17(4): 1–7.

REVIEW QUESTIONS

1. List the properties of x-rays.

   a.
   b.
   c.
   d.
   e.

2. The largest source of radiation exposure to the public is through

   a. building materials.
   b. medical and dental examinations.
   c. nuclear power plants.
   d. televisions.

3. The main job of the National Council on Radiation Protection and Measurements (NCRP) is to

   a. define occupational radiation exposure limits.
   b. enforce radiation safety laws.
   c. establish radiation protection regulations.
   d. compile data on radiation exposure.

4. Radiation is a risk-free medium used to diagnosis medical and dental problems.

   a. True
   b. False

5. Each state has its own bureau for regulating radiation practices.

   a. True
   b. False

Radiographic Imaging for the Dental Team,
by Sally Mauriello. J.B. Lippincott Company,
Philadelphia © 1995.

2

Infection Control in Dental Radiography

Upon the completion of this chapter, the student should be able to:

1. Understand the rationale for performing infection control procedures in dental radiography.

2. Describe the levels of disinfection and sterilization required in the radiography operatory.

3. Describe the two most common modes of disease transmission in radiography.

4. Describe the components of an infection control policy in dental radiography.

5. Discuss an acceptable infection control protocol that could be used in radiography.

6. Describe current federal guidelines governing infection control in the radiography area.

7. Discuss appropriate procedures that should be used in the removal of contaminated waste from the radiography area.

Transmission of infectious diseases is a major concern in dentistry. The radiography area presents infection control problems because of the potential for operator contamination and cross-contamination to other patients and office workers. Constant movement by the operator from the oral cavity to the exposure controls outside of the operatory to the darkroom, and finally, to film mounting increases the risk of a break occurring in the "chain of asepsis." Thus, the likelihood of exposing the operator as well as other patients to infectious disease is increased.

Recognition of appropriate procedures that should be used to disinfect and sterilize the radiography operatory and instruments will help to decrease the transmission of harmful microorganisms. The operator is responsible for providing a safe environment when radiographs are to be exposed as well as for rendering a radiograph with good diagnostic quality. Therefore, this chapter will discuss the components of infection control that should be used in the radiography area.

AGENCIES DEVELOPING GUIDELINES AND RECOMMENDATIONS

Several federal, state, and professional agencies govern health professions in the handling of bloodborne **pathogens.** The Occupational Safety and Health Administration (OSHA) has played a leading role in the protection of the employee who works with bloodborne pathogens. Although dental radiographers do not commonly come into contact with blood, they are unable to expose **radiographs** without coming into contact with saliva, which OSHA defines (1991) as "a potentially infectious material." Therefore, stringent procedures should be followed in radiography to prevent the contamination and cross-contamination of infectious diseases. The modes of transmission most likely to occur in radiography are direct contact with an infectious lesion or a passive contamination resulting indirectly from an infected counter or processor.

Other agencies that are important in setting regulations are the Environmental Protection Agency (EPA) and Food and Drug Administration (FDA). The EPA regulates surface disinfectants. Thus, effective agents will carry an EPA approval seal. The FDA is responsible for monitoring the marketing of chemicals used to disinfect and sterilize objects in the radiography area.

Agencies responsible for making recommendations are the American Dental Association (ADA), the Center for Disease Control (CDC), and the Office Sterilization and Asepsis Procedures (OSAP). The ADA plays an important role in coordinating the regulations and recommendations set forth by the various agencies. The CDC played a major role in developing the "Universal Precaution" policy. OSAP concentrates on disseminating infection control information to the practicing dentist in a usable format to encourage compliance in the dental office.

These agencies are a valuable information resource in developing and maintaining a high level of infection control in the dental practice.

DISINFECTION AND STERILIZATION IN THE DENTAL OFFICE

A good "rule of thumb" to use in infection control is to never disinfect when you can sterilize. Based on Spaulding's Classification of Inanimate Objects, surfaces that come into contact with intact mucous membranes, but do not enter normally sterile areas of the body, are classified as semicritical. In radiography, semicritical items (i.e., position-indicating devices) should be sterilized or treated with a high level of disinfection. Noncritical items, which are defined as surfaces that do not commonly touch mucous membranes, should be cleaned and disinfected after every use with a tuberculocidal intermediate level of disinfection (i.e., **tubehead** or lead-lined **collimator**).

Therefore, disinfection and sterilization procedures are required for nondisposable objects used during the exposure, processing, and mounting of radiographs. Disinfection should be performed using an EPA- and ADA-approved tuberculocidal intermediate-level disinfectant. The method should include the spray–wipe–spray technique. This allows the surface to first be cleaned and then for the disinfectant to work properly. Directions on the label should be carefully read and followed, because some chemical agents only clean and others only disinfect. Sterilization should include the use of steam or dry heat. If this is not possible, sterilization with ethylene oxide is an acceptable technique.

COMPONENTS OF INFECTION CONTROL FOR RADIOGRAPHY

Operatory

The first step in infection control is to determine the surfaces to be disinfected. In general, surfaces that can not be easily disinfected should be protected by a barrier—most commonly plastic or foil barriers. In the radiography operatory, these surfaces include the chair back, arm rests, headrest, and adjustment apparatus; the tubehead and arms holding the tubehead; the lead apron; and the knobs on the control panel (Figure 2-1(A-C)). The lead holder used for storing exposed

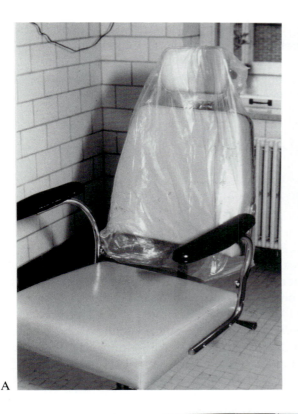
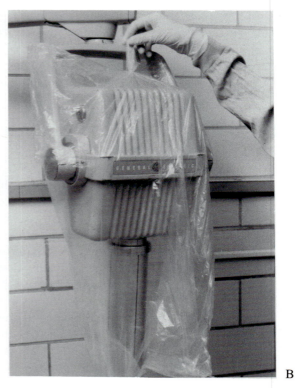
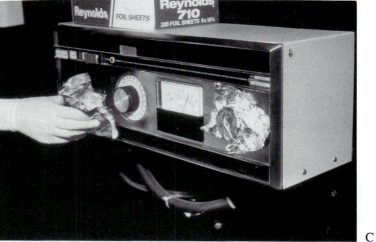

FIGURE 2-1 The proper use of barrier methods for infection control in (A) chair back, (B) unit, and (C) knobs on the control panel.

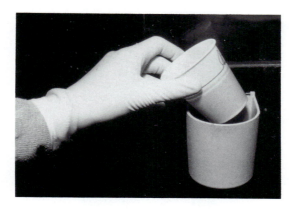

FIGURE 2-2 The use of a paper cup to line the lead receptacle that will hold exposed films.

films should be protected by inserting a paper cup or using another type of barrier (Figure 2-2). The exposure switch can be covered by foil or plastic, or can be converted to a foot control (Figure 2-3). Barrier methods are the method of choice on electrical switches because of the possibility of the cleaner and disinfectant causing an electrical short. On **extraoral** equipment, the **bite block** is the main piece of equipment that may come into contact with the mucous membranes. Therefore, the piece should be sterilized or protected with a plastic barrier (Figure 2-4). Other parts of the equipment that come into contact with the patient should be cleaned and disinfected.

Once the **radiography** operatory is set up, the film and film-holding devices should be prepared. The area should be disinfected and then a barrier method employed. This can be a paper sheet, paper towels, or plastic cover (Figure 2-5). If the paper products are not backed with an impervious material, the countertop must be disinfected after its use. Prior to beginning the procedure, secure all the supplies that may be needed during radiographic procedure in order to decrease the chance of cross-contamination. For example, anticipate the type of film-holding devices, cotton rolls, and bitewing tabs that may be needed if a patient has an edentulous area. *If supplies are needed during the procedure, remove the used gloves prior to obtaining them or ask for assistance from someone not involved in the procedure.* The use of over-gloves (food handler's gloves) are also appropriate. They slip over contaminated gloves and can be used to open drawers, doors, or containers to prevent cross-contamination. Films and film-holding devices should be placed on the barrier used. Once the procedure is completed, the barriers should be discarded. Surfaces not protected by barriers should be cleaned and disinfected. Nondisposable film holders should be sterilized after each use. During the clean-up procedure, the exam-

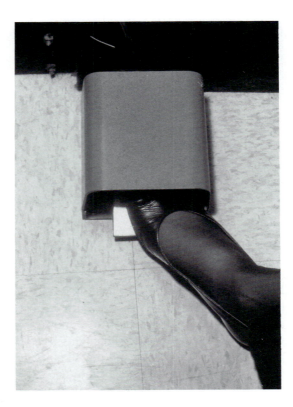

FIGURE 2-3 An exposure switch can be controlled by a foot pedal to maintain infection control.

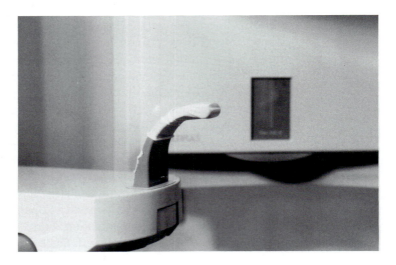

FIGURE 2-4 The bite block on an extraoral unit should be protected with a disposable plastic covering.

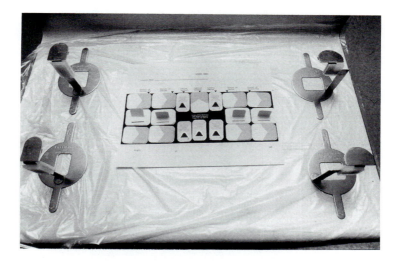

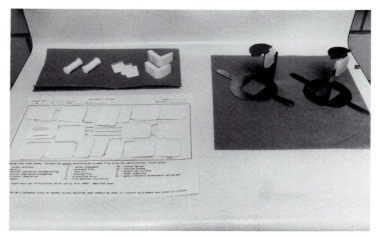

FIGURE 2-5 Two examples of countertops that have been properly disinfected and set up for a radiographic procedure.

ination gloves should be discarded and heavy-duty protective gloves used. A sink should be located in or close to the radiography area. Ideally, water controls should be operated by foot pedals or a knee lever (Figure 2-6). Hands should always be washed prior to donning gloves and immediately after removal.

Darkroom

The **processor** is probably one of the most difficult and crucial areas to disinfect. Regardless of whether a manual or an automatic processor with a daylight loader is used, films should always be "clean" or

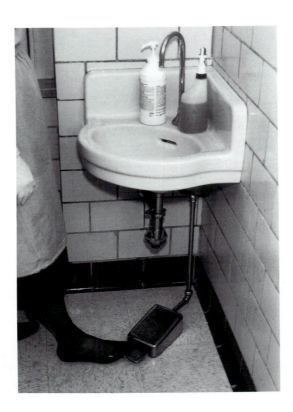

FIGURE 2-6   For infection control, the water flow in a sink can be controlled by foot pedals.

uncontaminated prior to beginning processing. To accomplish this step, the operator will be required to remove the "dirty" **film packets** from the container that is used to hold exposed films without contaminating clean gloved hands. For example, if a paper cup has lined the lead receptacle used to hold exposed films, then grasp the cup on the outer edges to prevent contamination of the clean gloved hands. The operator should then proceed to the darkroom or processing area. As in the operatory, the work counter in the darkroom should be disinfected and protected with a barrier during the processing procedure. Film packaging and processor type will determine the method of infection control that should be used during processing. If the film packet was pre-packaged in a plastic infection control envelope or barrier envelope, then the plastic envelope should be opened and the film packet dropped on a "clean" surface (Figure 2-7). The contaminated envelope should then be placed in an empty paper cup. After all the film packets have been removed from the plastic, the gloves should be removed with the inside out. If desired, hands could be washed to remove excess powder

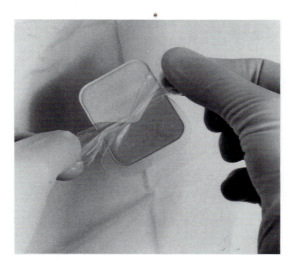

FIGURE 2-7 An uncontaminated film packet
is removed from its prepackaged plastic
envelope before processing.

remaining from the gloves or don clean gloves. At this point, the
uncontaminated film packets can be opened and the film placed in the
daylight loader and processed. If a manual processor is used, the film
packets can be opened and placed on the film rack for processing, as
discussed in Chapter 6. Once the films are processed, the contaminated
packets should be placed in a container marked with a biohazard sign.

Film packets without a barrier envelope present a problem in processing with a daylight loader. If the films placed in the processor are
contaminated, they will exit the processor contaminated. Therefore, it
is imperative to put uncontaminated films in the processor. One method
for achieving this goal is to place the paper cup of exposed films into a
daylight loader that has been lined with paper towels. Since it is virtually impossible to disinfect the cuffs in the daylight loader, the cup
should be placed in the daylight loader through the removable filter
window (Figure 2-8). Replace the filter and insert clean gloved hands
through the hand portals (Figure 2-9). (Hands can be double-gloved at
this point to allow for handling of contaminated films with the first set
of gloves. The second set of gloves can be used for handling uncontaminated film.) Film packets should be opened, and the film removed
by pulling the black paper wrapping out until the film drops on the
paper towel (Figure 2-10). Care should be taken to keep the film from
touching the contaminated polyvinyl film packet. Once this step is
completed, the contaminated gloves should be removed inside out to
prevent cross-contamination (Figure 2-11). The uncontaminated films

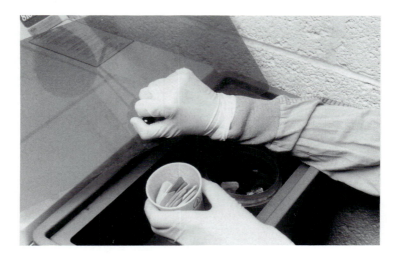

FIGURE 2-8 The proper placement of the cup holding
contaminated film packets into the daylight loader is through
the removable filter window.

can then be placed into the processor. Once all the films have been
placed in the processor, the contaminated film packets should be removed from the daylight loader through the filter window.

Contaminated films can be treated with a disinfectant before processing by using the spray–wipe–spray technique, and then allowing
the disinfectant to dry for the length of time recommended by the
manufacturer's instructions. Films can also be immersed in disinfectant
solutions for the recommended length of time to remove bioburden.

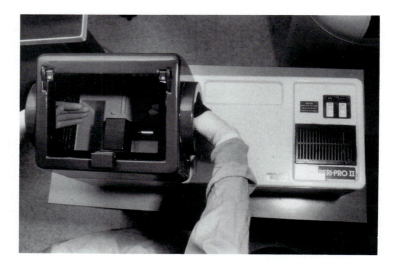

FIGURE 2-9 Clean gloved hands inserted through the portals.

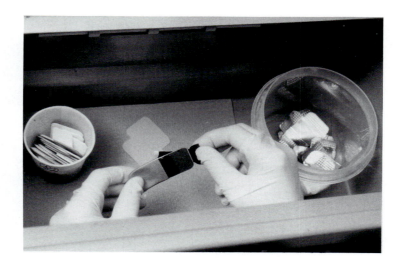

FIGURE 2-10 Clean film is being removed from the
contaminated packet and dropped on a paper towel.

Either technique would be appropriate and acceptable for reducing
contaminants prior to processing, but can be performed *only* on polysoft film packets. Paper film packets will not protect the film from
disinfectant damage due to immersion.

Processed films should be removed from the processor with gloved
hands and placed in a film mount (Figure 2-12). Ideally, the mount of

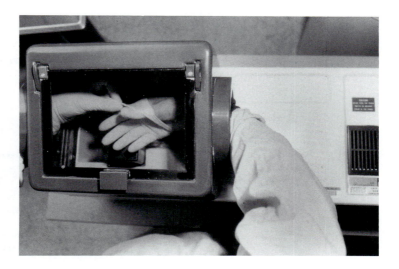

FIGURE 2-11 The proper way to remove contaminated gloves
is to turn them inside out. This prevents cross-contamination.

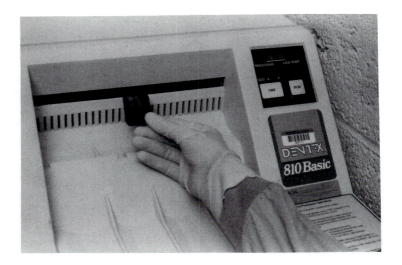

FIGURE 2-12   Processed films should be removed with gloved hands.

choice would be one that could be disinfected (i.e., a mount with a plastic covering or plastic windows) (Figure 2-13).

Operator Protection

In addition to providing a "clean environment," the operator should also be aware of procedures to insure personal safety. This is for the benefit of the patient *and* the operator. As mentioned earlier, the first line of protection is to wash the hands before donning the examination gloves. A mask is not required, but is strongly encouraged because of an occasionally overactive Wharton's salivary duct. Eyewear is also optional. Protective clothing should be worn and disposed of in the

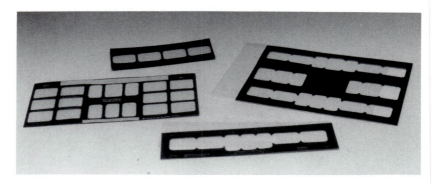

FIGURE 2-13   There are various types of films mounts that can be disinfected.

proper receptacle for separate laundering. A second line of protection is immunization against hepatitis B and routine testing for tuberculosis.

DEVELOPMENT OF AN INFECTION CONTROL PROTOCOL

Every dental office should have an infection control protocol to use in dental radiography. It will not only help ensure that a proper procedure is being used, but will also help to orient new staff to the appropriate protocol for that office. An easy approach for developing a protocol would be to devise a checklist. Steps should be defined for four primary areas: preparation of the operatory, exposure of the films, processing of the films, and disposal/clean-up of the operatory.

DISPOSAL OF HAZARDOUS MATERIAL IN THE RADIOGRAPHY AREA

Both the lead foil backing found in the film packet and the silver accumulated in the processing chemicals are hazardous materials to the environment. Therefore, it is important to dispose of these materials properly. The lead foil can be saved or the silver reclaimed and sold to scrap metal companies. These wastes should be disposed of according to federal, state, or local regulations.

SUMMARY

Infection control in radiography is an integral component in patient care. Prevention of disease transmission is the responsibility of the operator, and asepsis should be maintained at all times during exposure, processing, and mounting of radiographs. By using proper disinfection and sterilization techniques, barrier methods, and protective measures for the operator, the health professional can insure a safe environment for both the operator and patient.

BIBLIOGRAPHY

AUTIO KL, ROSEN S, REYNOLDS NJ, BRIGHT JS. Studies on Cross-Contamination in the Dental Clinic. *JADA* 1980; 100: 358–361.

COTTONE JA, TEREZHALMY GT, MOLINARI JA. *Practical Infection Control in Dentistry*. Philadelphia: Lea and Febiger, 1991.

KATZ JO, COTTONE JA, HARDMAN PK, TAYLOR TS. Infection Control in Dental School Radiology. *J Dent Educ* 1989; 53: 222–225.

WATHEN WF, KOLSTAD RA. *Kodak Dental Products.* Infection Control in Modern Dental Practice. Rochester, NY, 1992.

WHITE SC, GLAZE S. Interpatient Microbiological Cross-Contamination after Dental Radiographic Examination. *JADA* 1978; 96: 801–804.

REVIEW QUESTIONS

1. Disease transmission in radiology will most likely occur from

    a. direct contact with an infectious lesion.
    b. contamination from an infected counter top.
    c. contamination from an infected processor.
    d. all of the above.
    e. none of the above.

2. The components of an infection control protocol in dental radiography include

    a. operatory.
    b. darkroom.
    c. operator.
    d. a and c only.
    e. all of the above.

3. Both the lead foil and silver found in the processing chemicals should be treated a hazardous or contaminated waste.

    a. True
    b. False

4. Film-holding devices are considered semicritical items that require a low level of disinfection.

    a. True
    b. False

5. The product used for disinfection should be a tuberculocidal intermediate-level disinfectant approved by _____ and _____.

Radiographic Imaging for the Dental Team,
by Sally Mauriello. J.B. Lippincott Company,
Philadelphia © 1995.

3

Radiation Biology and Protection

Upon the completion of this chapter, the student should be able to:

1. Identify and define both traditional and metric radiation units of measurement.

2. Describe the effects radiation may have on molecules, cells, and organisms.

3. Describe common effects of radiation on humans.

4. Describe and apply the basic principles of radiation protection.

5. Describe the effects of radiation therapy on patients.

6. Apply professional judgment in using patient selection criteria for radiation exposure.

7. Provide patients with risk estimation information concerning radiation exposure.

In order to practice radiation safety, operators must understand the basic principles and tools of radiation biology and protection. These include the basic units of measurement, the effects of radiation, judgment in selection criteria, radiation protection, and risk estimation.

By classifying radiation in terms of units of exposure, exposure data can be compared and related to the side effects experienced by humans. Several terms are used to define radiation units. There are traditional terms used for these units of measurement. In addition, the updated metric system units called SI (Système Internationale d'Unités) are now being used more widely.

Unit of Exposure. The traditional unit of exposure, called the **Roentgen (R),** is defined as the measurement of exposure of air. One R is the amount of x or gamma radiation that will ionize one cubic centimeter of air. This defines the intensity of the radiation on an object. The SI unit normally associated with the Roentgen is the **Coulomb per kilogram (C/kg).** One R equals 2.58×10^{-4} C/kg.

Absorbed Dose. Absorption of radiation is measured by the **rad (radiation absorbed dose),** which is defined as the radiation energy imparted or absorbed in a mass. The SI unit for this term is the **Gray (Gy).** One rad is equal to 100 gy.

Dose Equivalent. The unit defined as the dose equivalent is the **rem (Roentgen-Equivalent-Man).** This unit is used to compare the biological effects of different types of radiation exposure. The **quality factor (QF)** is a number that helps relate different types of radiation (such as gamma or x-radiation) to similar effects in biological systems. The QF is related to the **relative biological effectiveness (RBE),** which is determined by measuring the damages produced by different types of radiation. The rem is determined by multiplying the QF by the rad. The SI unit associated with rem is the **Sievert (Sv).** One rem equals 100 Sv.

Linear Energy Transfer. LET is the amount of energy that is given up by ionizing radiation along a specified measure of length as it passes through the tissue. This concept allows us to place a numerical value on the type of radiation according to the tissue damage it causes. Usually, the higher the LET, the more damaging the biological effect.

The radiation to which we expose our patients are at fairly low levels. Some typical doses used in dental radiography are shown in Table 3-1.

EFFECTS OF RADIATION ON MOLECULES

Exposure of atoms to x-ray photons can damage a molecule by removing electrons from the atoms, thereby creating an **ion pair** (a negatively charged electron and a positively charged atom). This ability to create

TABLE 3-1
Typical exposures at skin entry ($\mu c/kg^{-1}$)

D Speed Film

Projection	70 kVp	80 kVp	90 kVp
Max molar	116	77.4	64.5
Max anterior	77.4	51.6	38.7
Mand molar	77.4	51.6	38.7
Mand anterior	58.1	38.7	32.3
Molar BW	77.4	51.6	38.7

E Speed Film

Projection	70 kVp	80 kVp	90 kVp
Max molar	58.1	38.7	36.1
Max anterior	38.7	25.8	21.9
Mand molar	38.7	25.8	21.9
Mand anterior	28.4	19.4	18.1
Molar BW	38.7	25.8	21.9

Source: Gibb, S.J. et al., *Dentonaxillofacial Radiology,* Volume 17, Number 1, 1988, pp. 15–23. Reproduced with permission from the Editor of *Dentomaxillofacial Radiology,* the International Association for Dentomaxillofacial Radiology, and the publisher Butterworth-Heinemann, Ltd.®

ions is the reason x-rays, gamma rays, and some other radiations are known as **"ionizing radiations."** It is ionization that causes harmful effects in the biological systems by creating free radicals (or ions) that can change the structure of molecules and induce the primary biological damage. The water molecule represents about 75% of the body's total number of molecules. As such, it is involved in the greatest number of interactions when the body is exposed to x-ray photons. These interactions are usually referred to as the **"radiolysis of water."** When the x-ray strikes the water molecule, hydrogen and hydroxyl free radicals can be formed. In addition, hydroperoxyl free radicals can occur and contribute in the formation of hydrogen peroxide (H_2O_2), which is poison to most tissues.

Radiation can have both direct and indirect effects on tissues. The **direct effect** occurs when a molecule is in the direct path of the radiation. The molecule is altered in its function and, subsequently, in its cellular structure. The **indirect effect** is caused when the impaired cell or molecule induces disruptions in the structure or function of regulatory molecules. The radiolysis of water is an example of an indirect effect.

One of the most significant molecules affected by radiation exposure is deoxyribonucleic acid (DNA). This molecule carries the genetic code for each cell in the human body. Three basic types of functional changes can result from DNA damage because of radiation exposure: (1) mitotic delay (cell division); (2) cell death; and (3) genetic damage. The latter two require low-to-moderate doses of radiation.

EFFECTS OF RADIATION ON CELLS

Radiation can affect all cells in the body. These effects are all in the **somatic effects** (damage that is manifested in the exposed individual) range, with the exception of the reproductive cells (ova and sperm). This means that although the cell can be damaged, it does not pass this damage on to its offspring cells. The period of time between the irradiation and the clinical appearance of any damage or side effects is called the **latent period.**

Genetic effect, on the other hand, is an effect in which the organism does pass along the damage to its offspring, thus creating mutations. The appearance of mutations does not necessarily occur in every subsequent generation, but can lie dormant, or recessive, for several generations.

Examples of radiation effects on the cells are apparent in the nucleus and in cell kinetics (turnover rate). The nucleus contains the chromosomes, which are believed to be the most sensitive sites in the cell to irradiation. Exposing the nucleus to radiation has been shown to inhibit cell division. Chromosome (DNA) **aberrations** can also occur.

Radiation effects in cell kinetics may be demonstrated by alteration of the mitotic cycle or cell death. Irradiation of the cell during mitosis causes a delay in the process of division; this reduces the size of the cell population. The delay in the division cycle is affected by the total dose, dose rate, and position in the cell cycle. A cell dies when it loses its ability for unlimited reproduction. This usually occurs after moderate radiation exposure in a cell that cannot complete the first few mitoses. This is termed reproductive death.

Recovery of the cell from radiation damage is usually higher if the radiation dosage is lower or if there are intervals (**fractions**) between exposures. Cell recovery is believed to involve primary repair to single DNA strands.

SENSITIVITY OF CELLS, TISSUES, AND ORGANS TO RADIATION

Several factors affect or modify the level of sensitivity a cell, tissue, or organ has to radiation exposure. Not all cells are equally sensitive to radiation. Cells that are most sensitive to radiation are ones that (1) are

TABLE 3-2
Radiation sensitivity of tissues and organs

High	Bone marrow
	Reproductive cells
	Intestines
	Lymphoid tissue
Moderately High	Oral mucosa
	Skin
Moderate	Growing bone
	Growing cartilage
	Small vasculature
	Connective tissue
Moderately Low	Salivary glands
	Mature bone
	Mature cartilage
	Thyroid
Low	Liver
	Optic lens
	Kidneys
	Muscle
	Nerves

immature (must undergo future growth and development); (2) are dividing rapidly (have frequent cell division); (3) are not specialized in their function; or (4) have a long mitotic history (many divisions over time). The exception to this rule is the lymphocyte, which is a highly specialized cell in the immune system. This cell does not divide, yet the small lymphocyte is considered one of the most sensitive to radiation exposure.

Examples of the relative sensitivity of some tissues and organs is shown in Table 3-2. Rubin and Casarett have divided cell sensitivity to radiation into the following 5 categories:

1. *Vegetative intermitotic cells* are the most sensitive to radiation. These cells regularly divide over a long period of time and include basal cells of the oral mucous membranes and the erythroblast.

2. *Differentiating intermitotic cells* are less sensitive than the vegetative intermitotic cells because they do not divide as often. An example of these is the inner enamel epithelium of developing teeth.

3. *Multipotential connective tissue cells* have moderate sensitivity to radiation. Examples of these cells are fibroblasts and mesenchymal cells.

4. *Reverting postmitotic cells* have a low radiosensitivity. These cells usually do not divide regularly, have relatively long lives, and are fairly specific in their functions. Ductal cells in the salivary glands, liver, kidneys, and thyroid are examples of these.

5. *Fixed postmitotic cells* are the least susceptible to radiation effects. These cells are highly specialized and do not divide once they mature. These cells include neurons, striated muscle cells, and squamous epithelial cells close to the surface of the oral mucous membrane.

There are several factors which can effect the radiosensitivity of cells. These include:

1. *Dose rate.* Cells can have a greater potential for repair if the exposure (total dose) is over a longer period of time (low dose rate) rather than a shorter period of time (high dose rate). This is because there is a greater opportunity for repair before the total dose is delivered.
   Example: total dose = 15 Gy (1500 rads)
   high dose rate = 5 Gy/min
   low dose rate = 10 mGy/min

2. *Oxygen.* The presence of oxygen increases the damage because of radiation exposure. The oxygen atoms provide an increase in the creation of hydrogen peroxide radicals, which are very damaging to the cells.

3. *Linear energy transfer.* The higher the LET, the more damage that will occur in the biological system. Higher LET radiations (such as alpha particles) cause more damage because they are capable of creating more hydrogen peroxide radicals and inducing double strand breakage in the DNA.

4. *Chemical agents.* Some chemical agents can inhibit the indirect effects of radiation by taking up the free radicals and thus arresting the production of hydrogen peroxide. These compounds are known as **"radioprotectors."** There are also chemicals that can increase the radiation effects. These are known as **"radiosensitizers."**

Although it was believed at one time that low doses of radiation were not harmful, all radiation creates some biological damage. There is no "safe" dose of radiation. Dental radiation produces very little damage, but it is still necessary to keep the exposure as low as possible. The damage caused by radiation is affected by the sensitivity of the tissue (Table 3-2), the exposure rate, and the dose as is shown in a **dose response curve** (Figure 3-1).

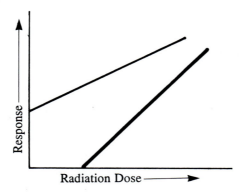

FIGURE 3-1 This dose response curve demonstrates the increased damage to the tissue as the radiation exposure increases. This linear-dose response relationship is represented as both a (A) nonthreshold dose and a (B) threshold dose.

The harmful effects of radiation can have a latent period ranging from a few hours to many years. The latent period depends on the total dose as well as the dose rate. When a large dose of radiation is given in a shorter period of time (shorter dose rate), the latent period will be shorter than if the dose is small and given over a longer period of time (known as fractionation). This concept is applied in radiation therapy by administering multiple small doses. This is thought to increase tumor destruction and give healthy tissue some repair opportunity. It also helps to decrease the side effects of radiation exposure.

Acute effects of radiation are usually the result of high doses of radiation (usually over the whole body). The symptoms of these "acute" effects may include nausea, vomiting, hemorrhage, diarrhea, fever, loss of hair, and death. **Chronic effects** of radiation are usually produced over a long period of time. These effects are usually shown as a decrease in the tissue to resist trauma and infection. The effects of radiation are considered to be *cumulative*. Tissues can repair themselves to some extent, but the damaging effects of repeated exposure can result in such health problems as cancers, premature aging, and cataracts.

The effects of radiation can be considered to be **stochastic** or **nonstochastic. Stochastic effects** are those where the risk of getting the effects is dependant upon the dose of radiation received. There is no known threshold below which the effects do not occur. An example of a stochastic effect is cancer. **Nonstochastic effects,** on the other hand, have threshold doses. It is believed that below these threshold doses, the effects do not occur. In addition, the severity of the effect is increased as the dose is increased. An example of this is erythema of the skin.

CRITICAL ORGANS

Although the risk associated with dental x-rays is minimal, some tissues and organs are exposed to more radiation when dental radiographs are taken. These are termed **"critical organs."** The doses required to produce significant effects on these critical organs is shown in Table 3-3.

1. *Skin.* Because the skin is exposed during dental radiography procedures, it is considered a critical organ/tissue. The effects of radiation on the skin can be seen as a reddening or erythema (similar to sunburn). This usually requires moderate-to-high doses of radiation.

2. *Thyroid gland.* The dose to the thyroid gland can be significant when taking dental radiographs if a thyroid collar is not used. This tissue is considered to be fairly radiation resistant in adults, but radiation sensitive in young children.

3. *Lens of the eye.* Although many experts no longer consider the lens of the eye a critical organ, significant radiation (greater than 2 Gy/ .02 rads) to the eye can result in cataracts. Using the paralleling technique can reduce exposure to the eye area.

4. *Bone marrow.* Significant changes in the bone marrow due to radiation exposure can result in leukemia. Since there are active bone marrow sites in the mandible and the skull, this should be taken into consideration with dental radiography.

TABLE 3-3
Critical organs: threshold dose

Organs	Dose (below which no effects are seen) (mGy)	(mrads)
Skin	250	2.5
Lens of the eye	2000	20.0
Thyroid gland	50	.5
Bone marrow	50	.5
Embryo or fetus	100	1.0

5. *Reproductive organs.* The reproductive cells are highly sensitive to radiation. However, the dose received during dental radiography exposure is almost unmeasurable. If the patient wears a lead apron, the dose is practically nonexistent.

6. *Fetus or embryo.* It is believed that the risk to the developing fetus during dental radiation exposure is nonexistent, but the exact amount of radiation that will produce damaging effects is unknown. The in utero effects are nonstochastic in nature, with a threshold of 10–25 cGy (1–2.5 mrads).

RADIATION PROTECTION

Two major concepts should be considered when beginning to study radiation protection. The first is the concept of *Maximum Permissible Dose* and the second is the *ALARA Principle.*

The **maximum permissible dose (MPD)** of whole body radiation should not exceed 5 rem (500 Sv) per year or 100 mrem per week for persons who are occupationally near radiation, such as allied dental health personnel and dentists. In addition, the radiographer should not receive more than 3 rem (300 Sv) in any given 13-week period. The MPD for a lifetime for radiation personnel should not exceed a dose of $(N - 18) \times 5$ rem. N is equal to the chronological age of the operator. Since there is no "safe" level of radiation exposure, each person in the dental office should strive to have no (zero) exposure.

The **ALARA (As Low As Reasonably Achievable) Principle** should be employed in all radiographic procedures. This principle emphasizes that the dose to the patient should be kept as low as reasonably achievable under the given set of circumstances.

When considering the concept of radiation protection, two sources of radiation to which both the patient and the operator are exposed must be discussed. These are the **primary radiation beam,** which exits the x-ray machine, and **scatter radiation,** which occurs when the primary beam strikes the patient (or any matter) and interacts to produce secondary radiation. Both types of radiation can contribute to exposure (Figure 3-2).

The three principles of radiation protection are (1) time; (2) distance; and (3) shielding. The time of exposure should be as short as possible. The distance between the source of radiation and the person should be as long as possible. And finally, shielding should always be used to protect the patient and operator from any unnecessary exposure. In order to maintain these principles of protection there are several precautions we can employ.

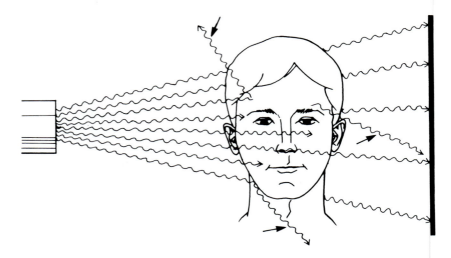

FIGURE 3-2 Scatter radiation occurs when the primary beam strikes the patient (or any matter) and interacts to produce secondary radiation.

Equipment and Operation

Filtration

The beam quality should be such that excessively high-energy and excessively low-energy radiation should be filtered out. This leaves only the portion of the x-ray beam that contributes to the production of a good, diagnostic radiograph. Certain filters remove both the excessive high and low portions of the x-ray beam (rare earth filters). Other filters, such as the aluminum filter, remove only the low-energy radiation. The beam **filtration** should comply with both state and federal regulations (Figure 3-3).

Collimation

Collimation provides the mechanism for limiting the area of tissue exposed to radiation. In addition, a smaller beam, which decreases the amount of scatter radiation produced, contributes to image quality. Collimation should comply with state and federal regulations. Restricting the beam to conform to the size of the x-ray film is highly recommended. The beam should be no larger than 7 cm (2.75 in.) in diameter at the patient's face. The use of rectangular PIDs or film holders, which collimate the beam to the actual size of the film, further reduce exposure.

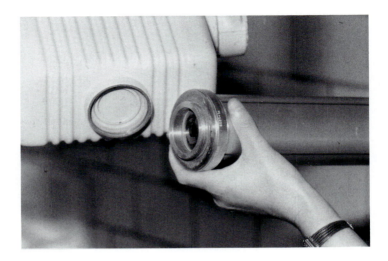

FIGURE 3-3 If you remove the PID from the x-ray tubehead, you can visualize both the aluminum filter and the collimator.

Technique and Processing

The technique used should produce quality radiographs. A technique chart should be posted at all exposure areas. Processing should follow the manufacturer's directions. Underprocessing to compensate for overexposure (or vice versa) should not occur (Figure 3-4).

Film Selection

The faster the film speed used, the less the exposure required to produce an image of the same density. The use of "E" speed film will

PROJECTION	mA	kVp	TIME in SECONDS	FILM TYPE
ANTERIOR	15	70	21/60	E
PREMOLAR	15	70	24/60	E
MOLAR	15	75	24/60	E
BITEWING	15	75	30/60	D
OCCLUSAL	15	75	30/60	D

TECHNICS CHART: GENDEX (GE) 1000

For **Large** Patients Add 5 Killovolts (kVP)
For Small Patients Reduce 5 Killovolts (kVP)

FIGURE 3-4 A technique chart should be posted at the exposure control panel.

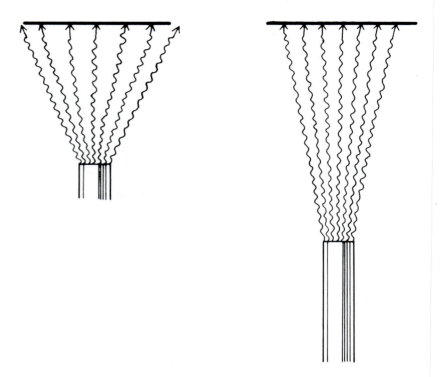

FIGURE 3-5   The longer the source to object distance, the less the exposure to the patient. This is due to a less divergent beam with less scatter radiation. Therefore, less tissue area is exposed.

reduce the patient's exposure by half. For extraoral radiography, the fast rare earth film-screen combination should be used.

Source to Film Distance

An extended distance between the radiation source (tubehead) and the patient, such as occurs when using a long **PID,** decreases exposure to the patient. This occurs because the longer the distance, the less the divergent the beam. The result is a smaller primary beam with less scatter, thereby exposing less tissue area. (Figure 3-5)

Timers

Timers (exposure buttons) should be electronic. The old mechanical timers are very inaccurate and can thus increase patient exposure. The exposure button should be placed outside of the x-ray exposure room to prevent the operator from walking in the room while the exposure is being made (Figure 3-6).

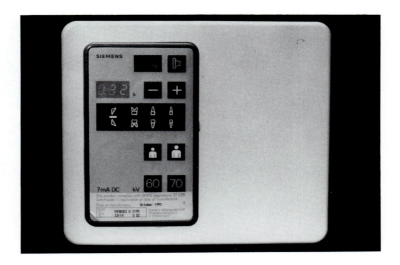

FIGURE 3-6 Timers (exposure buttons) should be located outside the operatory to avoid operator exposure.

Film-Holding Devices

Film-holding devices, such as the XCP or Precision Instrument, decrease the possibility of technique errors and thus reduce the need to retake radiographs. Film-holding devices allow us to align the film and the beam in the proper manner to produce a good quality radiograph. In addition, patients should never be allowed to hold the film in place with their fingers. This technique increases both patient exposure and the chance of technique error because of patient movement (Figure 3-7).

Kilovoltage

A range of 60–100 kVp is suitable for most intraoral radiography. The **kilovoltage** most suited for the diagnostic purpose should be used. High kVp is associated with lower contrast, lower entrance skin dose, higher deep tissue dose, and increased scatter. Low kVp contributes to higher contrast, higher entrance skin dose, lower deep tissue dose, and less scatter radiation.

Equipment Maintenance

Both the x-ray machine and processing equipment should be kept in proper working order. A quality assurance program to maintain the equipment can prevent malfunctions, thereby minimizing radiographic retakes. In addition, the x-ray tubehead should be adjusted periodically to prevent drifting. A drifting tubehead can severely hinder accurate radiographic technique, resulting in numerous retakes.

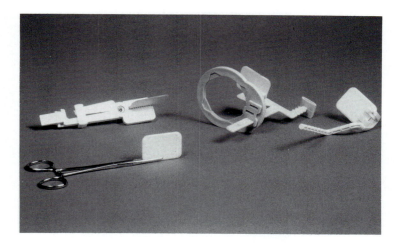

FIGURE 3-7   Several types of film-holding devices eliminate the need for patients to hold the film with their fingers.

Position Indicating Devices (PID)/Collimators

Ideally, rectangular, lead-lined cones should be used to decrease the amount of tissue exposure to the patient. These **Position Indicating Devices (PIDs)** collimate the beam to the approximate size of the film, thereby reducing patient exposure. If a rectangular PID is not available, a long, lead-lined open-ended cone can be employed. In addition, a film holding device, such as the Precision Instrument, can be used with the open-ended cone to achieve approximately the same effect as with rectangular collimation. Pointed, plastic cones are no longer used because of the extreme scatter radiation they produce because of noncollimation of the beam. In addition, their use is illegal in most states (Figure 3-8).

Patient Protection

Shielding

All patients should be covered with a lead apron, complete with a thyroid collar, during radiation exposure. In addition, the patient should not hold the film or the tubehead to provide stability. This can lead to unnecessary tissue area exposure (Figure 3-9).

Film Holding Devices

Film holding devices not only decrease retake errors, but by blocking the portion of the beam that does not reach the film can decrease the amount of tissue irradiated. This can be accomplished with several different types of film holding devices.

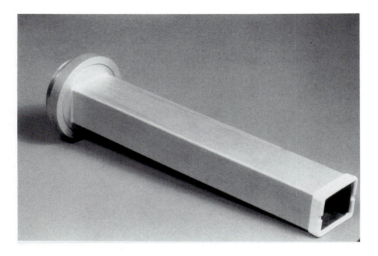

FIGURE 3-8 An example of a rectangular, lead-lined PID.

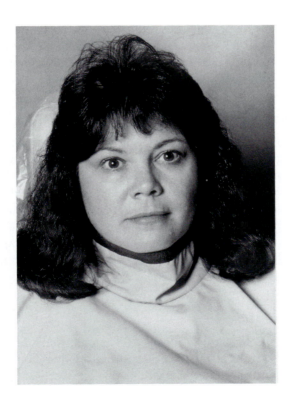

FIGURE 3-9 Patients should be covered with a lead apron and a thyroid collar.

Operator Protection

Operatory Construction and Shielding

The operatory should be constructed so that the operator may leave the room when making an x-ray exposure. If this is not possible, the operator should be provided with some type of appropriate barrier to stand behind during exposures. If no barrier is available, then the operator should stand at least 6 feet away and between 90 and 135 degrees from the primary beam. This is the area of least scatter radiation. Most construction provides adequate protection from scatter radiation to surrounding areas if materials such as plaster, cinderblock, or at least 2½ inches of drywall are used. Materials such as paneling alone do not provide adequate scatter protection. The National Council on Radiation Protection and Measurements can provide guidelines for construction (Figure 3-10).

Personnel Monitoring

All radiologic personnel should wear some type of radiation monitoring device. These usually are in the form of a clip-on badge containing a film or **thermoluminescent dosimeter (TLD).** At specified intervals, the badges are returned to the company to determine the amount of radiation exposure the person wearing the device has accumulated. These records can be kept to verify any cumulative radiation exposure (Figure 3-11).

Professional Judgment/Retake Policy

One of the most important factors in protecting the operator and the patient from excess radiation exposure is professional judgment. All patients should be questioned about their radiation exposure history. Women of reproductive age should be asked if they are pregnant. In addition, operators should use professional judgment in exercising all possible radiation safety techniques as well as in determining the appearance of an acceptable diagnostic radiograph. This can help establish a retake policy for the office and thus eliminate or reduce unnecessary radiographic retakes.

Patient Selection Criteria

One of the best means of reducing radiation dose to the patient is to carefully establish criteria as guidelines for selecting when and what type of radiographs will be taken. Selection criteria should be based on individual patient needs. The Basic Radiographic Selection Criteria was established by a joint effort of many professional dental associations (see Table 3-4).

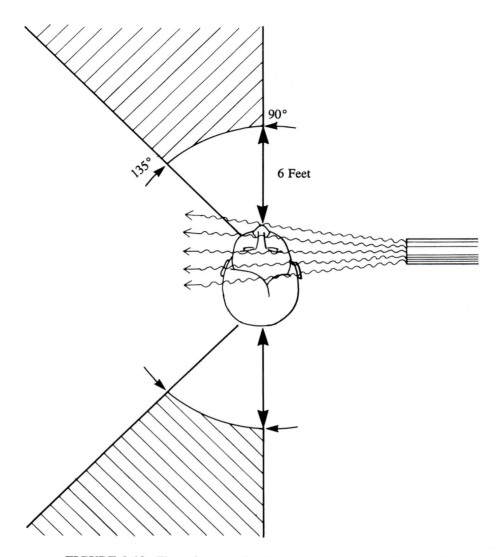

FIGURE 3-10 The safest area for the operator to stand during a radiation exposure procedure is at least six feet away from the primary beam at an angle between 90 and 135 degrees from the beam.

Radiation Therapy

Oral cancer constitutes about 4 percent of all malignancies. Therapies for oral cancer include surgery, radiation, chemotherapy, or a combination of these. Through either direct or indirect means, radiation therapy causes tissue changes that predispose the patient to ulcerations of the oral mucosa, dry mouth (xerostomia), dental caries, and osteomyelitis

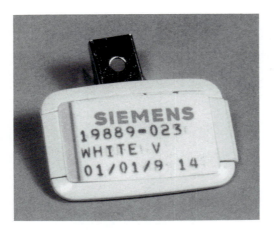

FIGURE 3-11   All radiologic operators should wear some type of radiation detection device. One type is a clip-on film badge.

(just to name a few). Prevention or treatment of these conditions requires a strict regimen both before and after radiation therapy. Depending on the patient's condition, some of the effects may last for a lifetime.

There are two means of therapy using radiation—external and internal (implantation). With external radiation, the extent of the injury due to radiation therapy depends on the size and the location of the tumor. In a "high posterior field," the nasopharynx, soft palate, and tonsillar areas are affected. In a "low anterior field," the tongue and the floor of the mouth are affected.

With internal radiation, such radioactive materials as Radon or radium, are used. This type of therapy often spares such structures as the salivary glands and the mandible from damage.

For most squamous cell carcinomas, the dose used in radiation therapy is between 6500 and 7500 rads (650000–750000 Gy). This dosage is divided into about 30 treatments (also known as fractions).

As the therapy progresses, several tissue changes occur. These include:

1. *Vascular changes.* Many times the smaller blood vessels are damaged by the radiation. This, in turn, can severely hinder the body's healing ability.

2. *Ulcerations of the Oral Mucosa.* This condition is known as mucositis. Radiation mucositis is very painful and usually begins early in the radiation therapy with redness and the gingiva is hemorrhagic with a white pseudomembrane covering it. Three to four weeks into therapy, white and yellowish ulcers appear on the gingiva. This

TABLE 3-4
Basic radiographic selection criteria*

The recommendations in this chart are subject to clinical judgment and may not apply to every patient. They are to be used by dentists only after reviewing the patient's health history and completing a clinical examination. *The recommendations do not need to be altered because of pregnancy.*

Patient Category	Child — Primary Dentition (prior to eruption of first permanent tooth)	Child — Transitional Dentition (following eruption of first permanent tooth)	Adolescent — Permanent Dentition (prior to eruption of third molars)	Adult — Dentulous	Adult — Edentulous
New Patient* All new patients to assess dental diseases and growth and development	Posterior bitewing examination if proximal surfaces of primary teeth cannot be visualized or probed	Individualized radiographic examination consisting of periapical/occlusal views and posterior bitewings or panoramic examination and posterior bitewings	Individualized radiographic examination consisting of posterior bitewings and selected periapicals. A full mouth intraoral radiographic examination is appropriate when the patient presents with clinical evidence of generalized dental disease or a history of extensive dental treatment.		Full mouth intraoral radiographic examination or panoramic examination
Recall Patient* Clinical caries or high-risk factors for caries**	Posterior bitewing examination at 6-month intervals or until no carious lesions are evident		Posterior bitewing examination at 6- to 12-month intervals or until no carious lesions are evident	Posterior bitewing examination at 12- to 18-month intervals	Not applicable
No clinical caries and no high-risk factors for caries**	Posterior bitewing examination at 12- to 24-month intervals if proximal surfaces of primary teeth cannot be visualized or probed	Posterior bitewing examination at 12- to 24-month intervals	Posterior bitewing examination at 18- to 36-month intervals	Posterior bitewing examination at 24- to 36-month intervals	Not applicable
Periodontal disease or a history of periodontal treatment	Individualized radiographic examination consisting of selected periapical and/or bitewing radiographs for areas where periodontal disease (other than nonspecific gingivitis) can be demonstrated clinically				Not applicable
Growth and development assessment	Usually not indicated	Individualized radiographic examination consisting of a periapical/occlusal or panoramic examination	Periapical or panoramic examination to assess developing third molars	Usually not indicated	Usually not indicated

Clinical situations for which radiographs may be indicated include:

A. Positive Historical Findings
1. Previous periodontal or endodontic therapy
2. History of pain or trauma
3. Familial history of dental anomalies
4. Postoperative evaluation of healing
5. Presence of implants

B. Positive Clinical Signs/Symptoms
1. Clinical evidence of periodontal disease
2. Large or deep restorations
3. Deep carious lesions
4. Malposed or clinically impacted teeth
5. Swelling
6. Evidence of facial trauma
7. Mobility of teeth
8. Fistula or sinus tract infection
9. Clinically suspected sinus pathology
10. Growth abnormalities
11. Oral involvement in known or suspected systemic disease
12. Positive neurologic findings in the head and neck
13. Evidence of foreign objects
14. Pain and/or dysfunction of the temporomandibular joint
15. Facial asymmetry
16. Abutment teeth for fixed or removable partial prosthesis
17. Unexplained bleeding
18. Unexplained sensitivity of teeth
19. Unusual eruption, spacing, or migration of teeth
20. Unusual tooth morphology, calcification or color
21. Missing teeth with unknown reason

Patients at high risk for caries may demonstrate any of the following:
1. High level of caries experience
2. History of recurrent caries
3. Existing restoration of poor quality
4. Poor oral hygiene
5. Inadequate fluoride exposure
6. Prolonged nursing (bottle or breast)
7. Diet with high sucrose frequency
8. Poor family dental health
9. Developmental enamel defects
10. Developmental disability
11. Xerostomia
12. Genetic abnormality of teeth
13. Many multisurface restorations
14. Chemo/radiation therapy

Source: Reprinted by permission from Eastman Kodak, Rochester, NY.

usually reaches a peak near the end of treatment. Within 2 to 3 weeks after completing therapy, the condition resolves itself.

3. *Oral Candidiasis.* This condition is a yeast infection that occurs because of an alteration in the saliva and oral bacteria. This may continue in a chronic form after therapy is complete.

4. *Salivary Gland Dysfunction.* Radiation leads to changes in the composition of the saliva and a decrease in the flow of saliva, usually because of compromised vasculature. The salivary flow can be reduced if all of the major glands are in the field of radiation. This produces a condition known as **xerostomia,** or dry mouth. One to two weeks after therapy begins, the saliva becomes viscose, decreases in flow, and increases in acidity. As a result, the saliva becomes ineffective as a cleaner, lubricator, and antibacterial and buffering agent. Plaque begins to build up and becomes an excellent medium for bacteria. The reduced salivary flow also hinders speech, swallowing, and mastication.

5. *Loss of Taste.* During the second week of therapy, the taste buds degenerate and atrophy. Most affected are bitter and acid tastes. This condition is usually temporary and may disappear within six months after therapy.

6. **Radiation Caries.** Changes in the saliva increase risk for caries. The decreased flow, increased acidity, and shift in oral flora all contribute to increased caries action. Usually the caries occur at the gingival margin. The patients risk for increased caries remains high throughout their lifetimes.

7. *Osteoradionecrosis.* Direct or indirect effects of radiation can make the bone virtually nonvital. This is seen most frequently in the mandible, usually following extraction, trauma, or infection. Clinically it is seen as exposed bone and is very painful. Usually this condition develops during the first year after radiation therapy, but it can occur anytime during the patient's lifetime.

8. *Limited Opening (**Trismus**).* Radiation of the mastication muscles or the temporomandibular joint can result in fibrosis of these areas. Because this can lead to a limited ability to open the mouth, it can have serious consequences for nutrition and oral hygiene.

Patient management during radiation therapy can be challenging. A complete and thorough evaluation of the dentition and periodontium should be documented because many changes can occur several years after therapy. Any urgent restorations or extractions should be completed prior to beginning therapy, along with the patient's scaling. Any trauma or infection present before therapy begins enhances the possibility of osteoradionecrosis occurring.

TABLE 3-5

Effective dose equivalents from dental x-ray techniques and probability
of excess fatal cancer risk per million examinations*

Technique	Dose millirems	Dose microSieverts	CA Risk per Million exams	Background equivalent
Panoramic—fast screens	1	10	0.25	½ day
Panoramic—par screens	2	20	0.5	1 day
Skull/Cephalometric images— fast screens[1]	2	20	0.5	1 day
Tomogram (8 cm × 8 cm field)[2]	1	10	0.25	½ day
FMX (E-Rectangular Collimation)	1.5	15	0.4	1 day
FMPAs (E-Rect) & 4 Bitewings (D-Round)	3.5	35	0.9	3 days
FMX (D-Rectangluar Collimation)	3.5	35	0.9	3 days
FMPAs (E-Round) & 4 Bitewings (D-Round)	5.5	55	1.75	4 days
FMX (D-Round Collimation)	10	100	2.5	1 week
Single PA or Bitewing (E-Rectangular Collimation)	0.1	1	0.025	2 hours
Single PA or Bitewing (D-Rectangular Collimation)	0.15	1.5	0.04	3 hours
Single PA or Bitewing (E-Round Collimation)	0.25	2.5	0.06	5 hours
Single PA or Bitewing (D-Round Collimation)	0.5	5	0.13	8 hours
4 Bitewings (E-Rectangular Collimation)	0.4	4	0.1	8 hours
4 Bitewings (D-Round Collimation)	2	20	0.5	1 day

* Based in part on data found in: White SC. Assessment of radiation risk from dental radiography. Dentomax-
illofac. Radiol., 1992; 21: 118–26. Additional extrapolations from National Council on Radiation Protection
and Measurements. (NCRP report; no. 100) 1989; 48, and Clark DE, Danforth RA, Barnes RW, Burtch ML.
Radiation Absorbed from Dental Implant Radiography: A Comparison of Linear Tomography, CT Scan, and
Panoramic and Intra-Oral Techniques. J. Oral Implantol, 1990; 16: 156–64.
Compiled by J. Ludlow DDS, MS, University of North Carolina School of Dentistry used with permission.

Patients should be thoroughly instructed in oral hygiene to decrease the possibility of caries and oral candidiasis. To aid in treating oral mucositis, patients can be instructed to rinse with a solution of baking soda and salt. This will ease the pain and lubricate the tissues. Oral candidiasis can be treated with a number of antifungal agents. Xerostomia responds well to artificial saliva substitutes or chewing sugarless gum to stimulate salivary flow. The increased risk in developing carious lesions can be prevented through home fluoride treatments using custom trays. The limited mouth opening that patients may experience can be treated through a series of exercises that aim at increasing or maintaining the intraoral opening. In addition, the patient should be encouraged to maintain good nutrition even though the taste sensation may be altered.

Scheduling treatment for patients undergoing radiation therapy can be very critical. The patient's oncologist should be consulted whenever dental treatment is anticipated, especially if radiographs may be needed. The dental team can play a vital role in enabling the radiation therapy patient to tolerate treatment and decrease the damaging effects.

RISK ESTIMATION

Often patients ask, "how much radiation am I being exposed to?" or, "what are my chances of developing cancer from dental x-rays?" These questions can best be addressed by using risk estimation. Table 3-5 addresses the risk of developing cancerous lesions from radiation. This type of information will often help to put into perspective the relative risks of being exposed to radiation.

SUMMARY

This chapter has introduced the major concepts concerning the effects of radiation exposure on human cells and tissues. In addition, the guidelines provided will allow the operator to apply sound, professional judgment in exposing patients to radiation. With the application of these concepts, patient exposure to radiation can be minimized.

BIBLIOGRAPHY

BENNETT J. Oral Care of Cancer Patients Undergoing Head and Neck Irradiation. *Dental Hygiene* 1979; 53(5): 209–212.

BOMBERGER A, DANNENFELSER BA. *Radiation and Health Principles and Practice in Therapy and Disaster Preparedness.* Rockville, MD: Aspen, 1984.

Bushong SC. *Radiologic Science for Technologists: Physics, Biology and Protection,* 3d ed. St. Louis: CV Mosby, 1984.

Council on Dental Materials, Instruments and Equipment. Recommendations in Radiographic Practices. *JADA* 1984; 109(5): 764–765.

Council on Dental Materials, Instruments and Equipment. Biological Effects of Radiation from Dental Radiography. *JADA* 1982; 105 (Aug): 275–281.

Council on Dental Materials, Instruments and Equipment. Recommendations in Radiographic Practices: An Update, 1988. *JADA* 1989; 118(1): 115–117.

Curry III TS, Dowdy JE, Murry Jr RC. *Christensen's Physics of Diagnostic Radiology,* 4th ed. Philadelphia: Lea & Febiger, 1990.

Frommer H. *Radiology for Dental Auxiliaries,* 5th ed. St. Louis: Mosby Year Book, 1992.

Gibbs SJ, et al. Patient Risk from Rotational Panoramic Radiography. *Dentomaxillofac Radiol* 1988; 17(1): 25–32.

Gibbs SJ, et al. Radiation Doses to Sensitive Organs from Intraoral Dental Radiography. *Dentomaxillofac Radiol* 1987; 16(2): 67–77.

Gibbs SJ, Pujol Jr A, Chen T-S, James Jr A. Patient Risk from Intraoral Dental Radiography. *Dentomaxillofac Radiol* 1988; 17(1): 15–23.

Goaz PW, White SC. *Oral Radiology Principles and Interpretation,* 2d ed. Philadelphia: CV Mosby, 1987.

Granier R, Gambini DJ. *Applied Radiation Biology and Protection.* New York: Ellis Horwood, 1990.

Hendee WR. *Health Effects of Low-Level Radiation.* Norwalk, CT: Appleton-Century-Crofts, 1984.

Horiot JC, Bone MC, Ibrahim E, Castro JR. Systematic Dental Management in Head and Neck Irradiation. *Radiation Oncology–Biology–Physics* 1981; 7(8): 1025–1029.

Keifer Jurgen. *Biological Radiation Effects.* New York: Springer-Verlag, 1990.

Langland OE, et al. *Panoramic Radiology,* 2d ed. Philadelphia: Lea and Febiger, 1989.

Langland OE, Sippy FH, Langlais RP. *Textbook of Dental Radiology,* 2d ed. Springfield, IL: Charles C. Thomas, 1984.

MATTESON SR, WHALEY C, SECRIST VC. *Dental Radiology,* 4th ed. Chapel Hill, NC: University of North Carolina Press, 1988.

MILES DA, VANDIS ML, JENSEN CW, FERRETTI A. *Radiographic Imaging for Dental Auxiliaries.* Philadelphia: WB Saunders, 1989.

NATIONAL COUNCIL ON RADIATION PROTECTION AND MEASUREMENTS. *Exposure of the U.S. Population from Diagnostic Medical Radiation.* NCRP Report No. 100, Bethesda, MD, 1989.

NATIONAL COUNCIL ON RADIATION PROTECTION AND MEASUREMENTS. *Exposure of the U.S. Population from Occupational Radiation.* NCRP Report No. 101, Bethesda, MD, 1989.

NATIONAL RESEARCH COUNCIL. *BEIR V: Health Effects of Exposure to Low Levels of Ionizing Radiation.* Washington, DC: National Academy Press, 1990.

NORTH CAROLINA DEPARTMENT OF ENVIRONMENT, HEALTH AND NATURAL RESOURCES, DIVISION OF RADIATION PROTECTION. *North Carolina Regulations for Protection Against Radiation.* Raleigh, NC, 1991.

SULLIVAN DM, FLEMING TJ. Oral Care for the Radiotherapy-Treated Head and Neck Cancer Patient. *Dental Hygiene* 1986; 60(3): 112–114.

WHITE SC. An Update on the Effects of Low-Dose Radiation. *AAOMR Newsletter* 1990; 17(4): 1–7.

REVIEW QUESTIONS

1. The unit of exposure of air is called

    a. Coulomb per kilogram.
    b. Gray.
    c. Rad.
    d. relative biological effectiveness (RBE).

2. The type of radiation effect that occurs when the molecule is in the direct path of the radiation and its function is altered is known as

    a. indirect effect.
    b. linear energy transfer.
    c. direct effect.
    d. radiolysis.

3. A radiation-damaged cell can pass along damage to offspring cells. This is an example of a

    a. somatic effect.
    b. genetic effect.

c. latent effect.

d. indirect effect.

4. List the three types of functional changes that can result from DNA damage due to radiation exposure.

   a. _____

   b. _____

   c. _____

5. Recovery of the cell from radiation damage is usually higher if the radiation dosage is lower or occurs in intervals.

   a. True

   b. False

6. List the "critical organs" for dental radiographic exposure.

   a. _____

   b. _____

   c. _____

   d. _____

   e. _____

   f. _____

7. List the formula for the Maximum Permissible Dose for radiation personnel.

   _____

8. What are the three principles of radiation protection?

   a. _____

   b. _____

   c. _____

Radiographic Imaging for the Dental Team,
by Sally Mauriello. J.B. Lippincott Company,
Philadelphia © 1995.

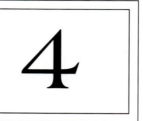

Radiologic Physics

Upon the completion of this chapter, the student should be able to:

1. Define and discuss the fundamental concepts of atomic structure.

2. Understand and discuss the concept of electromagnetic radiation.

3. Describe the x-ray tube and its main components.

4. Describe the x-ray generator and the process of x-ray production.

5. Explain the various interactions of x-rays with matter, and how they relate to x-ray production.

6. Describe the dental x-ray machine and explain its various components.

DEFINITION

Physics may be defined as the study of the relationship between matter and energy. Matter is anything that occupies space and has inertia. Inertia is the ability of objects to remain at rest if at rest, or to move if moving, unless affected by some outside force. Matter may be found in solid, liquid, gas, or plasma (stars) form. Everything in the universe is composed of matter. Common examples of matter are water, air, and wood.

Energy is the potential or ability to do work. Energy takes different forms, for example, mechanical, electrical, chemical, heat, light, and x-ray. Energy can also be converted from one form to another. For example, electrical energy is converted into light energy in the light-bulb; chemical energy is converted to electrical energy in a battery. Each of these energy conversions obeys the Law of Conservation of Energy. This law states that energy can neither be created nor destroyed. When it disappears in one form, it reappears in some other form.

Radiologic Physics is the study of those aspects of physics pertaining to the origin, nature, and behavior of x-rays and related types of radiation.

ATOMIC STRUCTURE

All matter is put together with the same building blocks. Matter is usually found in nature in impure or combined forms. For example, rock salt is a mixture of certain minerals of sodium chloride, magnesium chloride, and calcium sulfate. These minerals can be separated into their pure forms, such as pure salt (sodium chloride). If, in turn, the salt (sodium chloride) is broken down into smaller fragments, the smallest particle that is still recognizable as salt, is a **molecule** of salt. A molecule of salt is made up of two *atoms*—one of the elements is sodium and the other element is chlorine.

The **atom** is the smallest particle of an element that has the characteristic properties of that element. For example, a sodium atom retains everything about this element—its color, smell, chemical behavior, and so on. The structure of the atom has been best described using the model proposed by Neils Bohr in 1913. Bohr's model, also known as the quantum mechanical model, resembles a miniature solar system, with the sun at the center and the planets spinning about it (Figure 4-1). At the center of the atom lies a positively charged core **nucleus,** which makes up almost the entire mass of the atom. The nucleus contains **neutrons,** which have no charge, and **protons,** which are positively

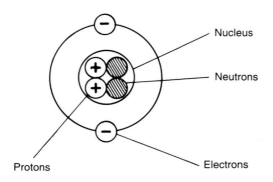

FIGURE 4-1 Model of the helium atom.

charged. Spinning about the nucleus are the **electrons,** which are negatively charged. The number of protons in the nucleus determines the identity of an element and makes it distinctly different from every other element. This number is characteristically the same for all atoms of a given element and is different from the atoms of other elements. The number of protons in the nucleus of the atom determines the **atomic number** of that element. (In neutral atoms, the number of protons is equal to the number of electrons.) The number of protons and the number of neutrons in the nucleus determines the atomic mass number of that element.

PERIODIC TABLE OF ELEMENTS

All of the elements can be arranged in an orderly series, called the periodic table of elements. The elements are arranged from the lowest atomic number to the highest. The periodic table is arranged in eight vertical groups and seven horizontal periods (Figure 4-2). The periods consist of elements with the same number of shells or orbits, but different chemical properties. The groups consist of elements with the same number of electrons in their outermost shell and have similar chemical properties.

Electron Binding Energy

Electrons are arranged in shells or orbits, and the strength of attachment of an electron to the nucleus is called the electron **binding energy.** As illustrated in Figure 4-3, the closest shell to the nucleus is the K-shell; the second closest is the L; and the third is the M, continuing in alphabetical order. The closer an electron is to the nucleus, the more tightly it is bound. Hence, its binding energy is higher. K-shell electrons have the highest, or strongest, binding energies. In addition, the

Group →	I	II										III	IV	V	VI	VII	VIII
1	1 H 1.00797																
																	2 He 4.0026
2	3 Li 6.939	4 Be 9.0122				**** Transitional Elements**						5 B 10.811	6 C 12.01115	7 N 14.0067	8 O 15.9994	9 F 18.9984	10 Ne 20.183
3	11 Na 22.9898	12 Mg 24.312										13 Al 26.9815	14 Si 28.086	15 P 30.9738	16 S 32.064	17 Cl 35.453	18 A 39.948
4	19 K 39.102	20 Ca 40.08										31 Ga 69.72	32 Ge 72.59	33 As 74.9216	34 Se 78.96	35 Br 79.909	36 Kr 83.80
5	37 Rb 85.47	38 Sr 87.62										49 In 114.82	50 Sn 118.69	51 Sb 121.75	52 Te 127.60	53 I 126.9044	54 Xe 131.30
6	55 Cs 132.905	56 Ba 137.34										81 Tl 204.37	82 Pb 207.19	83 Bi 208.980	84 Po [210]*	85 At [210]*	86 Rn [222]*
7	87 Fr [223]*	88 Ra [226]*															

(Left margin: **Period ↓**)

**For more details consult a chemistry text

FIGURE 4-2 Periodic table of elements.

greater the total number of electrons in the atom, the more tightly each electron is bound.

Table 4-1 shows examples of elements widely used in radiology, with their atomic numbers, atomic weights, K binding energies, and uses. Note that in Table 4-1, lead has the highest K-shell binding energy. Thus, it serves as an excellent barrier of protection against x-radiation. It takes high energies to penetrate lead, particularly when compared to aluminum. Because of lead's higher K-shell binding energy, more energy is required to dislodge one of its K-shell bound electrons and penetrate the element.

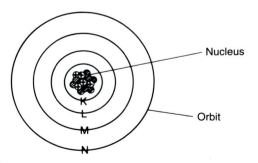

FIGURE 4-3 Arrangement of orbital shells.

TABLE 4-1
Chemical elements widely used in radiology, with their respective atomic numbers, atomic weights, and K binding energies

Element	Atomic Number	Atomic Weight	K-Shell Electrons Binding Energy	Use
Aluminum	13	27	1.560	x-ray filters and step-wedges
Iodine	53	127	33.17	x-ray contrast medium ("dyes")
Barium	56	138	37.44	x-ray contrast medium ("dyes")
Tungsten	74	184	69.53	x-ray targets in x-ray tubes
Lead	82	208	88.00	x-ray shields, aprons

X-RAYS (ROENTGEN RAYS)

The discovery of x-rays provided a new tool to help diagnose and treat disease. Today, x-rays are used in medicine, dentistry, scientific research, and industry. X-rays are a form of **electromagnetic radiation** similar to visible light, but with a shorter wavelength. All forms of electromagnetic radiation are grouped according to their wavelengths and are arranged in the electromagnetic spectrum as shown in Figure 4-4.

Electromagnetic radiation consists of wavelike fluctuations of electric and magnetic fields set up in space by vibrating electrons. A vibrating electric charge is surrounded by an electric field. If the charge does not move, the electric field at any given point is constant. If the

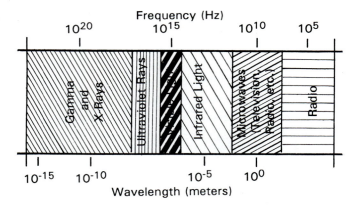

FIGURE 4-4 Electromagnetic spectrum.

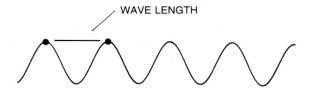

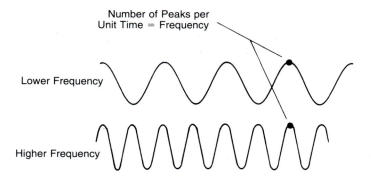

FIGURE 4-5 Wavelength and frequency of electromagnetic waves.

charge moves with uniform velocity, as happens when there is a steady flow of electrons, a magnetic field is also observed. If the charge is slowed down or accelerated, both the magnetic and the electric fields vary. The combined variation of electric and magnetic fields results in a loss of energy by the decelerating charge. This loss of energy is manifested in the form of electromagnetic radiation, or electromagnetic waves.

All electromagnetic waves travel at about the speed of light (3×10^8 meters or 186,000 miles per second in a vacuum or air). The main differences between the various electromagnetic waves are their **wavelength** and frequency. Wavelength is the distance between two positive peaks (or two consecutive negative peaks) of the wave form; frequency is the number of cycles per second that the wave passes a fixed point (Figure 4-5).

The radiation in the various sections of the electromagnetic spectrum range from radio, television, and radar waves to x-ray and gamma rays (see Figure 4-4). Radio, television, and radar waves have long wavelengths, low frequencies, and low penetrating abilities when compared to **x-ray** and **gamma rays,** which have short wavelengths, high frequencies, and the abilities to penetrate thick objects.

X-Radiation

X-rays can be produced when fast moving electrons experience sudden changes in velocity, either by changing direction or slowing down. This process can be brought about artificially in an x-ray tube. In a modern x-ray tube, electrons are accelerated across the tube by a high voltage applied between the **cathode** and the **anode.** When the electrons traveling at high speed reach the anode, and are suddenly stopped, their high kinetic energy is converted to x-rays and heat.

X-Ray Tube

X-rays are produced in an x-ray tube. X-ray tubes may vary in design and function, but they all share certain basic components. The main components of an x-ray tube are shown in Figure 4-6. They are the cathode, the anode, the **focusing cup,** and the glass envelope. The cathode is the negative electrode, and it consists of a **filament** coil of tungsten wire mounted in a concave metal cup known as the focusing cup. Tungsten is the material of choice because it has a high atomic number (lots of electrons) and a low melting point. During x-ray production, the filament is heated to incandescence (glowing hot) to literally boil off electrons. The focusing cup, a part of the cathode assembly, has a negative charge and is concave in shape. The filament is mounted inside the focusing cup. The focusing cup's negative charge and shape help to keep the electrons around the filament in a nice tight bundle. It also produces an electric field that focuses the electrons onto

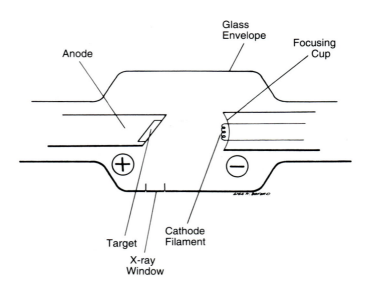

FIGURE 4-6 The main components of an x-ray tube.

a small area of the anode, which is known as the focal area or **target.** X-rays emerge from the focal area after the electrons strike it. The anode is the positive electrode, and it is made of a tungsten material embedded in copper. The copper serves to dissipate the heat generated during x-ray production. The efficiency of ordinary x-ray generating equipment is very poor. At 80 kilovolts, about 99.4 percent of all the energy that is put into the system for x-ray production is converted to heat. That is, only 0.6 percent of the input energy is converted to x-ray energy.

INTERACTIONS OF THE ELECTRON WITH TARGET ATOMS

Bremsstrahlung Production

Bremsstrahlung production occurs when a negatively charged electron approaches the positively charged nucleus and is deflected from its original path. This occurs because the electron experiences attraction from the positively charged nucleus. The change in direction experienced by the electron causes it to slow down. When the electron slows down, it loses energy. This loss of energy is manifested in the form of an x-ray photon (Figure 4-7). The energy given up is directly proportional to the energy of the photon and depends on the degree to which the electron is slowed down by the attraction of the nucleus. Bremsstrahlung is German for "braking radiation." Bremsstrahlung x-rays are heterogeneous or polyenergetic, that is, they have non-uniform energy. In the diagnostic range (x-ray energies used in medicine and dentistry to produce radiographic images), most x-rays are of bremsstrahlung origin.

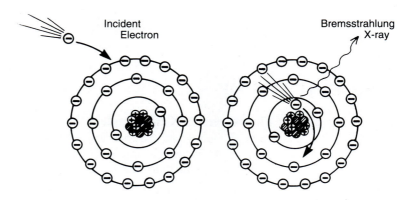

FIGURE 4-7 Production of bremsstrahlung x-rays.

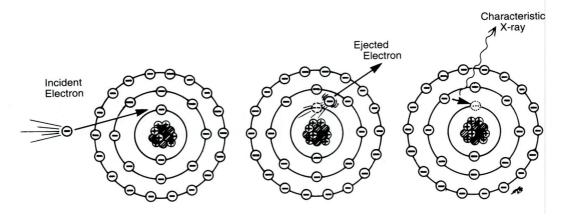

FIGURE 4-8 Production of characteristic radiation.

Characteristic Radiation

Characteristic radiation is the second process for x-ray production. It occurs when an incoming electron has sufficient energy to remove an electron from an inner shell of an atom in the target. In this case, the electron must have energy equal to or greater than the binding energy (energy holding electrons in place) of the electron in the target atom (Figure 4-8). After the electron is displaced from the target atom, the atom becomes unstable and is said to be in an excited state. Immediately, the vacancy left by the removed electron in the inner shell is filled by an electron moving inward from an outer shell in the atom. This is similar to removing the lowest book from a pile—all the others will move down. When this transition occurs, x-ray energy is produced or energy is given up in the form of x-radiation. The x-ray energy is equal to the difference between the binding energies of the two shells involved in the transition. Further, this energy is called characteristic x-ray because its energy is characteristic of the target element. In the diagnostic range, approximately 15 percent of the x-ray beam is characteristic in nature.

THE PROPERTIES OF X-RAYS

1. **Fluorescence:** X-rays produce fluorescence in materials such as calcium tungstate, lanthanum, and gadolinium oxysulfide. This property is utilized in intensifying screens (devices used to convert x-ray energy to light energy in a cassette) and x-ray image intensification (used in procedures where direct observation is necessary for examinations, such as barium studies, heart catheterization, and temporomandibular joint arthography).

2. Photographic Effect: X-rays produce a latent image on photographic film which can be developed to produce a visible image.

3. Penetrating and Invisible: X-rays are highly penetrating. They can pass through hard tissues, such as bone and enamel. X-rays cannot be seen, only detected.

4. **Ionizing:** X-rays have the ability to alter the atoms of the substances through which they pass by removing electrons from their atoms. This process is known as ionization and may have chemical and biological effects. The biological effects produced by ionization range from cell damage, or cell death, to cell mutations or changes. This property can be used in radiotherapy to kill malignant tumors. Cell mutations may lead to transformations of the affected cell into a cancer cell or may produce a genetic change.

5. Heterogeneous or Polyenergetic: X-rays have a range of energies and wavelengths. In diagnostic radiology, the useful range is from about 50 to 150 kilovolts.

6. Electrically Neutral: X-rays are not affected by electric or magnetic fields.

THE X-RAY GENERATOR

The principal parts of the x-ray generator are the autotransformer, high-voltage transformer, rectifier, and x-ray tube. However before these parts can be discussed, the concepts of **alternating (AC)** and direct current (DC) must be introduced. Current may be defined as the flow of electrons per unit time. Current is measured in **amperes,** which is defined as one coulomb quantity of electric charge flowing per second. There are two types of current: *direct* and *alternating*. Direct current is the flow of electrons in one direction; alternating current is the flow of electrons in two different directions. In the latter case, the electrons travel in one direction and then reverse direction.

Dental x-ray units are usually plugged into an ordinary household electrical outlet with a 110-volt source, but more powerful x-ray generating equipment requires the use of a 220-volt source. This source provides the *line voltage*. The line voltage is usually delivered in the form of alternating current. This is important since the **autotransformer** and high voltage **transformer** operate on alternating current.

Autotransformer

X-ray generators require the use of high and low voltage. Transformers can convert low voltage to high voltage and high voltage to low voltage. Transformers transfer electrical energy from one circuit to another without any moving parts. This process is known as *electromagnetic mutual induction.* The autotransformer, which connects to the high voltage transformer, alters the voltage coming in from the line voltage. The autotransformer is therefore a variable transformer, which allows the kilovoltage values to be changed as required for the different radiographic examinations.

The High Voltage Transformer

The high voltage transformer is also known as a step-up transformer. It converts low voltage to high voltage, which is used in diagnostic radiology. Remember that you start out with either 110 volts or 220 volts, but use approximately 70 kVp, or 70,000 volts, for an intraoral projection. The high voltage transformer boosts the voltage to 70,000 volts. When an x-ray machine has variable kilovoltage values, the different values are obtained by first altering the line voltage through the autotransformer. The autotransformer then sends the proper voltage value to the high voltage transformer for high voltage conversion.

Rectification

The electrical current produced in the high voltage transformer is in alternating form. Since x-ray tubes are designed to operate with direct current only, the alternating current coming from the high voltage transformer must be changed before it reaches the tube. The process of changing alternating current to direct current is known as **rectification.** A rectifier reroutes the current in such a way that the current reaching the x-ray tube always flows in the same direction—in this case from cathode to anode. Current may be rectified using one of three methods; **self-rectification** or self-half-wave rectification, half-wave rectification, or full wave rectification.

Most dental radiographic units self-rectify, that is the x-ray tube acts as its own rectifier. The high voltage is applied directly to the terminals of the x-ray tube, which is designed to allow current to flow from cathode (negative) to the anode (positive). When the current reverses itself, the anode becomes negative and the cathode positive. At that point, no current flows, because there is no electron cloud in the anode. If there were, the cathode would be severely damaged. When no current flows, that cycle of the alternating current is suppressed, resulting in a current with a half useful wave (Figure 4-9 a–b). Since most dental units are self-rectified, they produce only 60 impulses per second.

Dental x-Ray Tube

The tubes used for dental radiography consist of a stationary anode, cathode, and focusing cup. These elements are enclosed in a glass

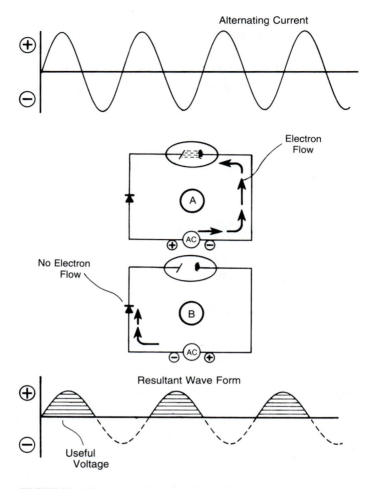

FIGURE 4-9 Alternating current being redirected by the rectifier. In (A), electrons flow from the cathode to the anode, but in (B), since the polarity reverses, the electrons cannot flow. The cycle of the wave is thus suppressed.

envelope, which contains a vacuum and is surrounded by cooling oil. The vacuum allows the electron stream to reach its target unobstructed without interacting with air molecules.

Filtration

Filtration is the process of removing nonproductive radiation from the x-ray beam. Filtration is very important because it reduces patient exposure to radiation. The three types of filtration are *inherent, added,* and *total.* Inherent filtration is provided by the materials of the tube and in the cooling oil. Added filtration is any additional filtration (e.g., **aluminum**) placed in the path of the beam before it exits the tube head. Total filtration is the sum of inherent and added filtration. Filtration affects the total exposure and quality of the x-ray beam. The exposure is decreased because low energy x-ray photons are removed from the beam. The quality increases because the average energy of the remaining x-ray photon in the beam is higher. The most widely used filter material in diagnostic radiology is aluminum. The National Council on Radiation Protection recommends 1.5 millimeters of aluminum equivalent filtration material for beams below 70 kilovolts and 2.5 millimeters of aluminum equivalent material above 70 kilovolts.

X-RAY INTERACTIONS WITH MATTER

When an x-ray beam passes through matter, its interaction with the molecules alters the beam and reduces its intensity. Some of the beam's energy is absorbed by the object the x-rays are traveling through; some is scattered. The process of beam energy reduction is known as **attenuation.** The most significant process by which x-rays are altered in diagnostic radiology are through classical (coherent scattering), **photoelectric,** and **compton** interactions.

Classical Interaction

Classical interaction occurs only when the x-ray photon possesses very low energy. The x-ray photon interacts with a tightly bound electron (an electron in the shell closest to the nucleus) without undergoing any change in wavelength. The photon is simply scattered without losing energy. This interaction has little or no importance in diagnostic radiology.

Photoelectric Interaction

During this process, the x-ray photon interacts with an inner-shell electron. The photon is completely absorbed, and the electron is ejected from the atom. The ejected electron is known as a photoelectron. Its kinetic energy is equal to the energy given up by the photon. Almost immediately after the electron is ejected from the atom, its shell vacancy is filled by an electron from a higher shell. In the process, characteristic radiation is emitted from the atoms that have been affected by the primary radiation coming from the tube (Figure 4-10). This interaction is important over most of the energy range used in diagnostic radiology, because it is a major factor in producing the contrast seen on radiographic film. Contrast is the difference between

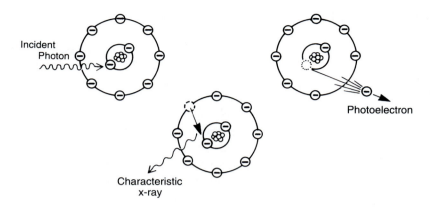

Incident
Photon

Characteristic
x-ray

Photoelectron

FIGURE 4-10 Photoelectric interaction.

radiographic densities, and density is what allows us to see objects of
different thicknesses in the human body.

Compton Interaction

This interaction can occur when an x-ray photon interacts with a
loosely bound electron and ejects it from the atom. The ejected electron
is known as a Compton electron. The x-ray photon imparts part of its
energy to the electron and scatters the rest (Figure 4-11). The number
of photons scattered in the forward direction, or the direction of the
film, increases as the average energy of the beam increases. In the
diagnostic range, photons scattered in the forward direction can reach
the film and add to background fog (a darkening due to radiation from
sources other than intentional exposure), thereby reducing image contrast. Scatter radiation which degrades image quality, makes no contribution to image formation.

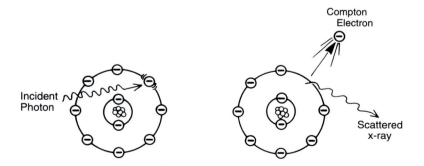

Compton
Electron

Incident
Photon

Scattered
x-ray

FIGURE 4-11 Compton interaction.

THE DENTAL X-RAY MACHINE

The basic dental x-ray machine consists of the tube head, adjusting arm, and control panel. The tube head houses the x-ray tube and, in some cases, the high voltage and filament transformers. The adjusting arm enables positioning of the tube head to line up the x-ray beam during radiographic procedures. The control panel houses the exposure regulating devices. These are the **milliamperage (mA), kilovoltage (kV),** and timer selectors. The mA selector controls the tube current and filament heat. The higher the mA value, the greater the number of electrons boiled off and the greater the tube current produced. The x-ray exposure is directly proportional to the mA. If the mA is doubled, the exposure is also doubled. Most dental x-ray units have fixed mA values or a limited selection of mAs. The typical mA values in dental radiography range from 7 mA to 15 mA. The kilovoltage selector controls the voltage applied across the x-ray tube. The kilovoltage determines the energy of the x-ray beam. The higher the kilovoltage, the higher the energy of the x-ray beam and the greater its penetrating power. The most common kilovoltage value used in dental radiography is 70. While some units are equipped with fixed kilovoltages, others offer variability by allowing selection of values from 50 to 90 kilovolts.

Timer Selector

The timer selector determines the duration of the exposure. That is, the timer controls the total time that the current passes through the x-ray tube and thus the time during which x-rays are emitted. Dental x-ray machines may have time selectors or impulse selectors. In a half-wave rectified machine, 60 impulses are produced every second, therefore 30 impulses (30/60) are equivalent to ½ of a second. Dental radiographic units use a **dead-man switch,** which is a switch or control that can maintain function only by continuous pressure by the operator. Milli-amperage, kilovoltage, and time must be properly balanced to produce images of optimum diagnostic value. The impact of these variables on image quality will be discussed in more detail in Chapter 12.

Designs

Manufacturers offer a wide variety of configurations for tube heads, control panels, and current types. One of the most significant changes in tube heads is mounting of the x-ray tube in the rear of the assembly (Figure 4-12). This recessed design allows the use of shorter cones, while maintaining an acceptable source-to-skin distance (SSD). Control panels may be equipped with conventional "knobs" or, in some cases, employ icons (Figure 4-13). These icons are preset timers referenced to the dental anatomy. In addition, some manufacturers offer

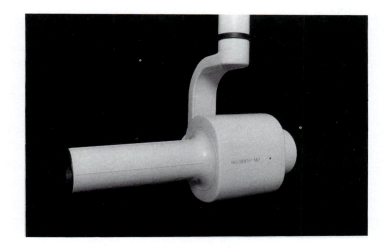

FIGURE 4-12 Recessed x-ray tube.

direct current constant potential voltage, in which a constant stream of x-radiation is generated instead of a series of pulses. This technology uses more efficient timers and results in a small radiation savings to the patient.

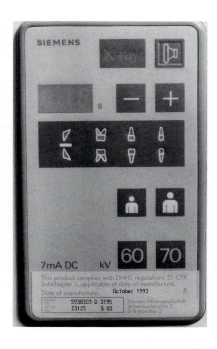

FIGURE 4-13 Control panel with icons.

SUMMARY

In 1985 Wilhelm Konrad Roentgen, a German physicist, discovered x-radiation while experimenting in his laboratory. This discovery, which changed the course of medical history and has had a tremendous impact on science and industry, provided the seeds for diagnostic radiology. A basic understanding of the physics of x-ray production is an important component of the education of radiology professionals. Operators who are well informed can follow the safest procedures for their patients and themselves, and consequently optimize the use of the equipment.

BIBLIOGRAPHY

Bushong SC. *Radiologic Science for Technologists: Physics, Biology, and Protection,* 4th ed. St. Louis: CV Mosby, 1988.

Curry III TS, Dowdey JE, Murry Jr RC. *Christensen's Physics of Diagnostic Radiology,* 4th ed. Philadelphia: Lea and Febiger, 1990.

Goaz PW, White SW. *Oral Radiology: Principles and Interpretation,* 3d ed. St. Louis: CV Mosby, 1994.

Sellman J. *The Fundamentals of X-ray and Radium Physics,* 7th ed. Springfield, IL: Charles C. Thomas, 1985.

Sprawls Jr P. *Physical Principles of Medical Imaging.* Rockville, MD: Aspen, 1987.

REVIEW QUESTIONS

1. The atomic number of an element is determined by the number of

   a. electrons.
   b. protons.
   c. neutrons.
   d. nucleus.

2. Radio, radar, television, and x-ray waves

   I.   have long wavelengths.
   II. have approximately the same frequency.
   III. are considered radiation.
   IV. travel at the speed of light.

   a. I and IV only
   b. I and III only
   c. III and IV only
   d. II and IV only

3. In the x-ray tube, x-rays emerge from the

    a. filament.
    b. cathode.
    c. anode.
    d. focusing cup.

4. Most of the x-rays produced in medicine and dentistry result from

    a. bremsstrahlung production.
    b. characteristic production.
    c. photoelectric interaction.
    d. Compton interaction.

5. Which of the following is *not* a property of x-rays?

    a. The ability to ionize.
    b. The ability to cause fluorescence.
    c. Invisibility.
    d. Deflection by magnets.
    e. Different wavelengths.

6. Which of the following interactions is most responsible for producing the contrast seen on radiographic film?

    a. Compton.
    b. photoelectric.
    c. classical.
    d. bremsstrahlung.

Radiographic Imaging for the Dental Team,
by Sally Mauriello. J.B. Lippincott Company,
Philadelphia © 1995.

5

Image Receptors

Upon the completion of this chapter, the student should be able to:

1. Define the term "image receptor."

2. Describe the construction and characteristics of dental radiographic film.

3. Distinguish between the characteristics and exposure considerations of D and E speed dental radiographic film.

4. Discuss the construction, use, and considerations of intensifying screens.

5. Describe the conditions and requirements for the storage and handling of dental radiographic film.

In order to produce good quality radiographs, one must understand the characteristics of image receptors and the factors influencing production of the image. A radiograph is basically an image of internal structures represented by various shades of gray. The terms *radiolucent* and *radiopaque* are vital in describing the image. **Radiolucent** areas are the black images on the film; **radiopaque** areas are the white images (Figure 5-1).

WHAT IS AN IMAGE RECEPTOR?

Dental radiographs record information about a patient on a medium that can be visualized and interpreted. They require an image receptor to receive the x-ray image after the x-ray photons have interacted and passed through the patient. Dental x-ray film is one such image receptor. Other types of image receptors used in everyday life include the television monitor and photographic film.

TYPES OF IMAGE RECEPTORS

The two most common types of image receptors in dental radiography are **direct exposure film** and **indirect exposure film** (also known as screen film). Of these, direct exposure film is more commonly employed. This type of film is used for periapical and bitewing radiogra-

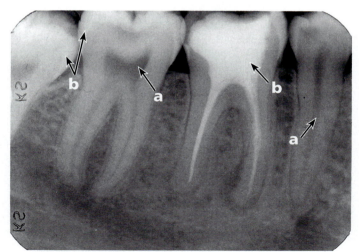

FIGURE 5-1 The areas labeled "a" are radiolucent. The areas labeled "b" are radiopaque.

phy, while indirect, or screen film, is used primarily for extraoral projections. The indirect exposure films are used in combination with a cassette film holder and screen.

FILM CONSTRUCTION

Since any contamination during the production of radiographic film would severely inhibit its ability to record a high-quality image, the film is produced under very strict and controlled conditions. Radiographic film has two basic components—the base and the emulsion. The emulsion surrounds the base (usually on both sides) and is held to the base by an adhesive layer (Figure 5-2).

Before 1960 the **base layer** was made of cellose acetate. Now, it is made of polyester, which is much more flexible. The base provides a semirigid foundation on which the emulsion is applied. This makes the film easy to handle. The base is nearly transparent with a slight blue tint to prevent eyestrain.

The **emulsion layer** contains the actual material with which the x-rays interact to record the radiographic image. The emulsion is composed of a mixture of gelatin and silver halide crystals. The gelatin, which supports the silver halide crystals, transmits light to aid in the exposure process. It is so porous that the processing chemicals can penetrate it during the processing procedure. The **silver halide** crystals are made up of approximately 95 percent silver bromide and 5 percent silver iodide crystals. These crystals, which are irregular in shape, are usually triangular and are responsible for recording the image seen in the developed radiograph (Figure 5-3). The x-ray photons, exiting the object being radiographed, strike the silver halide crystals. This causes a change in the crystals, which is referred to as the **latent (or invisible) image.** During processing of the film, the latent image becomes a true image that can be visualized after the processing. The size, number, and distribution of the crystals in the gelatin affect the quality and characteristics of the radiographic image.

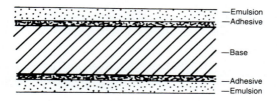

—Emulsion
—Adhesive

—Base

—Adhesive
—Emulsion

FIGURE 5-2 A representation of a cross-section of a dental x-ray film.

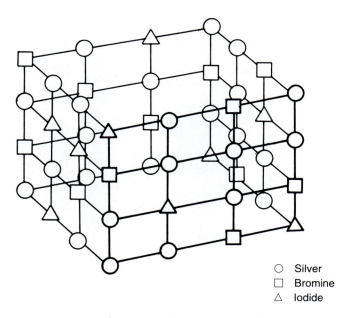

○ Silver
□ Bromine
△ Iodide

FIGURE 5-3 The silver halide crystal.

FILM CHARACTERISTICS

Radiographic images exhibit many characteristics, including fog, density, contrast, speed, resolution, and mottling. Fog and density can be caused by outside influences, but contrast, speed, resolution, and mottling are basically inherent characteristics.

Film **fog** can be seen as a radiographic image that is dull, washed out, and lacks contrast. It is caused by various factors, such as any increase in the time, temperature, or concentration in the processing solutions that deviate from the manufacturers recommendations. In addition, fog can be caused by contamination of the processing solutions, exposure of the film to unwanted radiation, light exposure, heat, chemical fumes, and age.

The contrast in a radiographic image is defined as the differences between the lights and darks in the image. Film that looks very gray has a low contrast or a long scale of contrast. Low contrast may result from an increase in kVp, poor processing conditions, or object size. Films that are black and white in appearance with very few grays are said to have high contrast or a short scale of contrast (Figure 5-4). In Figure 5-5, short and long scales of contrast are compared.

Image contrast can result from two factors—film contrast and subject contrast. **Subject contrast** occurs because patients have different anatomical builds. Some people are heavier, and some body parts are

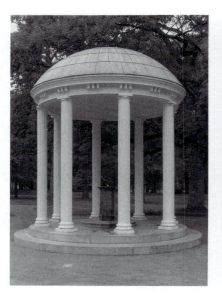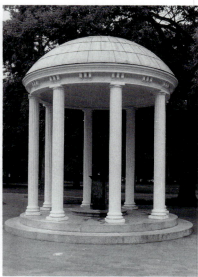

FIGURE 5-4 The picture on the right represents a high contrast image. The left picture represents one of low contrast.

thicker. Therefore the amount of radiation passing through the patient and reaching the film may vary from patient to patient. Factors that affect subject contrast are (1) kVp used, and (2) x-ray absorption by the subject, which depends on such factors as the thickness of the patient and the density of the tissue being radiographed. For example, enamel appears more radiopaque than the dentin because of its density.

Film contrast is an inherent characteristic, but it can be influenced by the film type, fog level, direct or indirect exposure, and the processing conditions. Any deviation from the manufacturers recommended processing directions can alter the film contrast.

Film **density** is defined as the blackness of the film. The precise numerical value of the density can be measured by a densitometer (Figure 5-6). In mathematical terms,

$$D = \log \frac{(I_o)}{(I_t)}$$

where: D is density

I_o is the original light transmitted to the film

I_t is the amount of light transmitted through a particular area of the film.

An example of a density measurement follows. When the radiograph allows only $\frac{1}{100}$ (or 1 percent) of the light to pass through, the ratio is

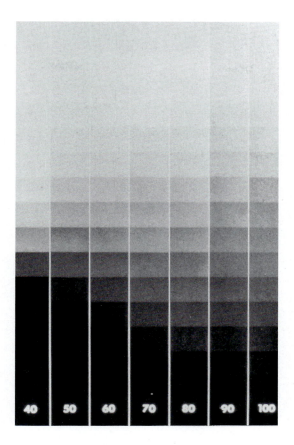

FIGURE 5-5 Short and long scales of contrast.

100 to 1. The logarithm of 100 (10^2) is 2. Therefore, the density of that area of the radiograph is 2. Densities on film can range in value from 0 (clear) to 4 (totally black). Densities that are considered to be diagnostically acceptable range from approximately .3 to 2.5. Factors that effect the density of a radiographic image include (1) the amount of radiation the film is exposed to (either by kVp or mA), (2) the processing factors, (3) the distance of the x-ray source from the patient, and (4) the thickness of the area being radiographed (for example, anterior versus posterior areas of the mouth). If the amount of radiation reaching the film decreases or the radiograph is underdeveloped, the resultant film will have a decreased density and appear lighter. In addition, if the distance from the x-ray source to the patient is increased or the thickness of the object being radiographed is increased, the x-ray will also have less density and appear lighter.

The relationship between the blackness, or density, on a film and the amount of x-ray exposure the film received can be measured and then

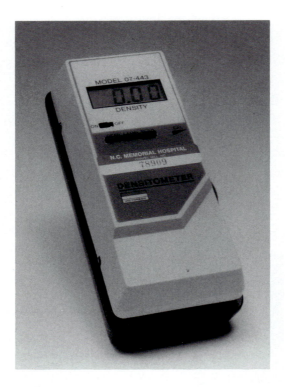

FIGURE 5-6 A densitometer can provide a numerical value for film density.

plotted as an **H and D Curve** (named after Hurter and Driffield), which is also known as a **characteristic curve** or representative curve (Figure 5-7). This relationship shows the effects that the amount of exposure has on the density of the film.

As previously stated, the density of the radiograph can be affected by the distance from the x-ray source to the patient and the image receptor. As x-rays travel a greater distance, they diverge to cover a larger area and become increasingly less intense. This relationship is governed by a concept known as the **Inverse Square Law.** If correct densities are to be maintained, the principles of the inverse square law must be observed. The inverse square law states that the intensity of the beam varies inversely to the square of the distance from the x-ray source to the object (Figure 5-8). For example, if you increased the distance of the x-ray source (the tubehead) by four times the original distance, the beam would cover an area, or be dispersed, 16 times ($4^2 = 16$) greater than that of the original area covered. In addition, its intensity would be only $\frac{1}{16}$ of the original. Therefore, the resulting image would be less dense, or lighter, but would cover a larger area.

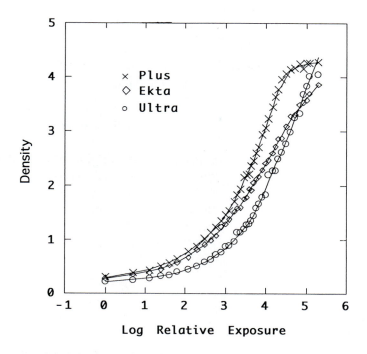

FIGURE 5-7 The H and D curve represents the relationship between the exposure of film and the density that is produced.

To compensate for this decrease in intensity, which occurs when we increase the PID (or cone) length on the x-ray tubehead, the machine settings must be adjusted so that a consistent density is kept on the radiographs. This can accomplished by adjusting the exposure time. If the original time and distance as well as the new distance is known, the

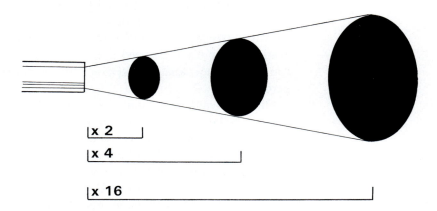

FIGURE 5-8 The inverse square law states that as the length of the beam increases, its intensity decreases and its size increases.

new time needed to maintain an acceptable density on the radiograph can be calculated by using the following formula:

$$\frac{\text{New Time}}{\text{Original Time}} = \frac{(\text{New Distance})^2}{(\text{Original Distance})^2}$$

$$\frac{\text{NT}}{\text{OT}} = \frac{(\text{ND})^2}{(\text{OD})^2}$$

Example: Suppose that the original PID on the machine is 6 inches long and the original exposure time is 18 impulses. If we change the PID to one that is 12 inches long, what should the exposure be in order to maintain the same density on the radiograph?

Solution: The formula would be:

$$\frac{\text{NT}}{\text{OT}} = \frac{(\text{ND})^2}{(\text{OD})^2}$$

$$\frac{\text{NT}}{18} = \frac{(12)^2}{(6)^2}$$

$$\frac{\text{NT}}{18} = \frac{144}{36}$$

$$\text{NT} = 18 \times 4$$

$$\text{NT} = 72 \text{ impulses}$$

Film speed is the sensitivity of the film as related to the size of the crystals in the film emulsion. The larger the crystals, the faster the film speed. The faster the film speed, the less the amount of radiation that is required to expose the film. Fast or high-speed films are very efficient because they respond to radiation exposure quickly. Therefore, they require less radiation to produce a radiographic image. Currently, in dentistry, two types of films—D speed, also known as Ultraspeed and E speed—are used. E speed is a faster or more sensitive film, which can reduce the radiation exposure to the patient by as much as 50 percent.

One disadvantage of using faster speed films is the size of the silver crystals in the emulsion. These larger crystals produce a grainier radiographic image. Accordingly, E speed film might give you an image that is not as appealing as that of a D speed film. Current research, however, indicates that there is hardly any detectable difference in the diagnostic quality between the images of D and E speed films.

Resolution relates to the ability of a film to record an in-focus, or true image. This is often seen as the ability of the radiographic image to discern the boundaries between two objects close together. An image that appears to be out of focus can be said to have poor resolution. Resolution is influenced by the crystal size in the emulsion. Therefore, faster speed films have lower resolution than their slower counterparts.

Radiographic mottle is often compared to "snow" on a television picture or static on a radio. Radiographic mottle is any undesirable variation in density caused by having too few photons creating the image. This characteristic is inherent in the system, but it can be somewhat influenced by the kVp, mA, and speed of the system. Using high mAs, low contrast, and a slow speed system can reduce mottle. Although conventional dental imaging does not deal with radiographic mottle, the use of digital imaging, (which will discussed in a later chapter) increases the possibility of having to deal with this imaging characteristic.

DIRECT VERSUS INDIRECT FILM

Direct exposure film, which is used for intraoral radiographs, is exposed when it comes in contact with x-ray photons. The emulsion on this film is usually thicker and has a higher concentration of silver halide crystals that can react directly with the x-ray photons. The resultant image is usually very sharp and displays great detail. This type of image is necessary for diagnosing caries and periodontal disease.

Direct exposure film is manufactured in D and E speeds. The most commonly used film at this time is D speed, but with the lower patient dosage and higher quality detail, E speed film is becoming more popular for all intraoral projections (Figure 5-9). In addition, Kodak has

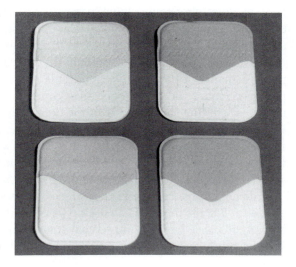

FIGURE 5-9 D and E speed films.

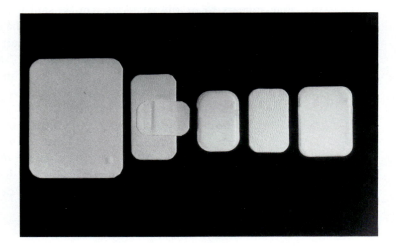

FIGURE 5-10 Film sizes (left to right): 4 (occlusal), 3 (long bitewing), 0 (pediatric), 1 (anterior), 2 (standard periapical and bitewing).

introduced the Ektaspeed Plus™ dental film, which is an E speed film with sharp, high-contrast images that are less dependant on processing conditions than the basic E speed film. Both D and E speed films are individually packaged in either single or double film packets. The sizes range from 0 (pediatric) to 4 (Figure 5-10).

Direct exposure film for dental radiographs is packaged in either paper or "polysoft" packets. The packets are colored coded to designate double and single packets as well as the film speed (Figure 5-11). The film inside is wrapped in black paper to help prevent accidental light exposure. The packet also contains lead foil to absorb the x-ray photons after they have passed through the film. In one corner, the packet has an embossed dot, which corresponds to the concave/convex dot impressed in the corner of the film. This dot enables the operator to properly mount the films once they are processed. If the films are mounted with the concave side of the dot facing the operator, the films will be viewed with the right side of the patient's mouth on the right side of the operator. If the films are mounted with the convex side of the dot facing the operator, the films will be viewed with patient's left side on the right side of the operator (Figure 5-12).

Indirect exposure film is also referred to as screen film. Outside of dentistry, it is the most widely used type of radiographic film. This film is exposed using intensifying screens housed in a cassette. Intensifying screens produce light when struck by x-ray photons. The light produced, in turn, exposes the film. The image is thereby formed. In dentistry, indirect exposure film is used for such extraoral radiographic procedures as panoramic and cephalometric radiography.

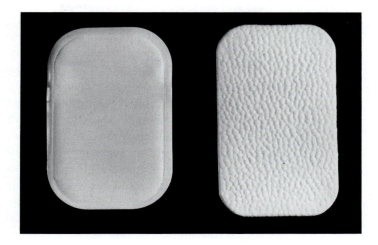

FIGURE 5-11 Film is supplied in both paper and polysoft film packets.

Indirect exposure film has the follow characteristics: (1) speed, (2) contrast, and (3) light spectrum response. Screen film is manufactured with different speeds or sensitivities, just like direct exposure film, and, as with direct exposure film, the thicker the emulsion and the larger the crystal size, the faster the film. Almost all screen films have an emulsion layer on each side of the base material. This double emulsion helps

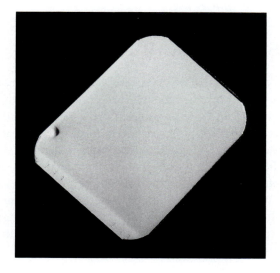

FIGURE 5-12 The embossed dot is useful in determining packet placement in the film holder and to aid in mounting the radiographs.

to increase the speed of the film without making the emulsion so thick on one side that light would have difficulty penetrating it.

Film manufacturers also produce screen films with different contrast levels. For black-and-white images, high-contrast film is preferred. For a grayer image, a low-contrast film is used.

The characteristic of greatest importance is the screen film's sensitivity to the color spectrum. Depending on what type of intensifying screens (fluorescent plates) are used in the cassette, care should be taken to match the light produced by the intensifying screen to the light sensitivity of the film. Some phosphors in the intensifying screens emit violet to blue light and should only be used with film that is sensitive to these colors. Other screens emit green light and should only be used with green light sensitive film. If the intensifying screen and film do not match, the image receptor speed will decrease and the amount of radiation used will have to increase. This defeats the benefits of the intensification process.

Exposure considerations for screen film include matching the intensifying screen and film to special procedures in the darkroom. Safelights must have a filter that matches the type of screen film being processed. Safelight filters used with intraoral film processing may fog some types of screen films. GBX-2 safelight filters (also known as Universal filters) can be used with most types of films used in medicine and dentistry today.

Although screen film provides an image with reduced patient radiographic exposure, the images have less detail than those exposed with direct exposure film. This must be considered when determining what type of film to use.

USE OF INTENSIFYING SCREENS

Usually less than 1 percent of the x-ray photons striking the film interact with the crystals to produce an image. When **intensifying screen** film systems are used, the x-rays strike the screen and cause the screen to emit light, which, in turn, interacts with the film to create a latent image (Figure 5-13). Approximately 30 percent of the x-ray photons striking the screen interact with it to produce light photons. Therefore, the intensifying screens increase the efficiency of the x-rays, thereby requiring fewer x-ray photons than direct exposure film. Thus intensifying screens create an image with lower patient exposure to radiation, but the image is not as clear as that produced by direct exposure.

Film is placed between two intensifying screens inside either a flexible or rigid cassette film holder (Figure 5-14). Intensifying screens have four basic layers: (1) the base, (2) the reflective coat, (3) the fluorescent layer, and (4) the protective layer (Figure 5-15).

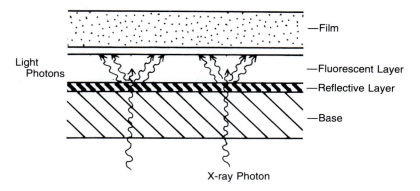

FIGURE 5-13 As the x-ray photons strike the intensifying screen, light photons are produced. These, in turn, expose the film.

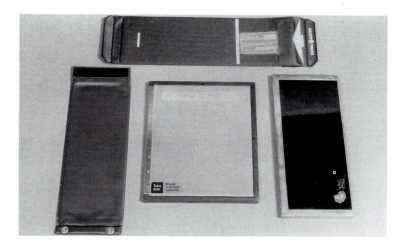

FIGURE 5-14 Rigid and flexible extraoral film cassettes.

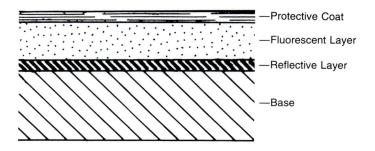

FIGURE 5-15 A cross-section of an intensifying screen.

The base serves the same purpose in the screen as it does in the film. It provides a rigid support for the fluorescent layer. Although it is usually made of a polyester material, cardboard and metal have been used.

The **reflective coat** is placed next to the base and serves to redirect light from the fluorescent layer back to the film. This increases the number of light photons reaching the film.

The **fluorescent layer** is the active part of the screen and contains the phosphors that convert the x-ray photons into visible light. The phosphors currently used in intensifying screens are calcium tungstate, barium lead sulfate, zinc sulfide, and the rare earth phosphors (gadolinium, lanthanum, and yttrium).

The **protective layer** is placed on the screen to make it more resistant to such damage as scratches and abrasions. In addition, this layer reduces the possibility that static electricity will be produced.

The most important characteristics of intensifying screens are speed and resolution. Screen speed is similar to the concept of film speed. It can be defined as the efficiency of the screen in converting x-ray energy to light energy. Several factors that may be inherent to the screen or under the control of the operator affect screen speed. Examples of these include phosphor crystal size, phosphor thickness, and variables in film processing (for example, increasing the developing time decreases the speed).

The resolution ability of a screen depends on crystal size, emulsion, and thickness. High-speed screens usually have lower resolution than slower-speed screens.

In the last several years, the screens' ability to convert x-ray energy to light energy has been made more efficient by the use of rare-earth elements. Rare-earth screens use phosphors, such as gadolinium, lanthanum, and yttrium. Because these screen elements are almost twice as efficient as calcium tungstate screens, patient exposure is reduced even more. Rare-earth screens usually emit light in the green color of the spectrum. As such, specifically matched film must be used with rare-earth screens to maintain their efficiency (Table 5-1).

FILM STORAGE AND HANDLING

To obtain the best quality radiographic image, the film should be stored and handled in a responsible manner. Improper storage and handling will contribute to poor quality images.

Since radiographic film is very sensitive to light, it should be stored and handled in the dark. Care should be given to ensure proper darkroom technique. Safelighting conditions should be observed. Rare-earth films will be fogged by a safelight with an amber filter. A red filter is safe for both green and blue light sensitive films.

TABLE 5-1
Radiography systems

System Components		Relative Speed*	Results
Intensifying Screens	Film Type		
KODAK LANEX Regular Screens	KODAK T-MAT G Film and KODAK T-MAT G Panoramic Film	400	excellent detail; high contrast
	KODAK T-MAT L Film	400	excellent detail; good soft-tissue visualization; wide range of densities
	KODAK T-MAT H Film and KODAK T-MAT H Panoramic Dental Film	400**	good detail; high constrast; use 2 films at once to obtain 2 original radiographs
	KODAK Ortho L Film	400	very good detail; good soft-tissue visualization
	KODAK Ortho G Film and KODAK Ortho G Panoramic Dental Film	400	very good detail; high contrast
KODAK LANEX Medium Screens	KODAK T-MAT G Film and KODAK T-MAT G Panoramic Film	250	excellent detail; high contrast
	KODAK T-MAT L Film	250	excellent detail; good soft-tissue visualization; wide range of densities
	KODAK T-MAT H Film and KODAK T-MAT H Panoramic Dental Film	250	good detail; high contrast; use 2 films at once to obtain 2 original radiographs
	KODAK Ortho L Film	250	very good detail; good soft-tissue visualization
	KODAK Ortho G Film and KODAK Ortho G Panoramic Dental Film	250	very good detail; high contrast
KODAK X-OMATIC Regular Intensifying Screens	KODAK X-OMAT RP Film	200	excellent detail; high contrast
	KODAK BLUE BRAND Film and KODAK BLUE BRAND Panoramic Dental Film	200	excellent detail; high contrast; manual processing
	KODAK SB Panoramic Dental Film	200	excellent detail; high contrast; 2-film technique to obtain two originals; manual processing
	KODAK EKTAMAT G Panoramic Film	100	for panoramic equipment using 8 mA or higher; excellent detail; high contrast
	KODAK EKTAMAT G Film	100	excellent detail; high contrast

* Medium-speed calcium tungstate and KODAK X-OMAT RP Film arbitrarily assigned a speed of 100. These relative speeds have been determined in accordance with ANSI PH 2.9-1974, but may vary in actual use depending on exposure, processing, and densitometry methods.

** System speed is 800 when only one film is exposed.

Source: Reprinted by permission from Eastman Kodak, Rochester, NY.

Temperature, humidity, and radiation (other than what contributes to the formation of the latent image) also affect the film. Because heat and high humidity increase the fog and decrease the contrast of film, radiographic film should be stored in a cool, dry place (no more than 68°F). Often references to refrigerating or freezing film are made to prolong its storage life, but film manufacturers do not recommend this practice. Radiographic film should not be stored or placed where it can encounter scatter radiation. Any scatter can cause film fog.

All film is shipped with an expiration date, which should be observed. Therefore, careful consideration should be taken when ordering large quantities of film, and film stock should be rotated so that the oldest film is used first. Aged film has increased fog and a loss of speed and contrast. Packages of extraoral film should be stored standing on their edges to lessen the possibility of film warping or the sheets of the film sticking together.

SUMMARY

This chapter has described image receptors and their respective characteristics. Film construction plays a vital role in image production. Film characteristics such as fog, density, contrast, resolution, speed, and mottling are factors that must be considered when storing, handling, exposing, and processing radiographic film.

BIBLIOGRAPHY

BUSHONG SC. *Radiologic Science of Technologists: Physics, Biology and Protection,* 3d ed. St. Louis: CV Mosby, 1984.

EASTMAN KODAK COMPANY. *The Fundamentals of Radiography,* 12th ed. Rochester, NY, 1980.

REVIEW QUESTIONS

1. The black areas on the processed radiograph are known as radiolucent.

a. True
b. False

2. Dental x-ray film is only one type of image receptor.

a. True
b. False

3. Dental x-ray film can be either direct exposure or indirect exposure film.

   a. True
   b. False

4. The film layer that contains the silver halide crystals is known as the

   a. base.
   b. protective layer.
   c. top coat.
   d. emulsion.

5. Films that are all black and white with very few grays are said to be

   a. very dense.
   b. high contrast.
   c. fogged.
   d. low contrast.

6. As x-rays travel further they become more intense.

   a. True
   b. False

7. The faster the film speed, the more radiation is needed to expose the film.

   a. True
   b. False

Radiographic Imaging for the Dental Team,
by Sally Mauriello. J.B. Lippincott Company,
Philadelphia © 1995.

6

Film Processing and the Darkroom

Upon the completion of this chapter, the student should be able to:

1. Discuss how the latent image is formed.

2. Identify the steps in film processing.

3. Describe the chemicals used in radiographic film processing and their functions.

4. Compare and contrast manual and automatic film processing.

5. Discuss the set-up and construction guidelines for a darkroom and safelighting.

6. Describe the equipment and procedures used in film duplication.

Processing of the radiographic image is one of the most important and critical steps in the production of high-quality and diagnostically acceptable radiographs. No matter how good the x-ray equipment works or how accurate the technical factors are, if the processing of the film is poor, the radiograph will be of poor quality. Processing involves not only knowledge of the radiographic film and chemistry used, but also the construction, care, and maintenance of the darkroom and its equipment.

Just like photographic processing, radiographic processing may be conducted in a darkroom using manual or automatic processing. Processing can also occur in daylight, if a **daylight loader** is attached to the automatic processor. The daylight loader allows the films to be unwrapped and fed into the processor outside of a darkroom (Figure 6-1).

This chapter will explore the formation of the latent image and how this image is transformed into a visible image through processing procedures. The processing chemicals, procedures in both manual and automatic processing, and film duplication will be discussed.

LATENT IMAGE FORMATION

In Chapter 5, the term **latent image** was defined as an invisible image present on the exposed but undeveloped film. To understand how the

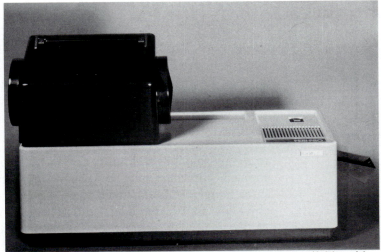

FIGURE 6-1 Many automatic film processors are available with daylight loaders.

latent image is changed into a visible image during the processing procedure, it is necessary to better understand the way the latent image is formed.

The silver halide crystal in the emulsion of radiographic film is composed of approximately 90 to 99 percent silver bromide and 1 to 10 percent silver iodide. This silver halide crystal is imperfect, and therefore, is very photosensitive. The silver halide crystal, which can be seen as a latticework of silver, iodine, and bromine, can display several types of defects. These defects include (1) a point defect, which occurs when a silver ion has moved out of its normal position in the crystal; (2) dislocation, which is a line of imperfection in the wall of the crystal; and (3) a **sensitivity speck,** which is produced by adding sulfur containing compounds to the emulsion. These compounds react with the silver halide to form silver sulfide. This area is located on the surface of the crystal and referred to as a sensitivity speck.

The silver is what gives us the dark areas on a developed radiograph. When a photon strikes the crystal, the energy absorbed gives an electron in the bromine ion enough energy to escape and lodge at the site of a crystal imperfection. In turn, it attracts a silver ion to neutralize it. The number of crystals affected this way depends on the number of photons striking a given area of the film. The accumulation of silver is what makes up the latent image on the film (Figure 6-2).

During developing, a chemical process reduces the silver ions to black metallic silver, which is deposited at the latent image site. The amount of blackness (density) on a developed film is a result of the amount of exposure of the film.

PROCESSING PROCEDURES

Whether x-ray film is processed in manual tanks or an automatic processor, four steps are involved: developing, fixing, washing, and drying. Each step plays a critical role in producing a good quality radiographic image.

Processing Chemistry

Processing solutions (chemistry) are manufactured as premixed or concentrated. The latter must be mixed with water. Processing chemicals can be bought in dry or liquid form, although the liquid form is most commonly used in the dental office. In addition, some solutions are manufactured with special chemicals that accelerate the procedure and reduce the processing time from the standard, time-temperature processing time of about 15 to 20 minutes to 4 to 8 minutes.

It is essential to follow the manufacturer's directions when storing, handling, and mixing the chemistry. Solutions should be changed ap-

Unexposed Crystal

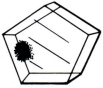

Exposed Crystal

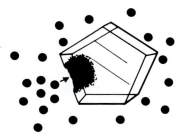

Exposed Crystal in Developer

FIGURE 6-2 During development, the silver halide crystals interact with the developer. Those crystals that were struck by x-rays during exposure react by separating into bromide (or iodide) and black metallic silver.

proximately every ten working days for manual processing and every 20 working days for automatic processing, depending on the volume of radiographs processed. Care should be taken to follow the manufacturer's directions concerning the temperature of the water and the amount used to mix the solutions. If these directions are modified, inconsistent image quality could result.

Certain general rules should be followed in the storage, handling, and mixing of manual-processing chemistry. These are:

1. Separate paddles should be used to stir the developer and fixer.

2. Cover the solutions in the tanks when not in use to prevent oxidation and evaporation.

3. Do not splash one solution into the other.

4. Clean tanks and covers before mixing and replacing solutions.

5. Store unused chemicals in a cool, dry place.

The **developer** is a chemical solution with active ingredients designed to change the silver halide crystals to metallic silver. This changes the latent image to a visible image. The characteristics of the

TABLE 6-1
Developing chemicals

Ingredients	Chemical	Activity
Reducing agents	Hydroquinone and phenidone	Changes the silver halide crystal to black metallic silver
Accelators	Calcium carbonate or potassium hydroxide	Swells the emulsion and provides an alkaline medium
Restrainers	Potassium bromide and potassium iodide	Blocks the action of the reducing agent on the unexposed crystals
Preservative	Sodium sulfite	Slows the oxidation and breakdown of the developer
Solvent	Water	Mixes the chemicals

developer include a strong, organic chemical odor, a yellow color, and a strong alkaline ph of about 10.4. The three factors influencing the development process are time, temperature, and the chemical activity.

The main ingredients found in the developer are (1) reducing agents, (2) accelerators, (3) restrainers, (4) a preservative, and (5) a solvent or vehicle (see Table 6-1).

- **Reducing Agents:** These chemicals "reduce" (or change) the exposed silver halide crystal to black metallic silver. They have little effect on the unexposed crystals on the film. The chemicals used as reducing agents are hydroquinone and phenidone. **Hydroquinone** blackens the crystal and is most responsible for bringing out the contrast. Hydroquinone, which is very sensitive to temperature changes, becomes inactive below 60°F and overactive above 70°F. **Phenidone** works quickly to develop the lighter areas of the film, providing the gray areas in the processed radiographs.

- **Accelerators:** These chemicals swell the emulsion and provide an alkaline medium. Since developers are only active at a high ph, accelerators allow the reducing agents to work. Without accelerators, the reducing agents would have little effect on the crystals. Accelerators are usually made of calcium carbonate or potassium hydroxide.

- **Restrainers:** Restrainers, also known as antifogging agents, block the action of the reducing agent on unexposed crystals. Without these chemicals, the processed radiographic film would be totally black. The chemicals used as restrainers are potassium bromide and potassium iodide.

■ Preservative: The preservative slows the oxidation and break down of the developer, thereby extending the life of the solution. Sodium sulfite is the chemical used as a preservative.

■ **Solvent:** The solvent is a vehicle to carry or mix the chemicals in the developer. It also helps to swell and soften the emulsion on the film, so that the chemicals can react with the crystals more effectively. Water is the basic solvent used.

After a radiographic film is removed from the developer, the unexposed silver halide crystals remain in the emulsion. If they remain there, they will eventually cause the film to discolor or darken. Therefore, these crystals need to be washed away and the emulsion needs to harden to prevent abrasion and scratches on the film. This is accomplished through a process known as fixation. The chemical solution used, which is known as the **fixer,** is a clear acidic solution (ph about 3.5 to 4.0). The fixing process, like the developing process, is affected by time, temperature, and chemical activity. The main ingredients in the fixer are (1) clearing agents, (2) acids, (3) a hardener, (4) a preservative, and (5) a solvent or vehicle (Table 6-2).

■ **Clearing Agents:** These chemicals change the unexposed silver halide crystals to soluble compounds that can be washed away. This helps to produce the gray and clear areas on the fully processed film. The chemicals used as clearing agents are ammonium thiosulfate or sodium thiosulfate.

TABLE 6-2
Fixing chemicals

Ingredients	Chemical	Activity
Clearing agents	Ammonium thiosulfate or sodium thiosulfate	Changes the unexposed silver crystals to soluble compounds so they can be washed away
Acid (or activator)	Acetic acid	Gives the fixer the proper pH and neutralize any remaining developer
Hardeners	Aluminum chloride (alum)	Toughens and shrinks the gelatin in the emulsion
Preservative	Sodium sulfite	Slows the oxidation or breakdown of the fixer
Solvent	Water	Mixes the chemicals

- Acids (or **activators**): These give the solution the proper ph and neutralize any remaining developer on the film. They also aid the other chemicals in their activities. Acetic acid or sulfur acid are the chemicals used.

- **Hardener:** A hardener helps to toughen and shrink the gelatin in the emulsion, which also helps to reduce the drying time needed at the completion of the processing. Hardeners are also present in the developer for some automatic processors to aid in transporting the film through the roller system. Aluminum chloride (alum) is used as the hardener.

- Preservative: Sodium sulfite is also used in the fixer to slow its decomposition or breakdown. If the fixer begins to break down, or deteriorate, the films will be cloudy and "tacky-damp."

- Solvent: As in the developer, water is the solvent used as the vehicle for mixing the chemicals in the fixer.

Washing the film in a bath of clear, circulating water is essential both after the removal of the film from the developer and after fixation. After the film is removed from the developer, it retains traces of the developing chemicals. These can contaminate the fixer solution if not removed. As a result, it is critical during manual processing to wash the films thoroughly after developing and before fixing. This step is not necessary in automatic processing.

After fixing, the film should again be thoroughly washed to remove any remaining chemicals. Otherwise, the radiographs will eventually discolor and fade.

Circulating water is used in the washing process to continually expose all surfaces to fresh water. This aids in removing all traces of the chemical solutions. Ideally, the flow rate of the water should be 2 to 3 gallons per minute in a 5 gallon tank. The temperature of the water bath should be approximately that of the developer.

Manual Processing Procedure

Manual processing is accomplished using tanks to hold the chemicals and water and hangers to hold the films. The films, which are attached to hangers, move from tank to tank according to a specific procedure known as the **time-temperature method.** This method is the most accurate for obtaining a good quality radiograph. The film is first immersed in the developer for a specific time, depending on the temperature of the solution. At the optimum temperature of 68°F, the film is left in the developer for approximately 5 minutes. The film is then washed for approximately 30 seconds and immersed in the fixer for twice the clearing time (that is, the time it takes for the visible image to

TABLE 6-3
Time/temperature chart[a]

Develop	Rinse	Fix	Wash
68 F, 5 min	30 sec	2–4 min	10 min
70 F, 4.5 min	30 sec	2–4 min	10 min
72 F, 4 min	30 sec	2–4 min	10 min
76 F, 3 min	30 sec	2–4 min	10 min
80 F, 2.5 min	30 sec	2–4 min	10 min

[a] These times and temperatures are specified using either D or E speed film and Kodak GBX fixer and developer.

appear on the film—not the total developing time), usually 2 to 4 minutes. Finally, the film is placed in the water tank for a 10-minute wash.

Processing solutions are manufactured to work most effectively within a small range of temperatures (Table 6-3). Very low or extremely high temperatures can render the solutions ineffective for processing.

For manual processing, the tanks are set up so that the developer is on the left, the water in the middle, and the fixer on the right (Figure 6-3). Typically, the water surrounding the developer and fixer tanks control the developer and fixer temperatures by increasing the hot or cold water flow.

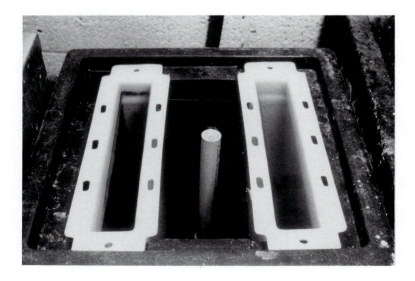

FIGURE 6-3 Manual processing tanks.

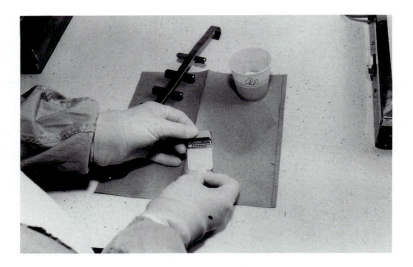

FIGURE 6-4 The films should be unwrapped by opening the film packets and pulling out the black paper.

Equipment that is needed to carry out manual processing includes (1) a timer to measure time in the developer, fixer, and water bath; (2) film hangers to hold the films during processing; (3) a thermometer to measure the developer temperature; and (4) a dryer to dry the films after they have been in the water bath. Films can also be air dried.

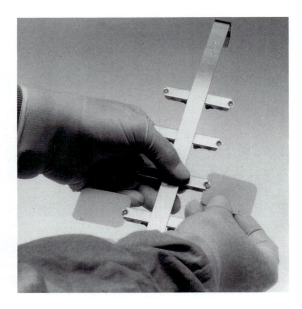

FIGURE 6-5 Once unwrapped, the film is clipped to a film rack.

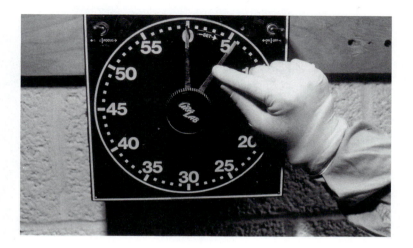

FIGURE 6-6 The timer should be set to accurately time the processing.

Prior to beginning the processing procedure, the solutions should be stirred and the temperature checked. The procedure for manual processing is as follows (Methods for carrying out this procedure using universal infection control are discussed in Chapter 2):

1. Unwrap films and securely clip them to the hanger. Be sure to handle the films only by the edges to avoid fingerprints (Figures 6-4 and 6-5).

2. Set the timer for the developing time specified on the time-temperature chart (Figure 6-6).

3. Immerse films in the developer using an agitating motion to break up any air bubbles around the film. Air bubbles can prevent the developer from fully reaching the film, thereby creating artifacts (unwanted densities superimposed on the film) (Figure 6-7).

4. At the end of the developing time, rinse the films in the water bath for 30 seconds (Figure 6-8).

5. Set the timer for twice the clearing time and immerse the films in the fixer tank (Figure 6-9).

6. After the fixing time has ended, place the films in the water tank for approximately 10 minutes. The water should continually circulate (Figure 6-10).

7. Films can be dried by placing the hanger in a dust-free area or in a film dryer (Figures 6-11 and 6-12).

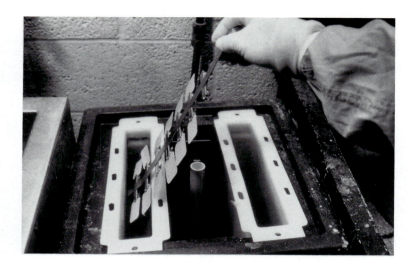

FIGURE 6-7 The films are immersed in the developer tank.

The developing procedure should not be judged by holding the films up to the safelight to determine the length of time the films should remain in the developer. The time-temperature method should be followed as outlined. If the films have to be viewed quickly during the treatment of a patient, the films can be viewed wet, in white (daylight) light, after they have been fixed for 2 minutes. But, the films must be returned to the fixer for the balance of the specified fixing time to ensure a long-lasting, high-quality radiographic image.

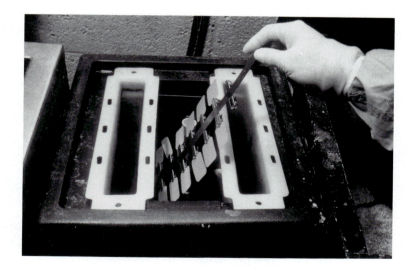

FIGURE 6-8 The films are removed from the developer and placed in the water bath to rinse prior to fixing.

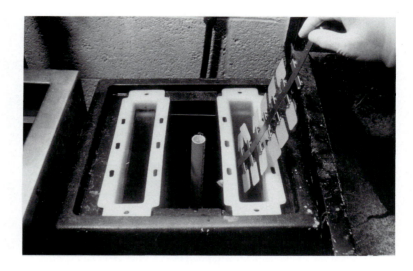

FIGURE 6-9 The rinsed films are immersed in the fixer tank.

Automatic Processing Procedure

Many dental offices enjoy the convenience of automatic processors. The total processing time, from developing to receiving the dried films, ranges from 90 seconds to 5 minutes. This is accomplished through special processing chemistry, higher temperatures (80 to 100°F), and an internal dryer (Figure 6-13).

The automatic processor uses a system of rollers to transport the film from the developer to the fixer, to the wash, and then to a dryer. The

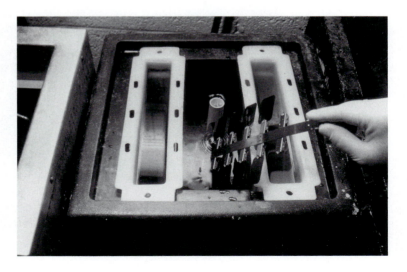

FIGURE 6-10 The films are rinsed in a bath of circulating water.

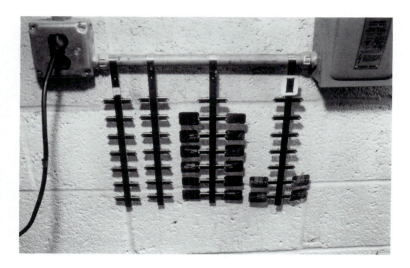

FIGURE 6-11   The films can be hung on a rack to be air dried.

rollers not only serve to carry the films but also to squeegee the solutions from the films in order to reduce contamination of one solution with another.

If maintained according to the manufacturer's instructions, automatic processors will produce consistent, high-quality processed radiographs. Typical maintenance includes checking the solution levels, temperatures, and water supply, as well as cleaning the tanks and

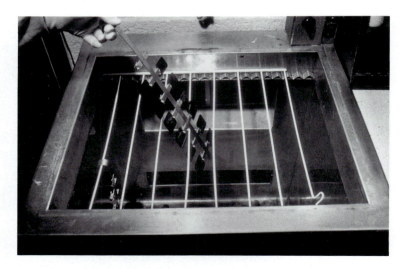

FIGURE 6-12   The films can be dried by placing them in a film dryer.

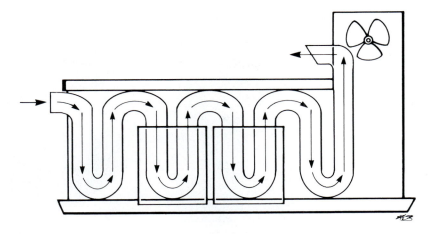

FIGURE 6-13 This drawing shows a cross-section of the rollers and tanks in a typical automatic film processor.

rollers. Cleaning films should be run through the processor at the beginning of each day to remove any contaminants on the rollers.

The chemistry used in automatic processors is different from the manual processing solutions. Only chemistry specifically made for automatic processors can be used, because it is manufactured to perform relatively quickly at high temperatures. Manual processing chemistry cannot withstand these demands.

The procedure for automatic processing is as simple as unwrapping the films and loading them one by one into the processor (Figure 6-14). If

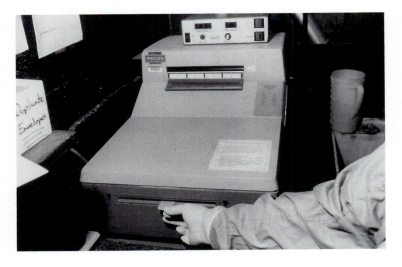

FIGURE 6-14 The film is loaded into the automatic film processor.

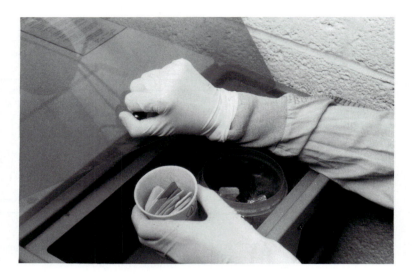

FIGURE 6-15 Daylight loader. See also Figure 6-1.

the processor is equipped with a daylight loader (Figures 6-1 and 6-15), it can be located outside of a darkroom. With a daylight loader, the films are unwrapped inside the loader and then fed into the processor.

Replenishment

The activity of the developer and fixer diminishes over time because of oxidation and multiple use of the solutions. When the solutions deteriorate, the films will take longer to develop and the contrast and speed of the film will be altered. The finished films will be light and have low contrast.

To maintain the activity of the solutions, as well as the level (or volume) of the solutions (some evaporates and some is carried out on the films into the water), replenishment is necessary. This requires that more solution be added to the original developer and fixer. The preparation of replenishment solutions should be carried out according to the manufacturer's directions. The main solutions usually serve as replenishing solutions as well. This should be done for both manual and automatic processing systems.

Replenishment cannot be carried out indefinitely because of oxidation and the accumulation of contaminants in the solution. Therefore, the solutions should be totally discarded and replaced at every 10 working days for manual processing chemistry and every 20 working days for automatic processing chemistry.

FILM TYPES AND PROCESSING CONSIDERATIONS

Both D and E speed films can be either manually or automatically processed, but E speed films are much more sensitive to processing conditions and can be excessively fogged in an automatic processor. As a result, the films may display less density and lower contrast.

Indirect exposure film (screen film) can be processed using either method. Most automatic processors are equipped to handle the larger, indirect exposure films, including panoramic and intraoral films.

DARKROOM

There are several factors in the construction, safelighting, and care and maintenance of the darkroom that can affect the final quality of the processed film. The construction and design of the darkroom should provide adequate space for the tanks, processing solutions, automatic processor (if applicable), and storage. Plumbing should include hot and cold water and drainage. The ventilation, humidity, and temperature should create an area that is cool and dry. Ideally, the temperature should not exceed 90°F and the humidity should be approximately 70 percent. High temperatures can fog the film and low humidity can cause static electricity that shows up as an artifact on the film. In addition, current OSHA requirements indicate that ventilation should be adequate to avoid chemical fume contamination.

The darkroom should be light tight. This means that when the lights are off, the room should be totally dark. Doorjambs, keyholes, and vents can be sources of light leaks into the room. Many offices use mazes or revolving doors to help prevent light leaks. To check for light leaks, simply turn the lights off, allow 2 to 3 minutes for your eyes to adjust, and then check if any light is entering the room.

The lighting in the darkroom should include a normal white light and a safelight. The safelight should be no closer than 4 feet from the automatic processor or wherever the films are unwrapped or removed from the cassettes. The most common safelight filters available are the Kodak GBX* and the Kodak ML-2*. The GBX is appropriate for both direct and indirect exposure films. The ML-2 filter can fog extraoral film and should not be used with them. The bulb used in the **safelight** should be no larger than 15 watts if it is shining down on the work surface. If the safelight is directed toward the ceiling, then the wattage can increase to 25. To determine if the safelight is safe (does not fog the films), place a penny on an opened film on the counter of the darkroom for several minutes. Then, process the film. If a visible image

*Eastman Kodak, Rochester, N.Y.

of the penny is on the processed film, the safelight filter or bulb is not safe.

Daylight loaders can be used both inside and outside darkrooms. Be sure that the white light in the room is not so bright as to fog the film when using the daylight loader.

The darkroom should be kept clean from contaminated trash, such as used film packets. In addition, avoid splashing chemicals or water on the countertops where films are handled. Chemicals or water that contact undeveloped film will show up as artifacts on the developed film. The darkroom should also be as dust free as possible, since dust can contaminate solutions and stick to wet films.

FILM DUPLICATION

Copies (or duplicates) of radiographs may be needed for several reasons, including sending radiographs to insurance companies so they can authorize treatment, referring patients to a specialist, and transferring records for patients who are moving or changing dentists. For these purposes, intraoral film packets can be purchased with double films in the packets. These provide two identical radiographs with each exposure. The alternative, which is duplicating the radiographs, avoids the use double film packets or exposing the patient to additional radiation.

Duplicating radiographs requires a film duplicator and duplicating film. The duplicator provides a light source (usually ultraviolet) to expose the film. This film differs from regular intraoral or extraoral film in that it has emulsion only on one side. In addition, the concept of exposure is different. The longer the film is exposed to the light source, the lighter—or less dense—the duplicate radiograph will appear. This can be valuable when duplicating radiographs that are either too dark or too light. These radiographs can be lightened or darkened to a certain extent depending upon how long the film is exposed during the duplication process.

Duplicating is carried out in the darkroom under safelight conditions. The films are placed on the duplicator, either alone or in a mount that will allow full contact with the film. Normal patient mounts are unsatisfactory for organizing the films on the duplicator; they allow a space between the original radiographs and the duplicating film that can result in a poor quality copy. Therefore, if a mount is used, it must allow the radiographs and the duplicating film to lie flush against one another. Clear mounts are acceptable for the duplication process.

After the radiographs have been placed on the duplicator (Figure 6-16), the duplicating film is placed over the radiographs with the emulsion side (usually gray or lavender) contacting the radiographs.

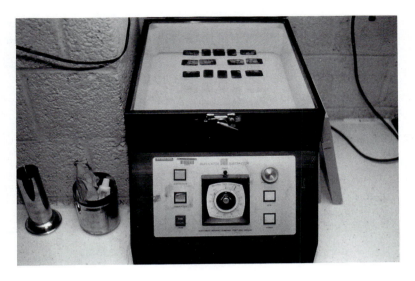

FIGURE 6-16 Film duplicator.

The duplicator is then activated for the time specified in the machine's directions. The duplicating film is then removed and processed in the normal fashion. If the resulting duplicate is not satisfactory, the process can be repeated to get a better copy without having to worry about re-exposing the patient.

SUMMARY

In this chapter, we have discussed the concept of radiographic film processing. It is essential that the operator understand the guidelines and underlying concepts in film processing, using the darkroom, and duplicating radiographs to avoid unnecessary patient re-exposure to radiation and to produce high-quality, diagnostically acceptable radiographs.

BIBLIOGRAPHY

CURRY III TS, DOWDEY JE, MURRY JR RC. *Christensen's Physics of Diagnostic Radiology,* 4th ed. Philadelphia: Lea and Febiger, 1990.

EASTMAN KODAK COMPANY, HEALTH SCIENCES DIVISION. *Exposure and Processing for Dental Radiography.* Publication No. N-413 P9974, Rochester, NY, 1990.

EASTMAN KODAK COMPANY, HEALTH SCIENCES MARKETS DIVISION. *The Fundamentals of Radiography,* 12th ed. Rochester, NY, 1980.

MATTESON SR, WHALEY C, SECRIST VC. *Dental Radiology,* 4th ed. Chapel Hill, NC: University of North Carolina Press, 1988.

McKINNEY WEJ. *Radiographic Processing and Quality Control.* Philadelphia: JB Lippincott, 1988.

REVIEW QUESTIONS

1. The silver halide crystal is made up of what 2 compounds?

    a. _____

    b. _____

2. List the steps in film processing.

    a. _____

    b. _____

    c. _____

    d. _____

3. The chemical in the developer that is responsible for blackening the crystals and bringing out the contrast is

    a. phenidone.
    b. calcium carbonate.
    c. hydroquinone.
    d. potassium bromide.

4. What is the solvent or vehicle used to mix the chemicals in the developer and fixer?

_____

5. Which solution is considered to be acidic?

_____

6. If the radiographic film is not washed properly, what will occur?

_____

_____

7. The optimum time and temperature for developing a radiographic film is

    a. 3 minutes/70°F.
    b. 5 minutes/68°F.
    c. 1 minute/85°F.
    d. 4 minutes/75°F.

8. When duplicating radiographic films, the longer the film is exposed to the light source, the lighter—or less dense—the duplicate radiograph will appear.

a. True
b. False

Radiographic Imaging for the Dental Team,
by Sally Mauriello. J.B. Lippincott Company,
Philadelphia © 1995.

7

Principles and Techniques of Imaging

Upon the completion of this chapter, the student will be able to:

1. Describe the rationale for using the shadowcasting principles.

2. Discuss shadowcasting principles in relation to dental radiography.

3. Apply shadowcasting principles to the imaging of oral structures.

4. Develop appropriate problem-solving solutions to various clinical situations dealing with the movement of the tooth or object on the radiographic film.

5. Describe three parameters that influence the appearance of the radiographic image.

The primary goal for dental radiographers is to produce a diagnostically acceptable x-ray film that is representative of the teeth or structures that are being radiographed. This involves not only the proper exposure settings, machine operation, and darkroom management, but competence in the technique of placing and exposing films in the oral cavity. Without a good radiographic technique, the most closely monitored processing conditions will be useless.

Good radiographic technique begins with the five basic principles that govern the accurate projecting of the tooth image or structure onto the radiographic film. These principles, called the shadowcasting principles, will dictate the size, shape, and location of the tooth image on the film. These principles are the building blocks for understanding the technical part of dental radiology and will be applied to all imaging techniques used.

SHADOWCASTING PRINCIPLES

Five shadowcasting principles should be followed when exposing radiographs. Each will be discussed, with a description of the principle and its proper application. Remember that our goal is to produce an x-ray image that closely resembles the object being radiographed.

1. *PRINCIPLE 1:* X-rays should be emitted from the smallest source of radiation (**focal spot** or **target**) as possible.

   To produce an image with sharp detail, it is necessary to produce an x-ray beam with parallel rays. The smaller the point at which x-rays are generated, the more parallel the x-rays will be (Figure 7-1). X-ray generation is discussed in Chapter 4. Thus, the smaller the focal spot, the better the **detail.** Focal spot size is determined by the manufacturer and can not be changed by the operator (Figure 7-2).

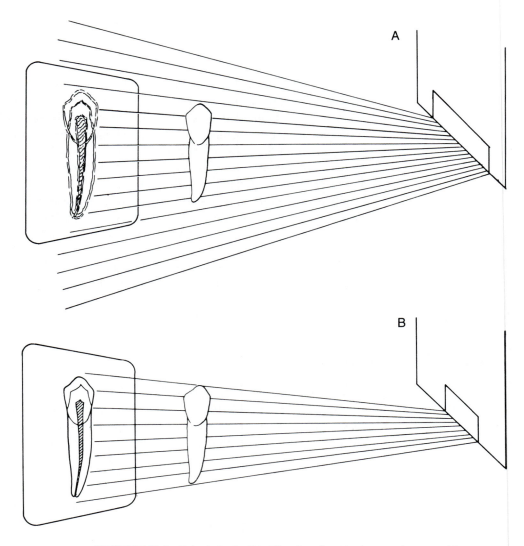

FIGURE 7-1 Principle 1. (A) The drawing depicts an image with poor detail due to the use of a large focal spot. (B) The image shows a small focal spot with a more detailed image.

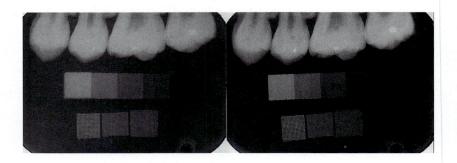

FIGURE 7-2 On the left, a phantom was exposed with a large focal spot and on the right with a small focal spot. Note the difference in detail.

2. *PRINCIPLE 2:* The x-ray source (focal spot or target) to object (oral structures) distance should be as long as possible.

This principle is accomplished through the use of a long position-indicating device or open-ended cone. The added distance results in an image with less magnification and sharper outline or border of the oral structure (Figure 7-3). This phenomenon occurs because the x-ray photons that interact with the film are straighter, or less di-

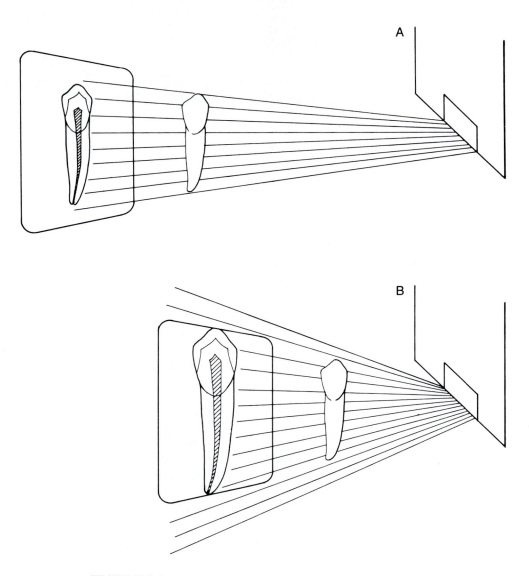

FIGURE 7-3 Principle 2. (A) The parallel photons provide an image with greater detail and less magnification when compared to the object in (B).

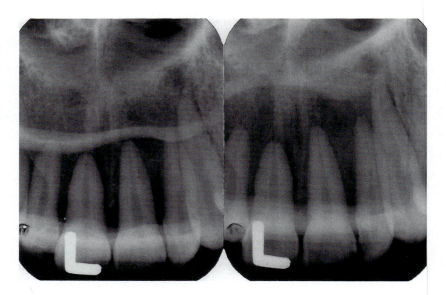

FIGURE 7-4 The object on the left (exposed with a long film to focal spot distance) shows an image of good detail compared with the image on the right (short film to focal spot distance), which is magnified and not distinct.

vergent. The straighter photons display a more accurate shadow or image on the film. At a short distance, a greater number of photons not parallel to the straight photons expose the film. This gives the image a spread out appearance. The information displayed by these photons make the image appear larger with less distinct borders. Thus, the shape and size of the object will be more accurate with a long focal spot to object distance (Figure 7-4).

3. *PRINCIPLE 3:* The object (oral structure) to film distance should be as short as possible.

   Placing the film as close to the object as possible decreases distortion by reducing magnification (Figure 7-5). As the object to film distance increases, the image becomes larger and fuzzy in appearance. Thus, a short object to film distance decreases magnification and enhances the sharpness of the image (Figure 7-6).

4. *PRINCIPLE 4:* The film and long axis of the object (oral structure) should be **parallel.**

   The long axis of the object and film should be as parallel to each other as possible (Figure 7-7). This decreases the amount of **distortion** to the radiographic image. A film not parallel to the long axis of the tooth will display magnification and distortion (Figure 7-8).

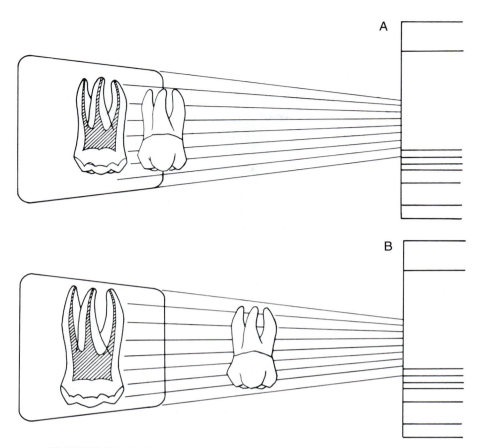

FIGURE 7-5 Principle 3. (A) The drawing depicts a close film to object distance with little magnification. (B) The increased film to object distance increases image magnification.

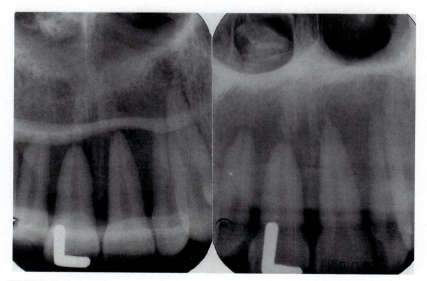

FIGURE 7-6 When compared, the object on the left shows the image of an object with a short film to object distance. The object on the right displays magnification due to the long film to object distance.

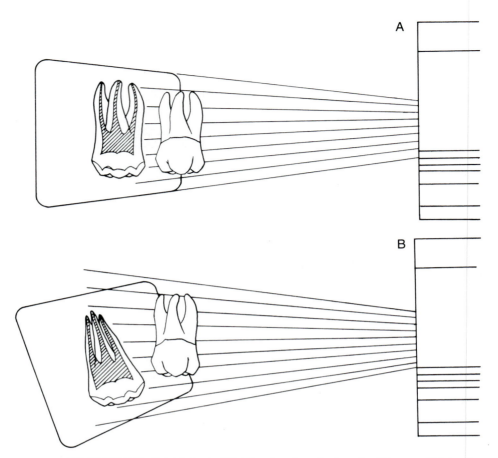

FIGURE 7-7 Principle 4. (A) The drawing depicts the film parallel to the long axis of the tooth. (B) The film is not parallel to the long axis of the tooth.

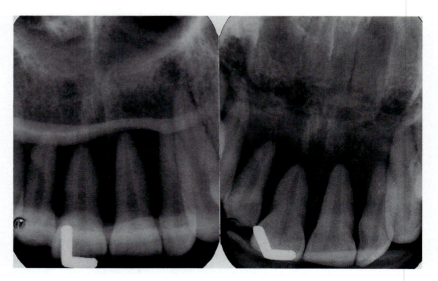

FIGURE 7-8 The x-ray on the left shows the image of an object with a parallel film and object. The x-ray on the right shows the distorted image of an object with an unparallel film and object.

5. *PRINCIPLE 5:* The x-ray beam should be placed **perpendicular** to the film.

This is accomplished by positioning the x-ray beam at right angles (perpendicular) to the long axis of the parallel film and object (Figure 7-9). If the x-ray beam is not perpendicular, the image will be distorted on the film and will not be representative of the object being radiographed. The distortion would manifest itself as a short, squatty structure (**foreshortening**) or a thin, stretched-out structure (**elongation**) (Figure 7-10).

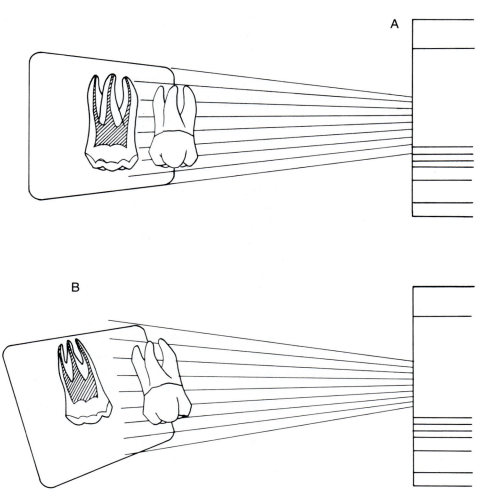

FIGURE 7-9 Principle 5. (A) The drawing depicts normal alignment of the film, tooth, and x-ray beam. (B) The drawing shows the beam not perpendicular to the tooth and the result is a distorted image.

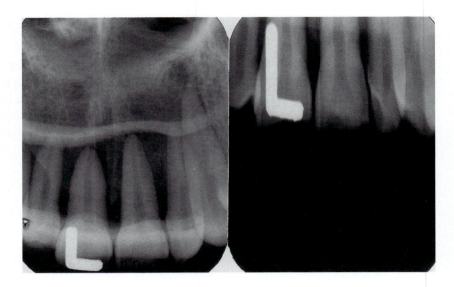

FIGURE 7-10   The x-ray on the left shows an image exposed with the beam perpendicular to the film. The x-ray on the right demonstrates the distortion that occurs when the beam is not perpendicular to the film.

THE RADIOGRAPHIC IMAGE

In addition to good radiographic technique, two other factors influence the radiographic image: the focal spot size and the penumbra (sometimes called the edge gradient). Both factors affect the appearance of the margin of the object by creating a fuzzy or unsharp edge.

As discussed in Chapter 4, the focal spot (target) is a small area located on the anode. Since x-rays are generated from more than one point on the focal spot, not all rays are parallel. Thus, the unparallel rays project the edge of the image in different areas (Figure 7-11). These areas are gray and represent the penumbra. The area of complete darkness is called the **umbra.** The smaller the focal spot, the smaller the penumbra. The penumbra is also controlled by the collimator.

Unfortunately, the smaller focal spot creates a dilemma in radiology. Due to the heat generated at the anode, it is necessary to have a large focal spot. Through the use of the **line-focus principle,** scientists have been able to overcome this problem. By angling the focal spot on the anode, the focal spot parallel with the central ray (effective focal spot) is smaller than the actual focal spot (perpendicular to the central ray). This principle is demonstrated in Figure 7-12. There is a limit to the degree of angulation that can be used to create the **effective focal spot.** Due to the self-absorption of photons on the anode side of the tube, an uneven **beam** intensity is produced. This varies depending on the angle of the focal spot and is referred to as the **heel effect.**

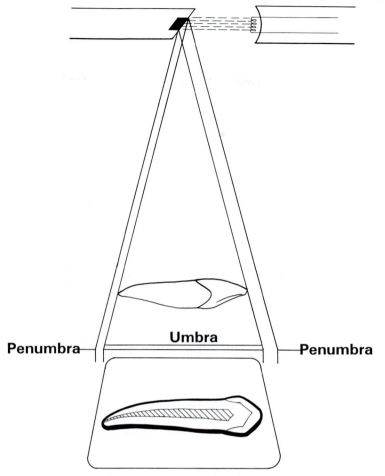

FIGURE 7-11   The development of the penumbra is due to the many points at which x-rays are generated on the focal spot.

PROJECTION GEOMETRY: MOVEMENT OF THE IMAGE

In some instances, you will be unable to project the object onto the film using the standard guidelines that we have discussed. A thorough understanding of the shadowcasting principles will help the radiographer develop alternative ways to project the image onto the film while the film and object remain in the normal position. This may be accomplished by altering the direction of the beam through adjustment of the **vertical** and **horizontal angulation,** thereby moving or casting the object image onto the film.

A change in horizontal angulation will shift the image right or left onto the film. If you direct the x-ray beam in the direction that you would like the tooth to move on the film, then the tooth image will shift in that direction. The following example will illustrate this principle. In Figure 7-13, the distal root of the mandibular third molar is not com-

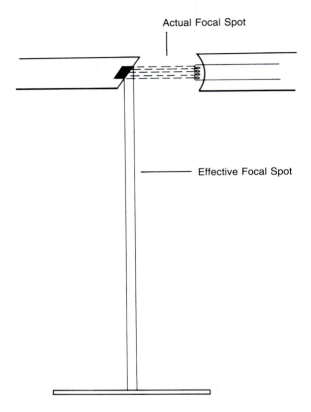

Actual Focal Spot

Effective Focal Spot

FIGURE 7-12 The line-focus principle. The beam appears to be generated from a small point source because of the angulation of the anode.

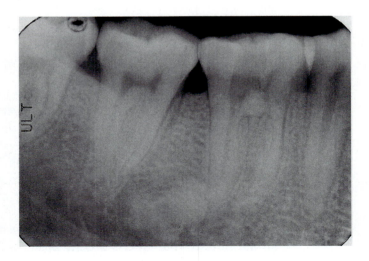

FIGURE 7-13 A mandibular molar projection with the distal of the third molar missing.

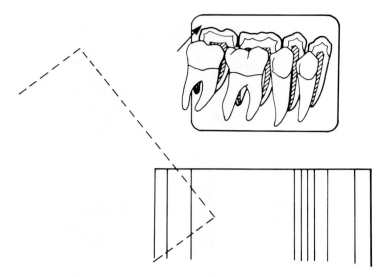

FIGURE 7-14 The drawing depicts the original tube angulation and resultant image for the molar projection. The dotted line projects the movement of the tubehead (beam directed mesially) and image (image moved mesially). The film remained in the same position.

pletely shown on the film. Since the operator was unable to move the film any further distal, a change in the horizontal angulation is necessary for the radiographer to project the **distal** root on the film. To accomplish this, the radiographer must direct the x-ray beam towards the mesial (Figures 7-14 and 7-15). The same principle applies to

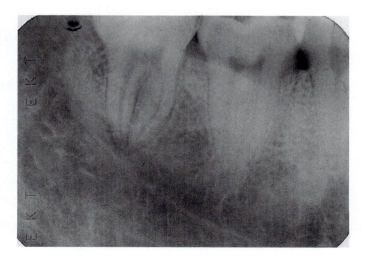

FIGURE 7-15 The x-ray beam was projected towards the mesial to project the entire third molar onto the film.

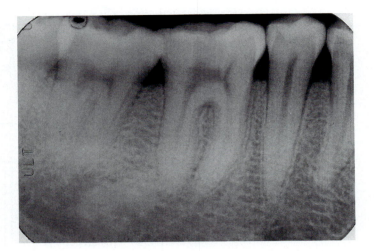

FIGURE 7-16 A mandibular premolar projection with the mesial portion of the first premolar missing.

projecting the **mesial** of the first premolar onto the film (Figure 7-16). To move the tooth to the distal, the beam should be directed distally (Figures 7-17 and 7-18). Obviously when the horizontal angulation is altered, the image will most likely display **overlapping** of the **interproximal** spaces. Usually these spaces can be opened on the **bitewing** projections.

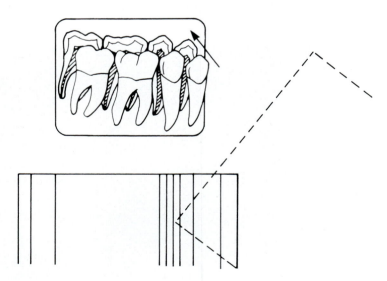

FIGURE 7-17 The beam should be projected towards the distal in order to project the entire first premolar onto the film.

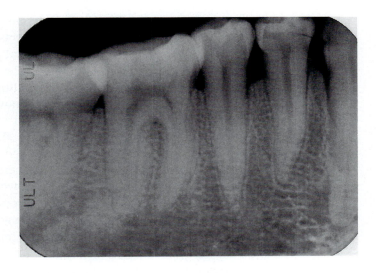

FIGURE 7-18   The entire first premolar can be projected onto the film by directing the beam towards the distal.

The vertical movement of the tooth follows the same principle. The image of the tooth can be moved up and down by adjusting the vertical angulation of the **beam.** To move the image on the film, the x-ray beam should be directed toward the desired movement of the tooth (Figure 7-19). Direct the x-ray beam in an upward direction to move the tooth

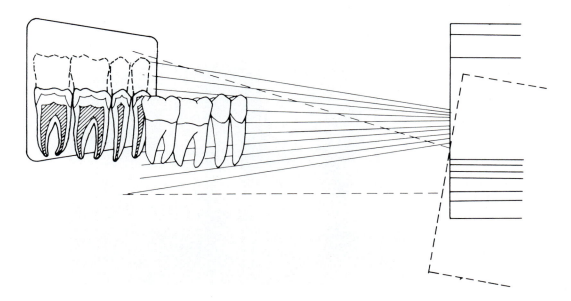

FIGURE 7-19   The tooth can be moved down on the film by adjusting the vertical angulation.

image to a higher position on the film. For example, a shallow **palate** could result in images with the apices of the roots missing on the film (Figure 7-20). To compensate for this anatomical constraint, an adjustment in the vertical angulation is required. The beam should be directed in a steeper **angulation** downward, pointing in the direction the radiographer wants the image on the film to move (Figures 7-21 and 7-22).

These applications are most often used in clinical situations that require imaging of the distal roots of mandibular third molars, impacted or unerupted third molars, mesial surfaces of mandibular first premolars, and rotated teeth. If the teeth are crowded and/or rotated, an adjustment in technique may be required to open the interproximal space (Figure 7-23). This adjustment would be achieved by modification of the horizontal angulation. Because the image of the tooth will move on the film if the horizontal angulation is changed, it will be necessary to position the film in a more mesial or distal direction. The position of the film is dependent on the direction of the x-ray beam needed to open the interproximal space. As an example, try to open the interproximal space between the first and second molar when the two teeth are severely rotated (Figure 7-24). You should direct the x-ray beam toward the distal to open the interproximal space with the film in a more posterior position in order to record the area of interest. Failure to do this will result in a film of the molar area, but without all of the molars present.

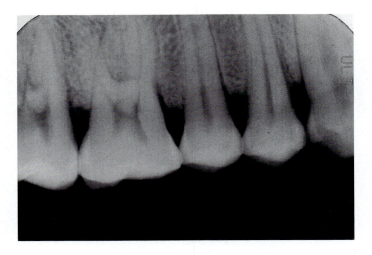

FIGURE 7-20   Root apices are missing because of a shallow palate.

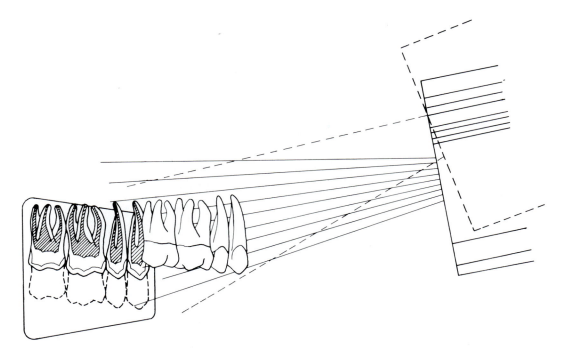

FIGURE 7-21 Normal tube angulation with apices missing. Readjustment of the beam pointing down would image the apices on the film.

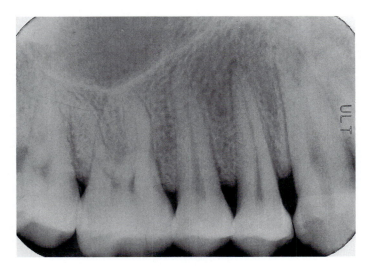

FIGURE 7-22 The apices are present because of the modification of the tubehead angulation.

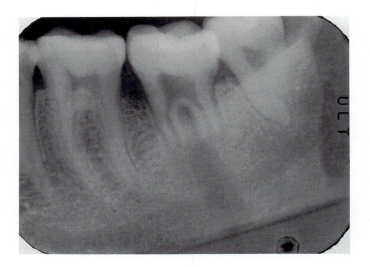

FIGURE 7-23 An x-ray of rotated teeth which result with interproximal overlap when standard horizontal positioning is used.

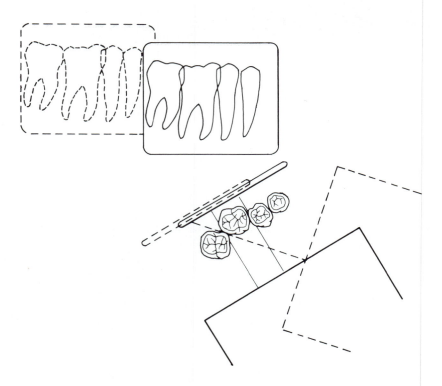

FIGURE 7-24 The drawing depicts tube angulation and imaging of teeth on the film. The dotted line represents the movement of the teeth on the film when adjustments in horizontal angulation are made to open the interproximal space.

PROJECTION GEOMETRY: PROBLEM-SOLVING TECHNIQUE ERRORS

Understanding the movement of the image through adjustment of the horizontal and vertical angulation will also assist the radiographer in solving errors in technique. After exposing radiographs on a patient, the films should be evaluated both for diagnostic purposes and technical merit. Missing crowns, missing roots, not having the correct teeth, and overlapped interproximal spaces may result in the need to re-expose the patient to obtain the needed diagnostic information. Thus, competence in exposing radiographs is a good way to decrease the exposure dose to the patient. The ability to technically evaluate films and determine the cause of errors will increase the competence of the radiographer.

Suppose a mandibular film was exposed and the roots of the molars were missing on the radiograph (Figure 7-25). The film was placed properly in the mouth, and the patient was biting on the film holder. What happened to the roots? In this case, the vertical angulation was not correctly directed to the film. To correct this error, increase the vertical angulation to the point where the x-ray beam is perpendicular to the tooth and film (Figure 7-26).

Another situation presents the maxillary central projection with the crowns missing (Figure 7-27). If packet placement was correct, then what could have caused this error? The answer is incorrect vertical angulation. The beam was directed to steep, thus projecting the crowns of the teeth downward in the direction of the beam. To correct this

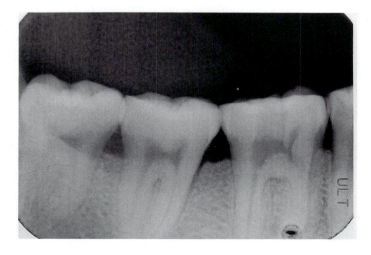

FIGURE 7-25 A properly placed mandibular molar projection with the root apices missing.

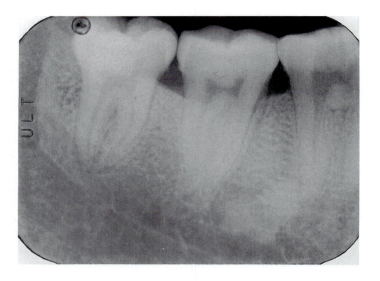

FIGURE 7-26 An x-ray showing the root apices after tubehead adjustments were made.

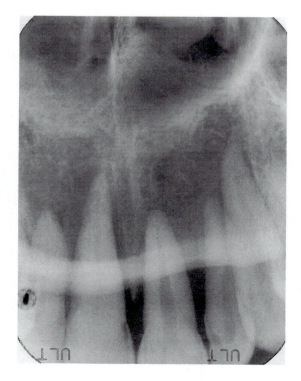

FIGURE 7-27 Maxillary central projection with crowns projected off of the film.

length of the root. What adjustments should be made on the retake to get the needed information?

a. Increase the vertical angulation with the beam directed toward the crown of the tooth.
b. Decrease the vertical angulation with the beam directed toward the root of the tooth.
c. Change the horizontal angulation directing the beam more mesial.
d. Change the horizontal angulation directing the beam more distal.
e. Lower the tubehead.

Radiographic Imaging for the Dental Team,
by Sally Mauriello. J.B. Lippincott Company,
Philadelphia © 1995.

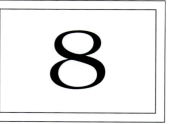

Intraoral Radiographic Procedures

Upon the completion of this chapter, the student should be able to:

1. Describe the two primary types of projections used in an intraoral technique.

2. Discuss the preparation of the operatory, film, and patient for making intraoral exposures.

3. Describe the four steps used in intraoral radiographic imaging.

4. Discuss the radiographic technique for using the Precision and Rinn XCP film-holding devices.

5. Describe the radiographic technique and rationale for exposing periapical and bitewing projections.

Intraoral radiography involves the placement of the film inside the patient's mouth, with the x-ray source generated outside. Because the goal of radiography is to produce an image that resembles the object being radiographed as closely as possible, the operator must be competent in radiographic techniques. This chapter discusses the primary projections used in intraoral radiography, preparation of the operatory, film, and patient, and two acceptable intraoral techniques.

INTRAORAL PROCEDURES USED IN DENTISTRY

The ideal radiographic technique would incorporate *all* of the shadowcasting principles discussed in Chapter 7. Unfortunately, a technique has not yet been devised that meets these requirements. Research has shown that the **paralleling technique** displays the most accurate image, with the least amount of radiation exposure to the patient. In some situations (i.e., a small mouth, shallow palate, tori, etc.), the operator may have to utilize other techniques. Appropriate solutions are discussed in Chapter 11.

In addition to the paralleling technique, the American Dental Association recommends use of a film-holding device that aligns the x-ray beam perpendicular to the film. Devices that meet this criteria are Precision* or Rinn* XCP instruments. Use of these instruments requires accurate film placement in the oral cavity. The horizontal angulation, vertical angulation, and centering of the beam are predetermined by the film-holding device. Although these instruments are the film-holding devices of choice, it is not always possible to adapt these to every patient. In those circumstances, the radiographer must recognize the limitations of the device and convert to a technique that requires manual determination of the horizontal angulation, vertical angulation, and beam centering. Therefore, it is necessary to understand the basic principles required to expose a **radiograph** using the shadowcasting principles. The technique using a styrofoam biteblock is discussed in Chapter 7. Mastery of this technique or a similar paralleling technique is recommended for use in conjunction with the Precision or Rinn XCP instruments.

TYPES OF INTRAORAL PROJECTIONS FOR A FULL SERIES

Two types of projections are commonly performed in **intraoral radiography.** The first, called a **periapical projection,** gets its name from

---

*Rinn Corporation, Elgin, IL.

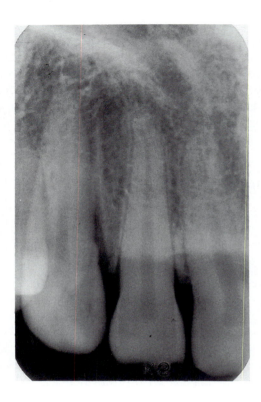

FIGURE 8-1   Radiograph of periapical projection.

"peri," meaning around, and "apical," meaning the end or apex of the root. Thus, the primary purpose for exposing this type of **projection** is to view the alveolar bone area around the apex of the root (Figure 8-1). The second type of projection is called a bitewing projection. Because of the position of the film in the mouth, the crowns of the teeth from both arches (maxillary and mandibular) are projected on the film at one time (Figure 8-2). The purpose of this projection is to view the sides or proximal surfaces of the teeth and the alveolar **crestal bone.** The bitewing is best suited for this purpose because there is very little distortion due to the slight vertical angulation used for this projection.

Bitewings can be exposed in both the anterior and posterior part of the mouth, but the posterior bitewing is the projection most frequently used. Anterior bitewings are not taken as frequently because of the ease with which the anterior teeth can be examined clinically for caries by using **transillumination.** Posterior bitewings can be exposed with the film turned horizontally or vertically. The horizontal bitewing is most often used unless there is 5 mm or more of bone loss. When this occurs, a vertical bitewing is indicated to allow the projection of the crest of the alveolar ridge to show on the film.

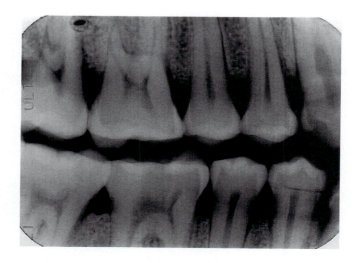

FIGURE 8-2 Radiograph of bitewing projection.

An intraoral **full mouth examination** of radiographs is composed of both periapical and bitewing projections. On the average adult, a full series of 18 to 20 films are needed to radiograph the entire mouth. Generally, there are fourteen periapicals and four to six bitewings, but this may vary with the school or dental office. Six periapicals are taken of the anterior region of the mouth. The specific projections are maxillary right lateral/canine, maxillary central, maxillary left lateral/canine, mandibular right lateral/canine, mandibular central, and mandibular left lateral/canine. There are eight periapicals taken in the posterior region of the mouth. These are maxillary and mandibular right and left premolar projections (four films) and maxillary and mandibular right and left molar projections (four films) (Figure 8-3). Usually, there are four posterior horizontal bitewings (right and left premolar and

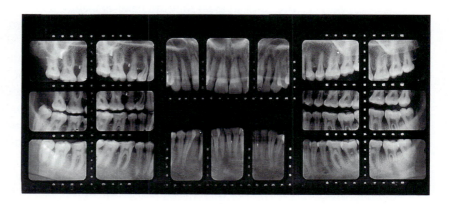

FIGURE 8-3 Mounted full-mouth series with horizontal bitewings.

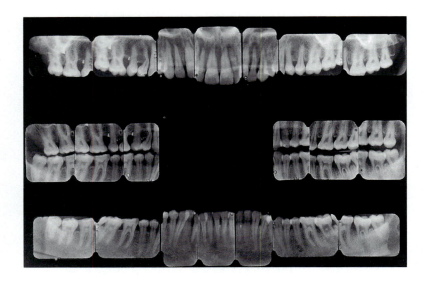

FIGURE 8-4   Mounted full-mouth series with vertical bitewings.

molar) or four to six posterior vertical bitewings (canine-premolar, premolar-molar, and molar). (Figure 8-4)

PREPARATION OF OPERATORY, FILM, AND PATIENT

Before exposing films on the patient, the operatory must be prepared for patient use. The proper infection control procedures should be followed as described in Chapter 2. This should include the chair, tubehead, console, workstation, and operator. The patient should be seated and draped with a lead apron and thyroid collar (Figure 8-5). Once the patient is seated, the headrest should be adjusted against the occipital lobe so that the head is steady and movement will not occur during the radiographic procedure. This, in turn, will prevent motion being displayed on the radiograph. The films should be placed on a layout sheet or something comparable that states each of the projections to be exposed. By placing the film on the layout sheet with the corresponding projection, the operator will be able to prevent accidental exposure of the same area twice (Figure 8-6). In the same manner, a paper cup or container for exposed films should be available so that films can be placed in it immediately after exposure to prevent **double exposure** of the film (exposing the same film twice) (Figure 8-7).

Dental film comes in several different sizes (see Chapter 5, Figure 5-10). Size 0 is small film (22 mm × 35 mm) used primarily for pediatric patients. Size 1 film (24 mm × 40 mm) is approximately the

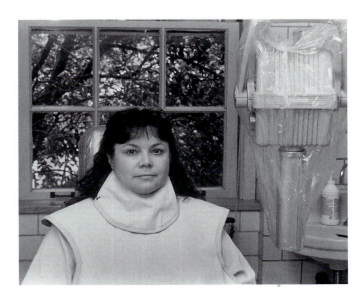

FIGURE 8-5 A draped unit with patient wearing apron, and thyroid collar.

same length as size 2 film (32 mm × 41 mm), but narrower. The size 1 film is used primarily for all lateral/canine projections and mandibular central projections because its smaller width more easily accommodates the curvature of the arch. Other uses of size 1 film include the premolar projection during the vertical bitewing survey if six films are

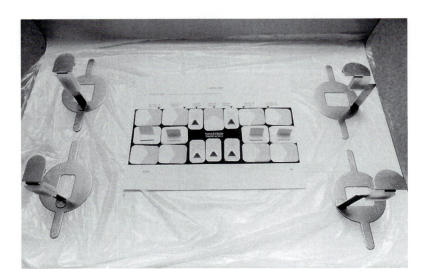

FIGURE 8-6 Layout sheet with film.

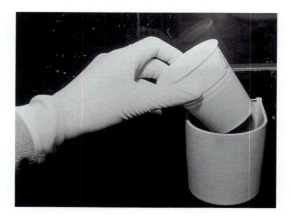

FIGURE 8-7   Cup for exposed film.

required and for horizontal bitewing surveys on children too small for size 2 film. Size 2 film, the standard film for adults, is used for the remaining projections (bitewings, the maxillary central projections, and all posterior projections). Size 3 film is a long narrow film (28 mm × 55 mm) used for a single bitewing projection on one side of the mouth. Lastly, size 4 film (57 mm × 76 mm) is an occlusal film used for special projections.

As mentioned previously, a paralleling device or **position indicating device (PID)** that aligns the **cone** to the film is the technique of choice (Rinn XCP or Precision Instruments). If the patient is unable to tolerate this device, then a film-holding device that uses the paralleling principle should be the second choice. An example of this would be a styrofoam biteblock. If the bisecting angle technique must be used, then such film-holding devices as Rinn* bisecting angle instruments (BAI), snap-a-ray, Stabe, or a hemostat with a rubber biteblock can be used. The use of the digital/finger method of holding the film should be avoided at all cost. Even though the x-ray dose is small, it can be reduced further by using a film holder. Once the film holder has been selected, the instruments should be placed on a paper towel or plastic cover that can be discarded after use.

STEPS OF RADIOGRAPHIC IMAGING USING THE PARALLELING TECHNIQUE

Four steps should be taken when exposing a film using the paralleling technique (unless you are using a film-holding device that aligns the PID). These steps should occur sequentially, starting with packet placement, vertical angulation, and horizontal angulation, and ending with cone centering. Each step is necessary to produce an accurate radiographic image. As mentioned previously, the position-indicating devices automatically determine the vertical angulation, horizontal angulation, and cone centering.

STEP ANALYSIS FOR PERIAPICAL PROJECTIONS USING THE PRECISION INSTRUMENTS AND RINN XCP INSTRUMENTS

The Precision Instrument will be demonstrated for packet placement and cone alignment. The Rinn XCP instruments are used in exactly the same manner. Bitewings will be demonstrated using the **bitewing tab** and XCP holder. Instructions for anterior, posterior, and vertical bitewings will be given.

The format used in this section follows a step analysis presentation. First, the step to be performed will be stated. It will be followed by the rationale for performing the step and the solution to any problems that may be encountered. Instructions will be stated for a normal mouth, with a discussion of special need patients (i.e. gagging, **torus,** etc.) presented in Chapter 9.

The orientation of the film will vary based on the area of the mouth being exposed. All anterior films will be placed in a vertical direction; posterior films in a horizontal direction. Bitewings will be both horizontal and vertical (Figure 8-8). The exposure side of the film is the

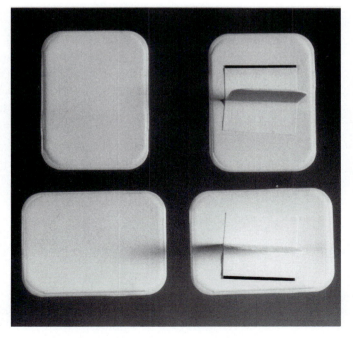

FIGURE 8-8   A film placed in vertical and horizontal directions, as well as vertical and horizontal bitewings.

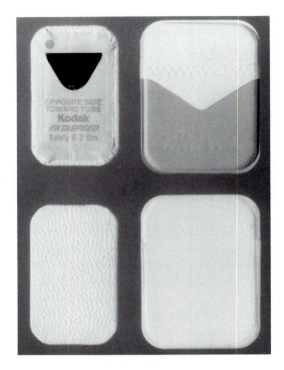

FIGURE 8-9   Exposure side and back side of film.

side without the flap. In one corner of the film, there is a raised bump or embossed dot. Size 1 film has the bump designated by a black circle on the back or nonexposure side of the film (Figure 8-9). The bump should always be placed in the slot of the film holder. This will place the bump at the incisal edge of the image, which will prevent it from interfering with diagnostic interpretation.

RADIOGRAPHIC TECHNIQUE

Ᵽ *Maxillary Central Projection*

Step 1 Film Packet Placement for the Central Projection

Secure the maxillary central instrument and assemble it with the correct bite block (long, narrow, plastic block). Place the bite block on the instrument with the thin portion of the block towards the film (Figure 8-10). The film is placed in the holder clasps on the Precision instruments. If the Rinn instruments are

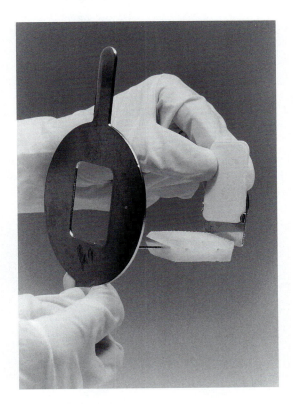

FIGURE 8-10 Position of the bite block on the Precision Instrument.

used, the film is placed in the bite block slot (Figure 8-11). For the purposes of this text book, the patient is positioned with the occlusal plane perpendicular to the floor. Note that the head does not have to be in this position when using the paralleling technique.

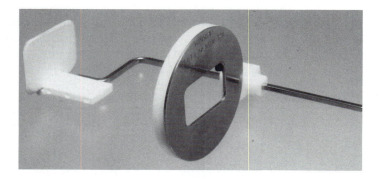

FIGURE 8-11   Film placement in the bite block on Rinn instruments.

Procedure A   Place the size 2 film in the film holder or bite block slot with the bump down in the slot. The exposure side of the film should be facing the x-ray beam (Figure 8-12).

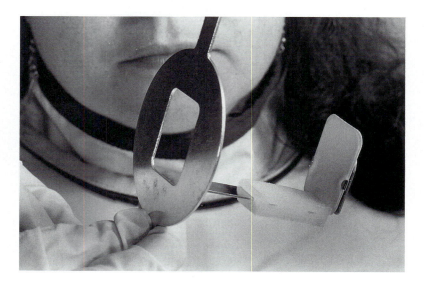

FIGURE 8-12   Size 2 film is placed in Precision PID for maxillary central projection.

Problem   A narrow palate limits the proper placement of the size 2 film in the maxillary central region. Under this condition, use the lateral/canine film holder.

Procedure B   Stand in the seven o'clock position while grasping the **faceplate** of the instrument with one hand. Ask the patient to open and, with the opposite hand, raise the upper lip. Tip the film holder so that the film is parallel with the floor. Put the film holder into the mouth in the area of the tongue. Reposition the film so it is as perpendicular to the floor as possible. Position the film behind the maxillary centrals with the incisal edges of the maxillary centrals in contact with the bite block and then ask the patient to close to stabilize the already positioned film holder in the mouth (Figure 8-13).

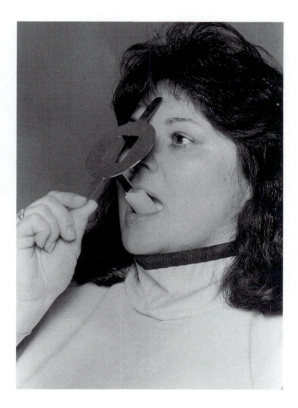

FIGURE 8-13 Precision PID positioned for maxillary central projection.

Rationale   Teeth placed at the end of the bite block will position the film so that it is aligned parallel to the long axis of the maxillary centrals.

Problem   The maxillary centrals are missing or broken. Position the film and stabe in the same manner, but insert a cotton roll in the area where the teeth are missing or broken. If the patient is asked to bite the film into position, the film will be in the wrong place.

Procedure C   Adjust the film holder so that the shadows or images of the maxillary centrals are projected in the center of the film. Have the patient bite to secure the instrument and stabilize the faceplate with the hand (Figure 8-14).

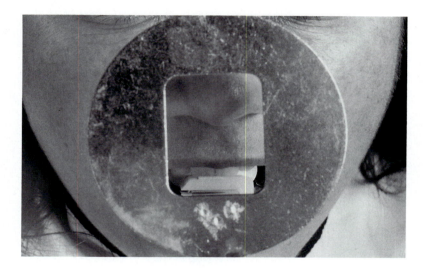

FIGURE 8-14   Precision PID positioned for maxillary central projection and stabilized with the hand.

Rationale   The teeth of interest should be centered on the film so the appropriate structures will be visible on the processed film for diagnosis.

Step 2 Align the PID (cone) to the faceplate.

Procedure A Grasp the back of the tubehead with one hand and the end of the PID with the other hand. The operator should then stand at the eight o'clock position and align the PID at a 90 degree angle to the faceplate. It is imperative to have the PID resting against the entire faceplate or have the PID equidistant from the faceplate—no more than ¼ inch away (Figure 8-15).

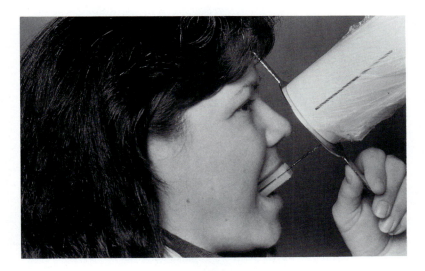

FIGURE 8-15 The PID (cone) projection must be properly aligned to the faceplate.

Helpful Hint: Alignment of the PID can be accomplished by sliding it onto the faceplate from the side or by positioning the PID from the front of the faceplate.

Rationale When the beam is aligned at a right angle to the film, then the image projected on the film will not be distorted and will be of good diagnostic quality.

Problem If the beam is not aligned against the faceplate or equidistant to it, then an instrument cut (**cone cut**) will occur. This is when the beam is partially blocked to the film (Figure 8-16). See Chapter 18.
     The remaining projections will follow the same presentation. Therefore, only the packet placement step will be discussed.

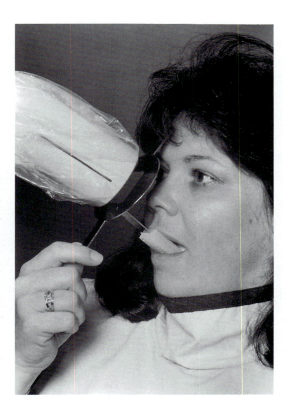

FIGURE 8-16 The PID (cone) is aligned incorrectly so that it is not equidistant to the faceplate.

⌘ *Maxillary Lateral/Canine Projection*

Step 1 Film Packet Placement for the Lateral/Canine
Projection

Procedure A Place the size 1 film in the lateral/canine film holder or bite
block slot with the bump down in the slot. The exposure side of
the film should be facing the x-ray beam.

Procedure B Holding the faceplate, stand in the eight o'clock position and
ask the patient to open. Retract the lip with the free hand and
place the free end of the bite block against the incisal edges of
the lateral and canine. Have the patient close and stabilize the
instrument with the hand (Figure 8-17).

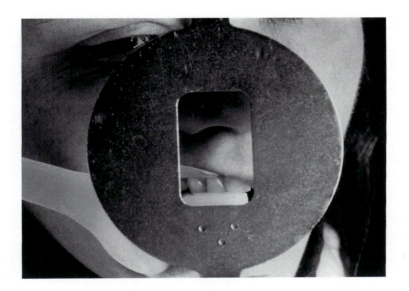

FIGURE 8-17 The proper position of the Precision PID for
maxillary lateral canine projection.

Procedure C View the teeth through the opening in the faceplate. If the
canine and lateral are not visualized, then adjust the instrument
until the desired teeth are present.

𝕞 *Maxillary Premolar Projection*

Step 1 Film Packet Placement for the Premolar Projection

Procedure A Place the size 2 film in the film holder or bite block slot with the bump down in the slot. The exposure side of the film should be facing the x-ray beam.

Procedure B Grasping the faceplate, stand at six o'clock and position the free end of the bite block against the occlusal surfaces of the maxillary premolars. Rotate the faceplate forward so that the edge of the film packet is positioned behind the lateral/canine on the opposite side of the mouth. This will ensure imaging the mesial of the first premolar (Figure 8-18).

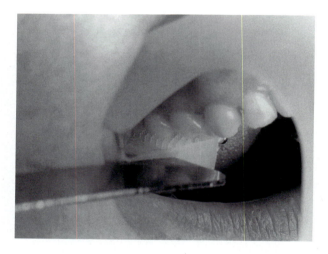

FIGURE 8-18 The proper position of the Precision PID for maxillary premolar projection. The edge of the film is behind the opposite canine.

Procedure C View through the opening in the face plate to check for the appearance of the appropriate teeth. Ask the patient to bite and stabilize the instrument with the hand (Figure 8-19).

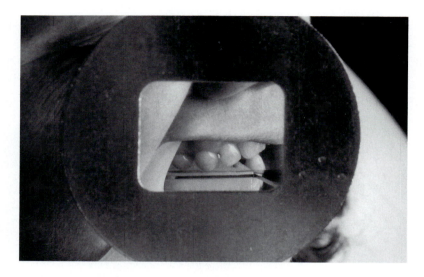

FIGURE 8-19 The proper position of the Precision PID for maxillary premolar projection, stabilized with the hand.

⚕ *Maxillary Molar Projection*

Step 1 Film Packet Placement for the Molar Projection

    Procedure A   Place the size 2 film in the film holder or bite block slot with the bump down in the slot. The exposure side of the film should be facing the x-ray beam.

    Procedure B   Grasping the faceplate, stand in the seven o'clock position and place the free end of the bite block against the occlusal surfaces of the molars (Figure 8-20).

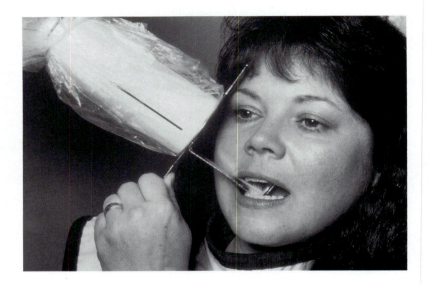

FIGURE 8-20   The proper position for Precision PID for maxillary molar projection.

Procedure C   Ensure that the second molar is in contact with the center of the bite block, allowing the film to be centered for the first, second, and third molars. Ask the patient to bite and stabilize the instrument with the hand (Figure 8-21).

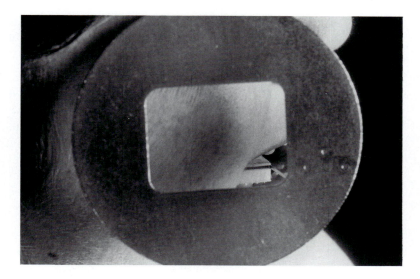

FIGURE 8-21   The proper position for Precision PID for maxillary molar projection and stabilization of the instrument by the hand.

☒ *Mandibular Central Projection*

Step 1 Film Packet Placement for the Mandibular Central
Projection

Procedure A   Place the size 1 film in the film holder or bite block slot with
the bump down in the slot. The exposure side of the film should
be facing the x-ray beam. Grasp the faceplate of the anterior
size 1 instrument and rotate it for placement in the mandibular
arch.

Procedure B   Standing in the seven o'clock position and ask the patient to
open and raise the tongue. Position the film at an angle under
the tongue with the free end of the bite block against the incisal
edges of the mandibular central incisors (Figure 8-22).

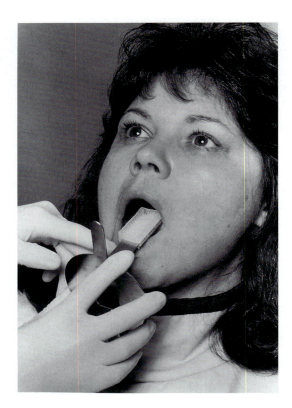

FIGURE 8-22   The proper position of the
Precision PID for mandibular central projection.

Procedure C As the patient closes, upright the instrument so that the film is parallel with the long axis of the teeth. Ask the patient to close and stabilize the instrument with the hand. Make sure the mandibular central incisors can be viewed through the opening in the faceplate (Figure 8-23).

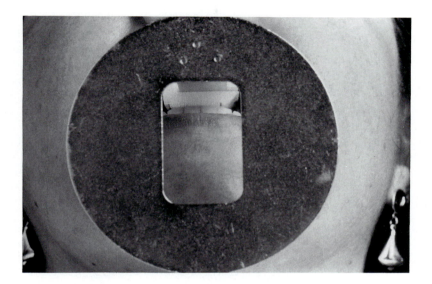

FIGURE 8-23 The proper position of the Precision PID for mandibular central projection.

⌘ *Mandibular Lateral/Canine Projection*

Step 1 Film Packet Placement for the Mandibular
Lateral/Canine Projection

> ***Procedure A***   Place the size 1 film in the film holder or bite block slot with the bump down in the slot. The exposure side of the film should be facing the x-ray beam. Grasp the faceplate and position for placement in the mandibular arch. Stand in the eight o'clock position and position the film under the patient's tongue, with the free end of the bite block resting on the incisal edges of the mandibular lateral and canine. As the patient closes, upright the film so that it is parallel with the long axis of the teeth (Figure 8-24).

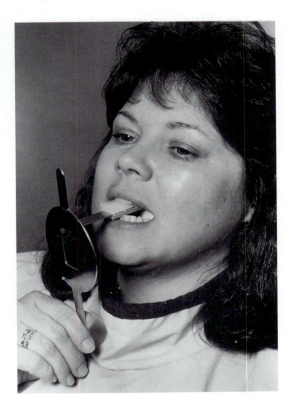

FIGURE 8-24 The proper position of the Precision PID for mandibular lateral/canine projection.

Procedure B Check to see if the mandibular lateral and canine can be viewed through the opening in the faceplate and adjust if necessary. If needed, have the patient stabilize the instrument with the hand (Figure 8-25).

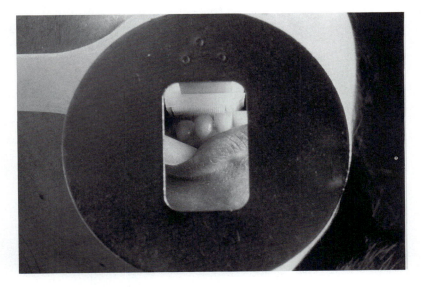

FIGURE 8-25 The proper position of the Precision PID for mandibular lateral/canine projection.

🦷 *Mandibular Premolar Projection*

Step 1 Film Packet Placement for the Premolar Projection

> ***Procedure A*** Place the size 2 film in the film holder or bite block slot with the bump down in the slot. The exposure side of the film should be facing the x-ray beam. Position the film holder for a mandibular projection. Standing in the six o'clock position, place the free end of the bite block against the occlusal surfaces of the premolars. Rotate the faceplate until the front edge of the film is positioned behind the lateral and canine on the opposite side of the mouth (Figure 8-26). This will ensure the imaging of the mesial of the first premolar.

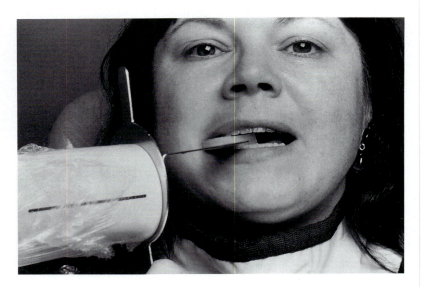

FIGURE 8-26 The proper position of the Precision PID for mandibular premolar projection.

Procedure B   Make sure the premolars can be seen through the opening in the faceplate. Have the patient bite and stabilize the instrument with the hand (Figure 8-27).

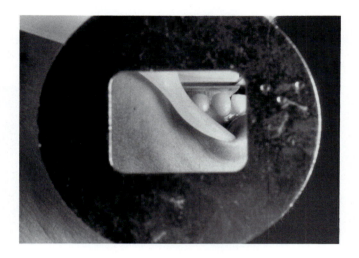

FIGURE 8-27   The proper position of the Precision PID for mandibular premolar projection.

𝕊 *Mandibular Molar Projection*

Step 1 Film Packet Placement for the Molar Projection

Procedure A Place the size 2 film in the film holder or bite block slot with the bump down in the slot. The exposure side of the film should be facing the x-ray beam. Position the film holder for a mandibular projection. Standing in the eight o'clock position, place the film under the side of the tongue and the bite block against the occlusal surfaces of the molars (Figure 8-28).

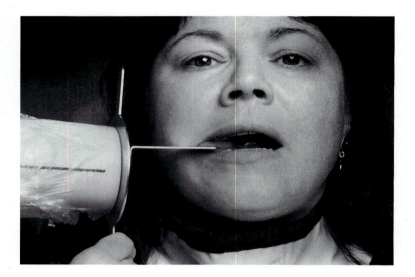

FIGURE 8-28 The proper position of the Precision PID for mandibular molar projection.

Procedure B Make sure to center the second molar on the film. Have the patient bite and stabilize the instrument with the hand (Figure 8-29).

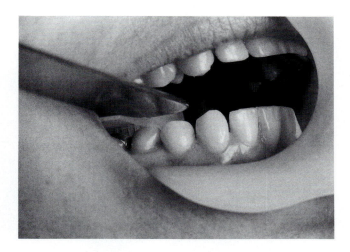

FIGURE 8-29 The proper position of the Precision PID for mandibular molar projection.

🦷 *Bitewing: Anterior Projection*

Step 1 Film Packet Placement for the Anterior Bitewing

> ***Procedure A*** With the size 1 film turned vertically, place the film in the bitewing holding device or place a bitewing tab on the exposure side of the film (Figure 8-30).

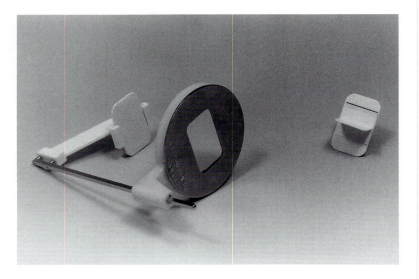

FIGURE 8-30 Anterior bitewing in XCP holder and bitewing tab.

Procedure B Place the film in the anterior portion of the mouth (center behind the centrals) and place the tab or holder against the incisal edges of the mandibular centrals. Have the patient bite (Figure 8-31).

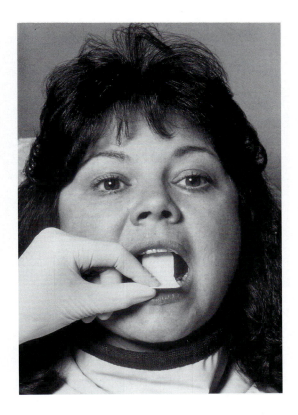

FIGURE 8-31 Anterior bitewing placed in mouth.

Problem While biting, the film may become bent and/or malpositioned. It will be necessary to push the film away from the teeth and have the patient bite on the edge of the holder or tab.

Rationale With the film away from the teeth, it will be possible to position the film so that it is parallel with the long axis of the teeth.

Step 2 Align the Vertical Angulation

      Procedure A   All bitewings are exposed with the vertical angulation preset at +10 degrees (Figure 8-32). If a film-holding device is being used, then the vertical angulation is determined by the position of the faceplate. The PID would be aligned to this.

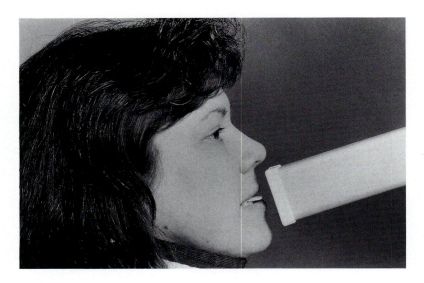

FIGURE 8-32 Alignment of vertical angulation.

      Rationale   This provides the optimal angulation to image proximal caries and the alveolar crestal bone.

Step 3 Align the Horizontal Angulation

> ***Procedure A*** Determine the direction needed to position the beam so that it passes through the interproximal space of the maxillary centrals. Once determined, align the PID so that it is in this position (Figure 8-33). If a film-holding device is used, align the PID to the faceplate.

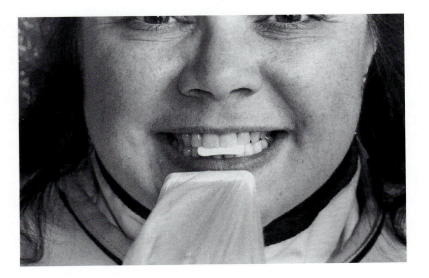

FIGURE 8-33 Align the PID (cone) for horizontal angulation with the anterior bitewing.

> ***Rationale*** This step is crucial for the bitewing projection. To clearly view the bone and proximal surfaces, the proximal space must be free of overlap.

Step 4 Center the PID (cone) on the Film

   Procedure A   Stand behind the tubehead and position the PID so that the x-ray beam will expose the entire film (Figure 8-34). Align the PID to the faceplate if a film-holding device is used.

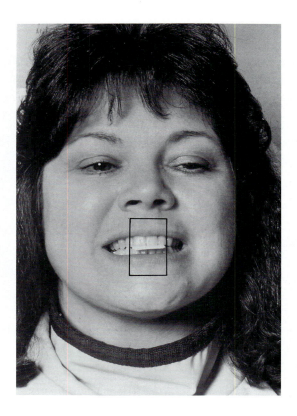

FIGURE 8-34   Center the PID (cone) for the anterior bitewing.

   Rationale   In order to prevent a conecut, the beam must expose the entire film.

⌷ *Horizontal Posterior Bitewings: Premolar*

Step 1 Packet Placement for the Premolar Bitewing

> ***Procedure A*** Place a size 2 film in a horizontal position in the film-holding device or attach a bitewing tab in the middle of the film.

> ***Rationale*** The horizontal position will allow for the imaging of normal bone levels and fit comfortably in the mouth.

> ***Procedure B*** Position the film so the front edge is behind the canine on the opposite side (Figure 8-35), the same as for the premolar periapical projection. Place the bitewing tab in contact with the mandibular premolars. Have the patient close while holding the tab in place.

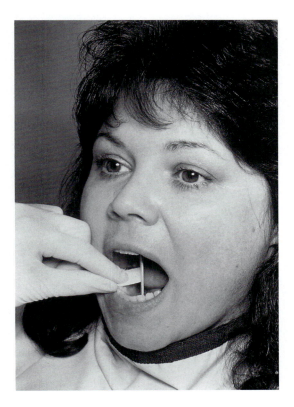

FIGURE 8-35 Proper placement of horizontal premolar bitewing.

> ***Rationale*** This film position will allow the imaging of the canine on the film. Stabilizing the tab against the occlusal of the mandibular premolars while the patient closes will prevent movement of the film.

Step 2 Align the Vertical Angulation

   Procedure A Preset the vertical angulation at +10 degrees. If a film-holding device is being used, then the vertical angulation is determined by the position of the faceplate. The PID would be aligned to this (Figure 8-36).

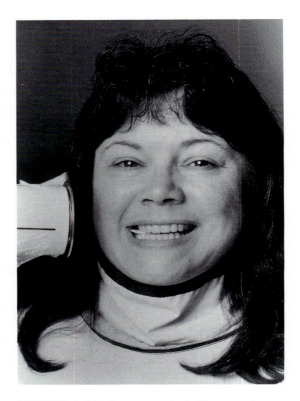

FIGURE 8-36 Proper vertical alignment for horizontal premolar bitewing.

   Rationale This provides the optimal angulation to image proximal caries and the alveolar crestal bone.

Step 3 Align the Horizontal Angulation

Procedure A Determine the direction needed to position the beam so that it passes through the interproximal space of the maxillary premolars. Once determined, align the PID so that it is in this position (Figure 8-37). If a film-holding device is used, align the PID to the faceplate.

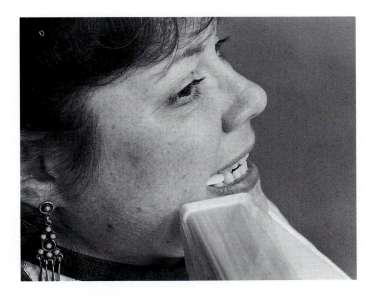

FIGURE 8-37 Proper horizontal alignment for horizontal premolar bitewing.

Rationale This step is crucial for the bitewing projection. In order to clearly view the bone and proximal surfaces, the proximal space must be free of overlap.

Step 4 Center the PID (cone) on the Film

    Procedure A   Stand behind the tubehead and position the PID so that the x-ray beam will expose the entire film (Figure 8-38). Align the PID to the faceplate if a film-holding device is used.

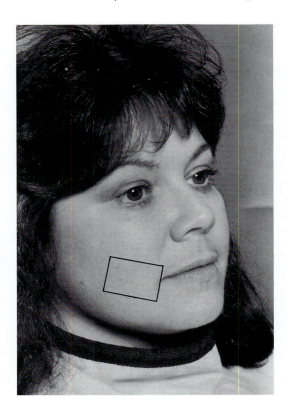

FIGURE 8-38 Center the cone for the horizontal premolar bitewing.

    Rationale   In order to prevent a conecut, the beam must expose the entire film.

ᗺ *Molar Bitewing*

Step 1 Packet Placement of the Horizontal Molar Bitewing

Procedure A   Place a size 2 film in a horizontal position in the film-holding device or attach a bitewing tab in the middle of the film.

Rationale   The horizontal position will allow for the imaging of normal bone levels and fit comfortably in the mouth.

Procedure B   Place the film in the mouth with the second molar centered on the film. Place the tab or biteblock against the occlusal surfaces of the mandibular molars (Figure 8-39). Have the patient bite while holding the tab in place.

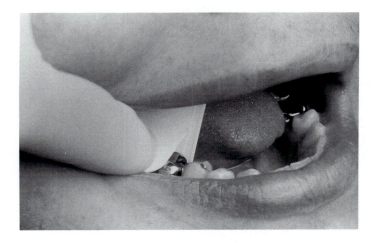

FIGURE 8-39   Proper placement of the horizontal molar bitewing.

Rationale   Holding the tab in place stabilizes the position of the film while the patient closes.

Step 2 Align the Vertical Angulation

  Procedure A Preset the vertical angulation at +10 degrees. If a film-holding device is being used, then the vertical angulation is determined by the position of the faceplate. The PID would be aligned to this (Figure 8-40).

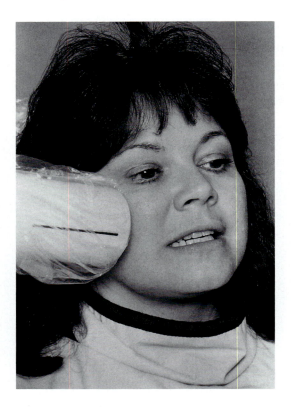

FIGURE 8-40 Proper vertical alignment for the horizontal molar bitewing.

  Rationale This provides the optimal angulation to image proximal caries and the alveolar crestal bone.

Step 3 Align the Horizontal Angulation

> ***Procedure A*** Determine the direction needed to position the beam so that it passes through the interproximal space of the maxillary first and second molar. Once determined, align the PID so that it is in this position (Figure 8-41). If a film-holding device is used, align the PID to the faceplate.

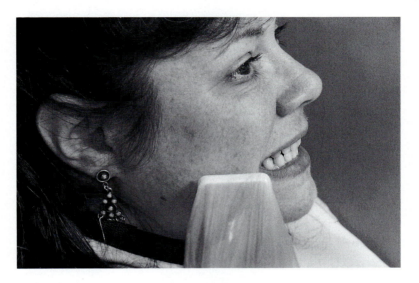

FIGURE 8-41 Proper horizontal alignment for the horizontal molar bitewing.

> ***Rationale*** This step is crucial for the bitewing projection. In order to clearly view the bone and proximal surfaces, the proximal space must be free of overlap.

Step 4 Center the PID (Cone) on the Film

Procedure A Stand behind the tubehead and position the PID so that the x-ray beam will expose the entire film (Figure 8-42). Align the PID to the faceplate if a film-holding device is used.

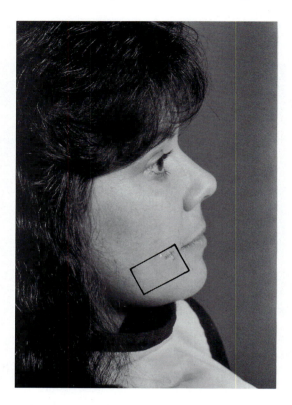

FIGURE 8-42 Center the cone for the horizontal molar bitewing.

Rationale In order to prevent a conecut, the beam must expose the entire film.

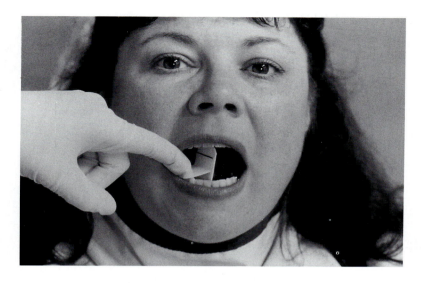

FIGURE 8-43 Proper placement of the premolar vertical bitewing with size 1 film.

VERTICAL POSTERIOR BITEWINGS: PREMOLAR AND MOLAR

The steps are identical to the horizontal bitewings except that the film is positioned in a vertical direction. This allows for the imaging of the alveolar bone in patients with 5 mm or more bone loss. Some patients will require the use of six posterior bitewings instead of four. In these situations, a size 1 film can be used for the most anterior film, then two size 2 films for the remaining projections. The size 1 film allows for easy placement in the canine/first premolar area of the mouth (Figure 8-43).

SUMMARY

The intraoral radiographic technique of choice should employ the paralleling principles, a position indicating device, and rectangular PID (cone). The two primary projections used in intraoral radiography are periapicals and bitewings. Steps for preparation of the operatory, film, and patient are discussed in detail. The radiographic techniques discussed in this chapter include both the Precision and Rinn XCP paralleling instruments. Various bitewing projections and the rationale for use are discussed in full.

BIBLIOGRAPHY

CURRY III TS, DOWDY JE, MURRY JR RC. *Christensen's Physics of Diagnostic Radiology,* 4th ed. Philadelphia: Lea and Febiger, 1990.

GOAZ PW, WHITE SW. *Oral Radiology: Principles and Interpretation,* 3d ed. St. Louis: CV Mosby, 1994.

MANSON-HING, LR. *Fundamentals of Dental Radiography,* 3d ed. Philadelphia: Lea and Febiger, 1990.

MATTESON SR, WHALEY C, AND SECRIST V. *Dental Radiology,* 4th ed. Chapel Hill, NC: University of North Carolina Press, 1988.

REVIEW QUESTIONS

1. List the two types of projections used in an intraoral full series.

2. List the correct sequence of steps used to expose an intraoral projection.

3. The film holding device of choice for exposing intraoral radiographs is the

   a. stabe.
   b. snap-a-ray.
   c. hemostat.
   d. Precision.
   e. all of the above

4. The appropriate projection to expose when the area of interest is the root apex is the

   a. periapical.
   b. bitewing.
   c. vertical bitewing.
   d. anterior bitewing.
   e. occlusal.

5. A projection used to view proximal surfaces and alveolar crestal bone is

   a. periapical.
   b. bitewing.
   c. occlusal.
   d. all of the above
   e. none of the above

6. A vertical bitewing is indicated when ____ mm of bone loss is present.

   a. 3
   b. 4
   c. 5
   d. all of the above
   e. none of the above

7. All anterior films are placed in a ____ orientation to the tooth.

8. The bump located on the film should always be placed in the slot of the film holding device.

   a. True
   b. False

Radiographic Imaging for the Dental Team,
by Sally Mauriello. J.B. Lippincott Company,
Philadelphia © 1995.

9

Alternative Radiographic Procedures

Upon the completion of this chapter, the student should be able to:

1. Name various alternative radiographic imaging techniques.

2. Determine clinical situations in which the use of these imaging techniques is appropriate.

3. Discuss the advantages and disadvantages of each of the imaging techniques.

4. Describe the procedure for exposing radiographs with each of the alternative imaging techniques.

INTRODUCTION

The American Dental Association has recommended that a film-holding device that aligns the beam to the film should be used with rectangular collimation. As discussed in Chapters 7 and 8, the instrumentation technique of choice in radiography is the paralleling technique. Therefore, the ideal technique to use when exposing radiographs would be a film-holding device that uses the paralleling technique and rectangular collimation. Unfortunately, not all mouths are anatomically the same. Thus, the "ideal" technique will not be appropriate for all situations. Therefore, the operator should be familiar with alternative techniques that may be needed if the preferred method is not possible. This chapter will discuss four imaging techniques that could be used to expose intraoral radiographs.

PARALLELING TECHNIQUE WITH THE STABE* AND RECTANGULAR COLLIMATION

The most desirable alternative technique is a styrofoam bite block film holder used with the paralleling technique and rectangular collimation (or circular cone with rectangular collimator attachment). The same shadowcasting principles are followed with the styrofoam bite block as with other paralleling devices. This technique has three advantages: (1) good imaging principles (it adheres to shadowcasting principles), (2) patient comfort (it is a lightweight device and is smaller than the film), and (3) it allows the patient to stabilize the film by biting instead of holding the device with the hand. The styrofoam bite block is also disposable. The primary disadvantage to using the styrofoam bite block is the lack of an extension arm to align the beam perpendicular (at a right angle) to the film.

The procedure for using the styrofoam bite block film holder with the paralleling technique follows four basic steps that will be repeated for each projection.

Step 1　Packet Placement. (Places the packet parallel to the long axis of the teeth and centers the teeth of interest on the film.)

Step 2　Vertical alignment of the beam. (Positions the beam perpendicular to or at right angles to the film and teeth.)

Step 3　Horizontal alignment of the beam. (Opens the interproximal space of interest.)

Step 4　Centering (enclosing) the beam on the film. (Exposes the entire film to the x-ray beam.)

These steps should be applied to *all* radiographic techniques that do not use a device to align the PID (cone).

---

*Rinn Corporation, Elgin, IL.

OPERATOR TECHNIQUE

ໝ *Maxillary Central Projection*

Step 1 Film Packet Placement for the Central Projection

Procedure A   With the raised bump in the lower right corner, place the size 2 film in the styrofoam bite block with the film aligned vertically and the tube side of the film facing the x-ray beam (Figure 9-1).

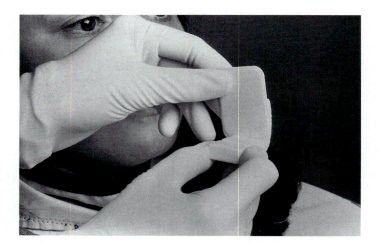

FIGURE 9-1   Styrofoam bite block with size 2 film placed vertically for an anterior projection.

Rationale   Placing the film with a vertical orientation will allow the film to adapt to the anterior portion of the mouth. In addition, the anterior teeth are longer than the posterior teeth. Therefore, the vertical alignment of the film will enable the entire image of the tooth and surrounding bone to be projected accurately and completely for a thorough diagnosis of the area.

Procedure B Grasp the bottom portion of the indented end of the styrofoam bite block between the thumb and forefinger. Stand to the side of the patient in the seven o'clock position. Ask the patient to open and with the opposite hand, raise the upper lip. Tip the styrofoam bite block so that the film is parallel with the floor. Put the film and styrofoam bite block into the mouth towards the area of the tongue. Reposition the film so it is as parallel with the long axis of the teeth as possible. Position the film behind the maxillary centrals with the incisal edges of the maxillary centrals resting beyond the indented end of the styrofoam bite block (Figure 9-2).

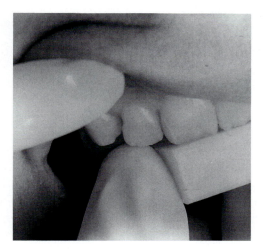

FIGURE 9-2 Packet placed against the incisal edges of the maxillary central incisors.

Rationale Teeth placed at the free end of the styrofoam bite block will position the film so that it is aligned parallel to the long axis of the maxillary centrals.

Procedure C   Adjust the film packet so that the shadows or images of the maxillary centrals are projected in the center of the film. Have the patient bite to secure the styrofoam bite block (Figure 9-3).

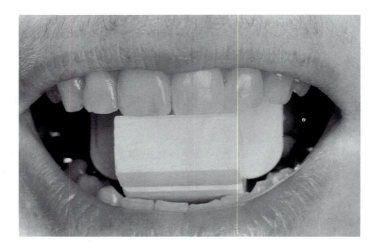

FIGURE 9-3   The patient should bite to stabilize the styrofoam bite block for the maxillary central projection.

Rationale   The teeth of interest should be centered on the film so that the appropriate structures will be visible on the processed film for diagnosis. Biting the styrofoam bite block will hold the film securely without requiring the operator or patient to hold the film with a finger (an unacceptable technique).

Step 2 Vertical Alignment of the PID (Cone)

Procedure   Grasp the back of the tubehead with one hand and the end of the PID (cone) with the other hand. The operator should then stand in the eight o'clock position and direct the beam at a 90 degree angle to the film (Figure 9-4).

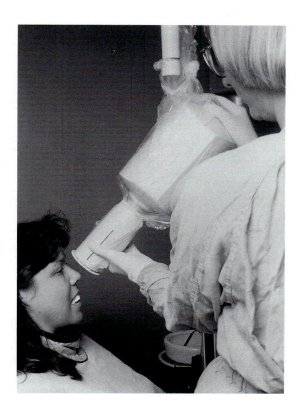

FIGURE 9-4   Adjusting the vertical alignment for the maxillary central projection.

Helpful Hint: Angle the bottom of the PID (cone) the same as the bottom line of the styrofoam bite block. The PID (cone) should be a direct extension of the bottom of the styrofoam bite block (Figure 9-5).

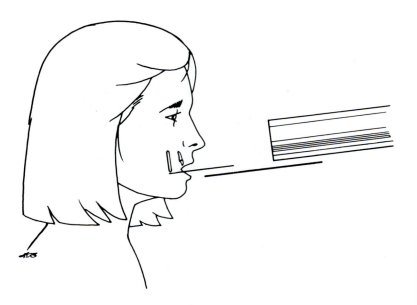

FIGURE 9-5   The drawing depicts alignment of the vertical angulation according to the bottom of the cone and bite block.

Rationale   When the beam is aligned at a right angle to the film, then the image will be accurately projected in a vertical dimension on the film, thus providing a film of good diagnostic quality.

Step 3 Horizontal Alignment of the PID (Cone)

Procedure The operator should stand behind the tubehead housing in the six o'clock position to the patient. Grasp each side of the tubehead with both hands. Direct the beam so that is passes between the contact area of the two teeth of interest. In this projection, the beam would be directed between the maxillary central incisors (Figure 9-6).

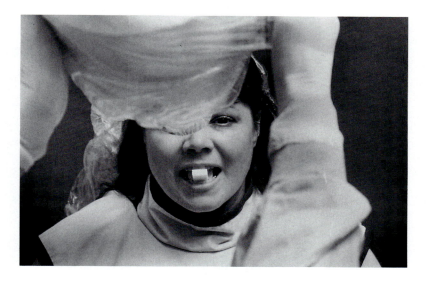

FIGURE 9-6 Proper horizontal alignment for the maxillary central projection.

Rationale Aligning the beam in this manner will allow this contact area to be opened and the roots to be projected accurately. The ability to evaluate these surfaces for dental disease will be improved.

Step 4 Centering the Beam to Expose the Entire Film

Procedure   The operator should be behind the tubehead housing in the six o'clock position. Without moving any of the previously adjusted angulations, grasp each side of the tubehead housing and lift it up so that the styrofoam bite block can be viewed from below the tubehead housing. Then, pull down on the tubehead until the bottom of the styrofoam bite block is no longer in view (Figure 9-7).

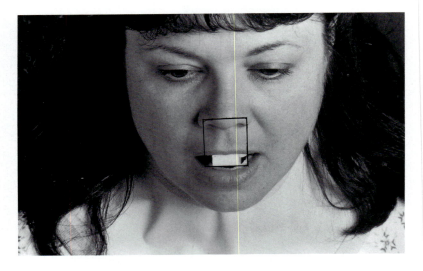

FIGURE 9-7   The highlighted area represents the area that should be covered (exposed) by the x-ray beam.

Helpful Hint: Take an object (pencil or finger) and line up the bottom of the styrofoam bite block and PID (cone). Do the same for one side of the film and the side of the PID (cone).

Rationale   In order for the image to be projected onto the film, the beam must expose (enclose) the entire film.

⏃ *Maxillary Right Lateral/Canine Projection*

Step 1 Film Packet Placement for the Lateral/Canine
Projection

Procedure Place a size 1 film in the styrofoam bite block using a vertical
orientation. Standing in the eight o'clock position, place the film
behind the maxillary lateral and canine with the incisal edges of
the maxillary lateral and canine resting by the indented end of
the styrofoam bite block (Figure 9-8).

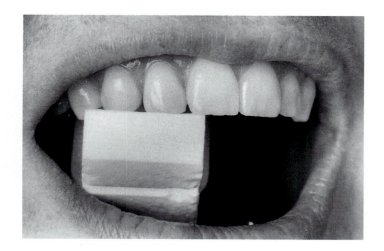

FIGURE 9-8 Packet placement for the maxillary lateral/
canine projection.

Rationale A size 1 film is recommended for this area of the mouth due to
the curvature of the palate.

Step 2 Vertical Alignment of the PID (Cone)

      Procedure   Standing in the eight o'clock position, align the PID (cone) so that the x-ray beam is projected at a right angle to the film (Figure 9-9).

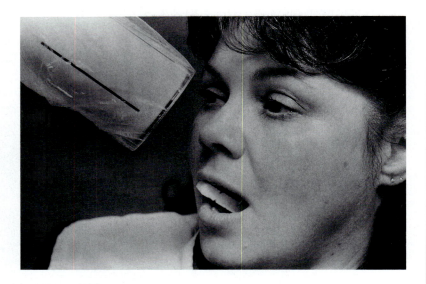

FIGURE 9-9 Proper vertical alignment for the maxillary lateral/ canine projection.

      Rationale   Directing the beam at a right angle to the film follows the shadowcasting principles.

Step 3 Horizontal Alignment of the PID (Cone)

> ***Procedure*** The operator should be behind the tubehead housing in the seven o'clock position to the patient. Raise the tubehead above the teeth of interest. Position the tubehead so the beam is directed between the maxillary lateral and canine (Figure 9-10).

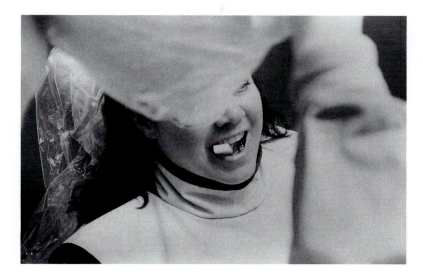

FIGURE 9-10 Proper horizontal alignment for the maxillary lateral/canine projection.

> ***Rationale*** Standing in this position will allow the operator to visualize the interproximal space to be opened.

Step 4 Centering the Beam to Expose the Entire Film

Procedure   Standing in the seven o'clock position, the operator should lower the tubehead until the film can not be seen (Figure 9-11).

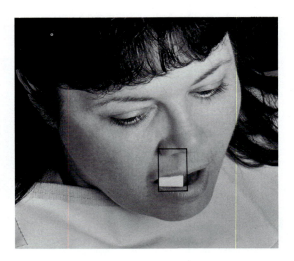

FIGURE 9-11   Cone centering for the maxillary lateral/canine projection.

Rationale   Covering the film with the x-ray beam will assure the image of the teeth of interest are on the film.

ᗰ *Maxillary Right Premolar Projection*

Step 1 Film Packet Placement for the Premolar Projection

Procedure Using a size 2 film, place the film in the styrofoam bite block horizontally and position the packet in the mouth to center the premolars on the film (Figure 9-12).

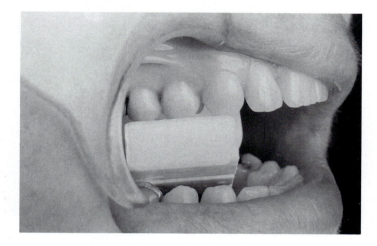

FIGURE 9-12 Packet placement for the maxillary premolar projection.

Rationale The film should be turned horizontally for easier placement in the palate.

Step 2 Vertical Alignment of the PID (Cone)

Procedure   The operator should stand in the six o'clock position to align the PID (cone) at a right angle to the film (Figure 9-13).

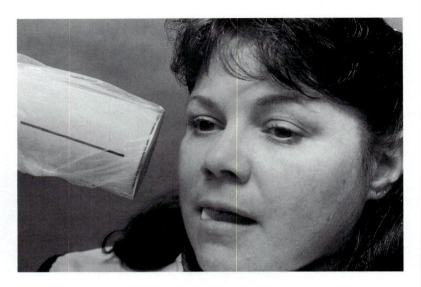

FIGURE 9-13 Proper vertical alignment for the maxillary premolar projection.

Rationale   Standing in this position will allow the operator to visualize the vertical orientation of the PID (cone) to the film.

Step 3 Horizontal Alignment of the PID (Cone)

Procedure The operator should stand behind the tubehead housing in the eight o'clock position to the patient. With the tubehead raised above the area of interest, direct the beam so that it passes between the interproximal space between the maxillary premolars (Figure 9-14).

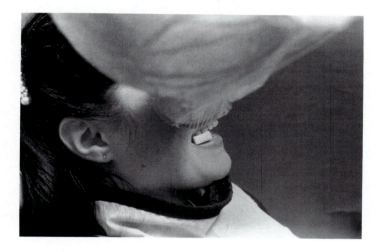

FIGURE 9-14 Proper horizontal alignment for the maxillary premolar projection.

Rationale Standing in this position will allow the operator to visualize the interproximal space between the teeth of interest. The PID (cone) can then be positioned appropriately.

Step 4 Centering the Beam to Expose the Entire Film

Procedure The operator should stand behind the tubehead housing in the eight o'clock position. The tubehead should be adjusted until the film and styrofoam bite block are no longer viewed (Figure 9-15).

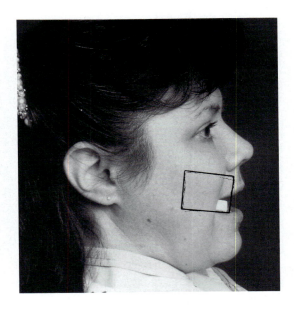

FIGURE 9-15 Cone centering for the maxillary premolar projection.

Rationale Standing in this position will enable the operator to lower the tubehead until the film can not be seen. At this point, the x-ray beam will expose the entire film and prevent a conecut.

☒ *Maxillary Right Molar Projection*

Step 1 Film Packet Placement for the Molar Projection

> ***Procedure***   The packet is placed horizontally in the styrofoam bite block. Placement of the film in the mouth should be no further forward than the distal half of the maxillary second premolar (Figure 9-16).

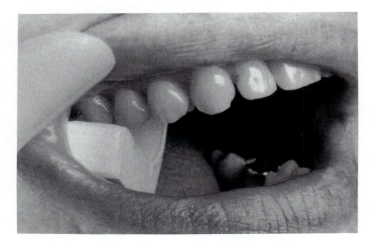

FIGURE 9-16   Packet placement for the maxillary molar projection.

> ***Rationale***   Positioning the film in this manner will allow for the imaging of the first, second, and third molars on the film.

Step 2 Vertical Alignment of the PID (Cone)

Procedure The operator should stand in the seven o'clock position to align the vertical angulation (Figure 9-17).

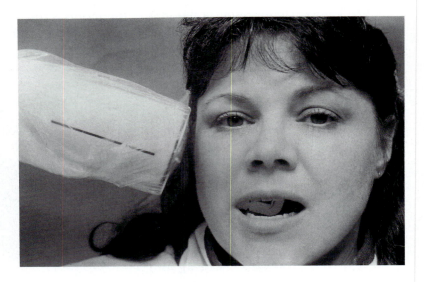

FIGURE 9-17 Proper vertical alignment for the maxillary molar projection.

Rationale Standing in this position will allow the operator to view the proper 90 degree angulation of the PID (cone) (x-ray beam) to the film.

Step 3 Horizontal Alignment of the PID (Cone)

Procedure   The operator should be in the nine o'clock position to the patient with the tubehead housing raised above the area of interest. The beam should be directed through the interproximal space of the maxillary first and second molars (Figure 9-18).

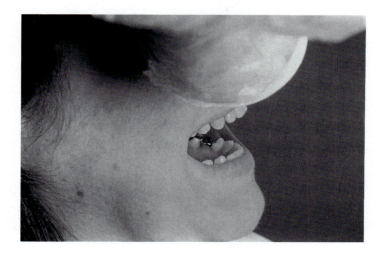

FIGURE 9-18 Proper horizontal alignment for the maxillary molar projection.

Rationale   Standing in this position will allow easy visualization of the interproximal space. It will be necessary to retract the patient's cheek with one hand while viewing the interproximal space.

Step 4 Centering the Beam to Expose the Entire Film

Procedure The operator should be behind the tubehead housing in the nine o'clock position. The tubehead should then be lowered until the film can no longer be viewed (Figure 9-19).

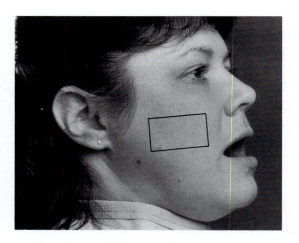

FIGURE 9-19 Cone centering for the maxillary molar projection.

Rationale Following this procedure will insure proper coverage of the film by the x-ray beam.

Exposing projections for the maxillary left would be identical to the right, except that the operator's positioning is reversed, that is the five o'clock position instead of the seven o'clock position.

⾙ *Mandibular Central Projection*

Step 1 Film Packet Placement for the Central Projection

> ***Procedure A*** Place a size 1 film in the styrofoam bite block in a vertical position. Then, turn the styrofoam bite block in a downward position for placement in the mandibular arch (Figure 9-20).

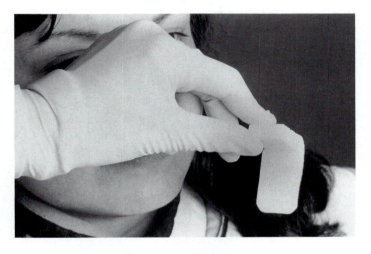

FIGURE 9-20 The mandibular position of styrofoam bite block with size 1 film placed vertically.

> ***Rationale*** Due to the curvature of the mandibular arch, a size 1 film is more easily adapted to the arch with the vertical orientation.

Procedure B Grasp the bottom portion of the indented end of the styrofoam bite block between the thumb and forefinger. Stand to the side of the patient in the seven o'clock position. Ask the patient to open and with the opposite hand, pull down the lower lip. Tip the styrofoam bite block so that the film is at a 45 degree angle to the floor. Put the film and styrofoam bite block into the mouth under the tongue. As the patient bites, upright the film so it is as parallel to the long axis of the tooth as possible. Position the film behind the mandibular centrals with the incisal edges of the mandibular centrals resting beyond the indention the styrofoam bite block (Figure 9-21).

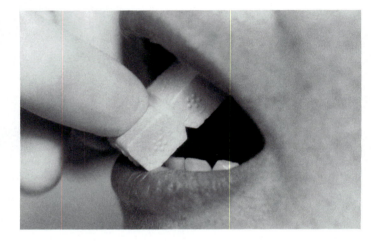

FIGURE 9-21 The teeth positioned on the bite block for the mandibular central projection.

Rationale Standing in this position allows for easy visualization of the floor of the mouth. Waiting to upright the film when the patient closes allows for the muscles in the floor of the mouth to relax. Thus the film can be better placed. Positioning the free end of the styrofoam bite block on the incisal edges allows for a parallel relationship between the teeth and film.

Procedure C   Position the film packet so that the shadows or images of the mandibular centrals are projected in the center of the film. Have the patient bite to secure the styrofoam bite block (Figure 9-22).

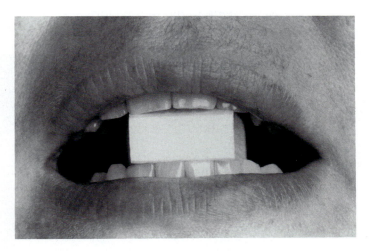

FIGURE 9-22   Packet placement for the mandibular central projection.

Rationale   The teeth of interest should be centered on the film so the appropriate structures will be visible on the processed film for diagnosis. Biting the styrofoam bite block will hold the film secure without requiring the operator or patient to hold the film with a finger (an unacceptable technique).

Step 2 Vertical Alignment of the PID (Cone)

Procedure Grasp the back of the tubehead with one hand and the end of the PID (cone) with the other hand. The operator should then stand at the nine o'clock position and direct the beam at a 90 degree angle to the film (Figure 9-23).

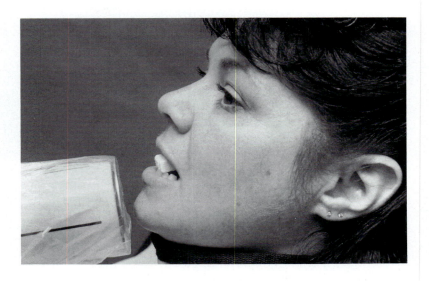

FIGURE 9-23 Proper vertical alignment for the mandibular central projection.

Helpful Hint: Angle the top surface of the PID (cone) the same as the top of the styrofoam bite block. The PID (cone) should appear as a direct extension of the top of the styrofoam bite block.

Rationale When the beam is aligned at a right angle to the film, then the image will be projected accurately on the film, thus providing a film of good diagnostic quality.

Step 3 Horizontal Alignment of the PID (Cone)

Procedure The operator should be standing in the six o'clock position to the patient behind the tubehead housing. The tubehead should be positioned below the teeth of interest. Grasp each side of the tubehead with both hands. Direct the beam so that it passes through the interproximal area of the two mandibular central incisors (Figure 9-24).

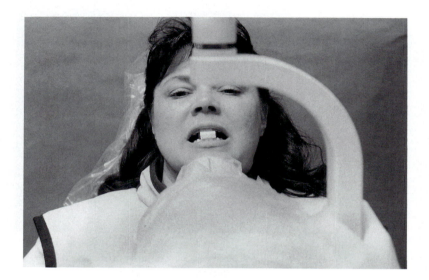

FIGURE 9-24 Proper horizontal alignment for the mandibular central projection.

Rationale Aligning the beam in this manner will allow this contact area to be opened and the roots to be projected accurately. The ability to evaluate these surfaces for dental disease will be improved.

Step 4 Centering the Beam to Expose the Entire Film

Procedure The operator should be behind the tubehead housing in the six o'clock position. Without moving any of the previously adjusted angulations, grasp each side of the tubehead housing and lift it up so until the top edge of the film can not be viewed from above the tubehead housing (Figure 9-25).

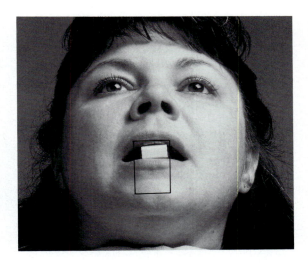

FIGURE 9-25 Cone centering for the mandibular central projection.

Helpful Hint: Take an object (pencil or hand) and line up the top of the styrofoam bite block and PID (cone). Do the same for one side of the film and the side of the PID (cone).

Rationale In order for the image to be projected onto the film, the beam must expose (enclose) the entire film.

☒ *Mandibular Left Lateral/Canine Projection*

Step 1 Film Packet Placement for the Lateral/Canine
Projection

Procedure Standing in the seven o'clock position, position the styrofoam
bite block and size 1 film following the same steps as for the
mandibular central projection. Position the film behind the
mandibular lateral and canine with the incisal edges of the
mandibular lateral and canine resting beyond the indention of
the styrofoam bite block (Figure 9-26).

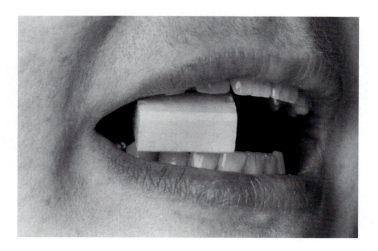

FIGURE 9-26 Packet placement for the mandibular
lateral/canine projection.

Rationale A size 1 film is recommended for this area of the mouth due to
the curvature of the arch and position of the tongue.

Step 2 Vertical Alignment of the PID (Cone)

Procedure   Standing in the six o'clock position, align the PID (cone) so that the x-ray beam is projected at a right angle to the film (Figure 9-27).

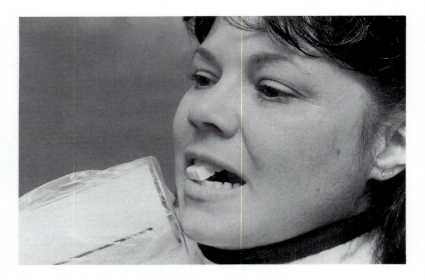

FIGURE 9-27   Proper vertical alignment for the mandibular lateral/canine projection.

Rationale   Directing the beam at a right angle to the film follows the shadowcasting principles and decreases the chance of elongating or foreshortening the image.

Step 3 Horizontal Alignment of the PID (Cone)

>***Procedure*** Standing in the seven o'clock position to the patient, lower the tubehead below the teeth of interest and direct the beam through the interproximal space of the mandibular lateral and canine (Figure 9-28).

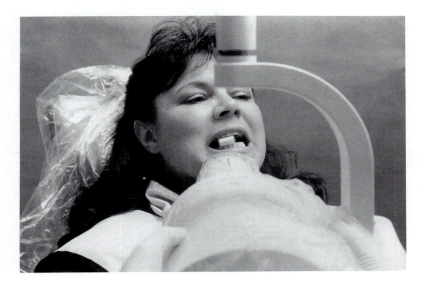

FIGURE 9-28 Proper horizontal alignment for the mandibular lateral/canine projection.

>***Rationale*** Standing in this position allows easy visualization of the interproximal space.

Step 4 Centering the Beam to Expose the Entire Film

Procedure   Standing in the same position behind the tubehead housing, raise the tubehead until the top of the film can no longer be seen (Figure 9-29).

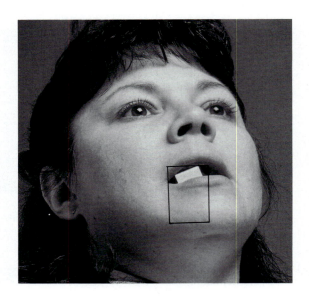

FIGURE 9-29 Cone centering for the mandibular lateral/canine projection.

Rationale   This will insure complete coverage of the film with the x-ray beam.

ꇙ *Mandibular Left Premolar Projection*

Step 1 Film Packet Placement for the Premolar Projection

Procedure   Using a size 2 film, place the film in the styrofoam bite block horizontally and break off the indented end of the styrofoam bite block. Position the packet in the mouth by grasping the edge of the film with the thumb and forefinger. Lay the back of the styrofoam bite block on top of the tongue and position the film so that it is centered behind the premolars. By rolling the film down, move the tongue away from the teeth and rest the free end of the styrofoam bite block against the occlusal surface of the premolars. Have the patient bite (Figure 9-30).

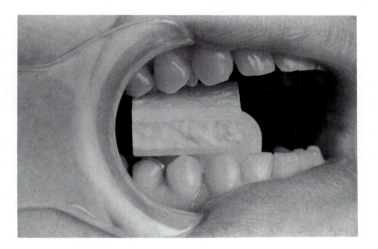

FIGURE 9-30   Packet placement for the mandibular premolar projection.

Rationale   The film should be turned horizontally for easier placement in the floor of the mouth. By rolling the film, the tongue can be easily displaced and the film positioned appropriately.

Step 2 Vertical Alignment of the PID (Cone)

Procedure   The operator should stand in the six o'clock position to align the PID (cone) at a right angle to the film (Figure 9-31).

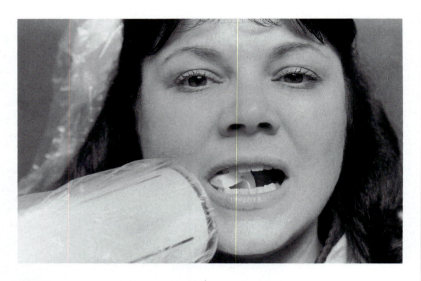

FIGURE 9-31   Proper vertical alignment for the mandibular premolar projection.

Rationale   Standing in this position will allow the operator to visualize the vertical orientation of the PID (cone) to the film.

Step 3 Horizontal Alignment of the PID (Cone)

Procedure   The operator should be behind the tubehead housing in the four o'clock position to the patient. With the tubehead lowered below the area of interest, direct the beam so that it passes through the interproximal space between the mandibular premolars (Figure 9-32).

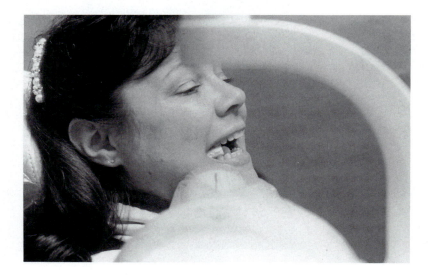

FIGURE 9-32 Proper horizontal alignment for the mandibular premolar projection.

Rationale   Standing in this position will allow the operator to visualize the interproximal space between the teeth of interest. The PID (cone) can then be positioned appropriately.

Step 4 Centering the Beam to Expose the Entire Film

Procedure The operator should be behind the tubehead housing in the four o'clock position. The tubehead should be adjusted until the film and styrofoam bite block are no longer viewed (Figure 9-33).

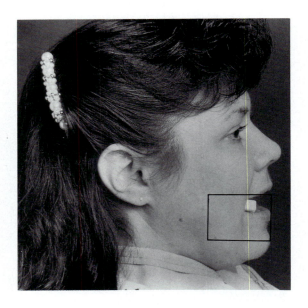

FIGURE 9-33 Cone centering for the mandibular premolar projection.

Rationale Standing in this position will enable the operator to raise the tubehead until the film can not be seen. At this point, the x-ray beam will expose the entire film and prevent a conecut.

☒ *Mandibular Left Molar Projection*

Step 1 Film Packet Placement for the Molar Projection

> ***Procedure*** Break off the indented end of the styrofoam bite block. The packet is placed in the styrofoam bite block in the same manner as for the premolar projection. Placement of the film in the mouth should be no further forward than the distal half of the mandibular second premolar (Figure 9-34).

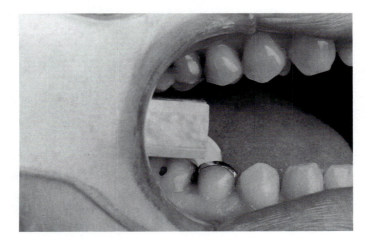

FIGURE 9-34 Packet placement for the mandibular molar projection.

> ***Rationale*** Positioning the film in this manner will allow for the imaging of the first, second, and third molars on the film.

Step 2 Vertical Alignment of the PID (Cone)

   Procedure   The operator should in the five o'clock position to align the vertical angulation (Figure 9-35).

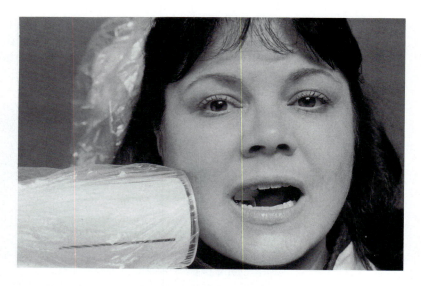

FIGURE 9-35   Proper vertical alignment for the mandibular molar projection.

   Rationale   Standing in this position will allow the operator to view the proper 90 degree angulation of the PID (cone) (x-ray beam) to the film.

Step 3 Horizontal Alignment of the PID (Cone)

Procedure The operator should be in the three o'clock position to the patient with the tubehead housing below the area of interest. The beam should be directed through the interproximal space of the mandibular first and second molars (Figure 9-36).

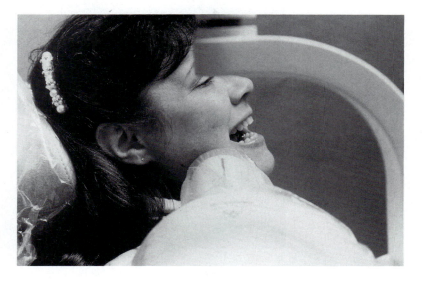

FIGURE 9-36 Proper horizontal alignment for the mandibular molar projection.

Rationale Standing in this position will allow easy visualization of the interproximal space. It will be necessary to retract the patient's cheek with one hand while viewing the interproximal space.

Step 4 Centering the Beam to Expose the Entire Film

Procedure   The operator should be behind the tubehead housing in the three o'clock position. The tubehead should then be raised until the film can no longer be viewed (Figure 9-37).

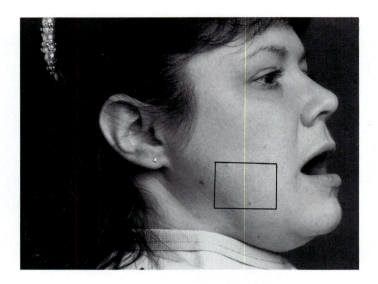

FIGURE 9-37   Cone centering for the mandibular molar projection.

Rationale   Following this procedure will insure proper coverage of the film by the x-ray beam.

Exposing projections for the mandibular right would be identical to the left except operator positioning is reversed, ie. the nine o'clock position instead of the three o'clock position.

BISECTING ANGLE TECHNIQUE

The bisecting angle technique was the first imaging method used to expose dental radiographs. Over the years, it has been discouraged because of the noncompliance of this technique with the shadowcasting principles. Still, some clinical situations, such as a small mouth, low palate, and large tori, warrant use of this technique. These are anatomical constraints that prevent the film from being placed parallel to the long axis of the tooth being imaged.

This technique has two advantages. First, the film is placed as close to the tooth as possible, thereby follows one of the shadowcasting principles. Second, when the film is closer to the teeth, the patient seems to be able to tolerate the film in the mouth more easily. Thus, it provides greater comfort for the patient.

The two disadvantages of the technique are distortion of the tooth and superimposition of the zygomatic arch over the apices of the maxillary molars (Figure 9-38). The increased likelihood of tooth distortion occurs primarily for two reasons. First, the technique does not adhere to two of the shadowcasting principles (the film is not parallel to the tooth and the beam is not perpendicular to the film). The amount of guesswork involved in determining the angle that bisects the tooth and film and then aligning the beam perpendicular to the bisecting line of this angle, increases the chance of a miscalculation. The teeth will commonly appear foreshortened (short and squatty) or elongated (long and stretched). The second disadvantage is the superimposition of the

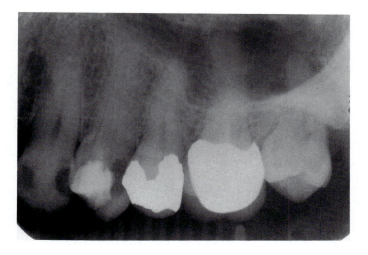

FIGURE 9-38 Note the foreshortened buccal root of the maxillary first molar and the zygomatic arch superimposed on the apices of the maxillary second molar.

zygomatic arch onto the maxillary molar apices. Because of the steep vertical angle required to image the maxillary molars using this technique, the shadow of the zygomatic arch is placed on top of the molar apices. This inhibits the accurate interpretation of the posterior area involving the molar root apices.

The actual technique involves two imaginary lines. The first passes through the long axis of the tooth to be imaged; the second follows the vertical axis of the film. The point at which the film and tooth join represents the apex of the triangle (Figure 9-39). The radiographer must then draw an imaginary line that would bisect the angle formed by the film and tooth. The tubehead or beam should then be directed so that it is perpendicular to that bisected line. Hence the name of the technique—"bisecting" the angle.

The film-holding devices that can be used for imaging this technique are the styrofoam bite block, hemostat, snap-a-ray,* and Rinn XCP bisecting angle instruments (BAI)* (Figure 9-40). The latter device will eliminate the need to align the PID (cone). An extension arm is attached at an angle to approximate a perpendicular line to the bisected angle. Using this device, the film holder is placed in the mouth with the film against the tooth. The extension arm then automatically indicates the position in which the PID (cone) should be placed (Figure 9-41). It should be noted that the size of the beam should be restricted to the rectangular shape of the film. This can be accomplished by using an

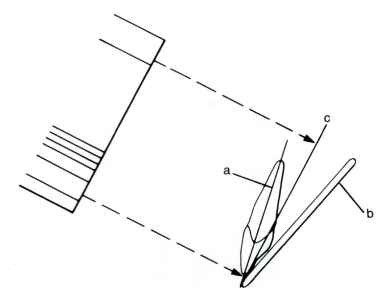

FIGURE 9-39 (a) This line represents the long axis of the tooth. (b) This line shows the long axis of the film. (c) This line shows the imaginary line that bisects the angle formed by the tooth and film.

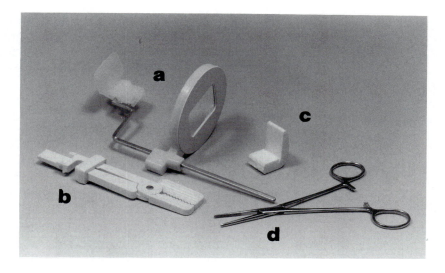

FIGURE 9-40 Various film-holding devices that can be used with the bisecting angle technique: (a) Rinn XCP bisecting angle instruments, (b) snap-a-ray, (c) styrofoam biteblock, and (d) hemostat.

imaging instrument that limits the size of the beam (i.e., by attaching a rectangular shaped disk to the end of a circular PID (cone) or by using a rectangular PID (cone). When using devices that do not have an extension arm, the vertical angulation of the PID (cone) must be visualized without an extension arm to align the beam.

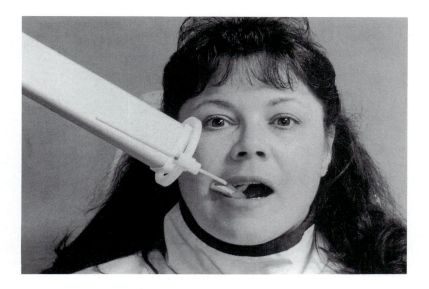

FIGURE 9-41 The Rinn BAI placed in the mouth with the extension arm aligning the beam to the film.

The primary advantage of using a styrofoam bite block with the bisecting angle technique is the ability of the patient to bite on the device and not have to hold or stabilize the film with the hand. The styrofoam bite block is also disposable. The primary disadvantage includes the absence of an extension arm.

Operator Technique

The following steps should be employed when using the styrofoam bite block for the bisecting angle technique.

Step 1   Break off the end of the styrofoam bite block at the indented line and place the film securely in the film slot (Figure 9-42).

Step 2   Place the film against the tooth to be radiographed with the film edge slightly below the incisal or occlusal surface. Have the patient bite gently until the styrofoam bite block is secure. The film should *not* be held with the finger (Figure 9-43).

Step 3   Draw an imaginary line from the long axis of the tooth and the vertical plane of the film. Join these two lines at the junction of the crown of the tooth and the film. This will form the angle to be bisected (Figure 9-43).

Step 4   Visualize an imaginary line bisecting the angle. Align the PID (cone) at right angles to the imaginary line bisecting the angle (Figure 9-44).

Step 5   Center the PID (cone) so that it will expose the entire film (Figure 9-44).

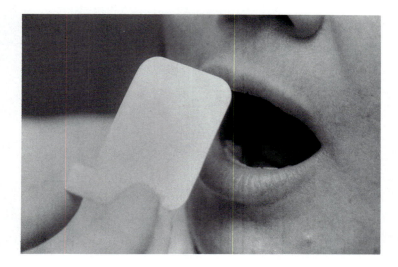

FIGURE 9-42 Film placement in the styrofoam bite block with the indented end removed.

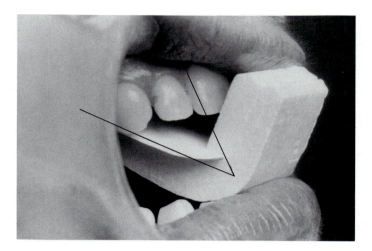

FIGURE 9-43 Styrofoam bite block placed in the mouth for the bisecting angle technique and stabilized by the teeth. The lines demonstrate the angle formed by long axis of tooth and film.

Some general guidelines that can be used to set the vertical angulation are given Table 9-1. The patient's occlusal plane must be parallel to the floor when following the suggested vertical angles in Table 9-1. Remember that patients have different anatomical features and will not always adhere to these guidelines.

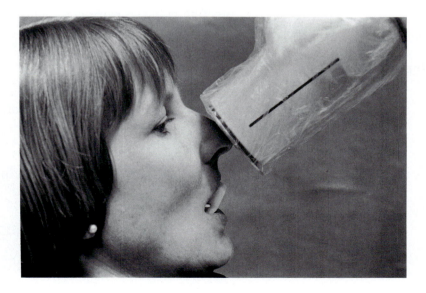

FIGURE 9-44 Vertical alignment of the beam at right angles to the imaginary line bisecting the angle formed by the tooth and film. Center the beam to expose the entire film.

TABLE 9-1
Guidelines for setting vertical angulation

Maxillary central	+55° to +65°
Maxillary lateral/canine	+45° to +50°
Maxillary premolar	+40°
Maxillary molar	+25° to +30°
Mandibular central	−30°
Mandibular lateral/canine	−30°
Mandibular premolar	−10°
Mandibular molar	0°

HEMOSTAT

The hemostat (Figure 9-45a) is a scissor-like device with locking handles that can be used to hold an intraoral dental film. It is ideal for patients who are unable to open their mouths very wide due to conditions such as **trismus,** broken jaw, and so on. The bisecting angle technique must be used when the film holder is the hemostat.

The primary advantage of this film holder is its small size. This makes it an invaluable device for patients who are unable to open their mouths very wide. Another advantage is that the hemostat can be sterilized. Disadvantages include the need for the patient to hold the instrument, thus exposing the hand to radiation, and possible inaccurate projection geometry with the use of the bisecting angle technique. In addition, this film holding device does not have an extension arm to align the PID (cone).

Operator Technique

The technique is the same as described previously for bisecting the angle using a styrofoam bite block, but the handle of the hemostat must be held stable by the patient.

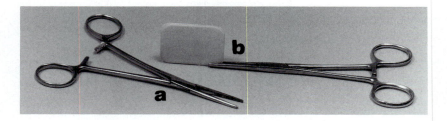

FIGURE 9-45 (a) The hemostat has locking handles. (b) Placement of film in the hemostat.

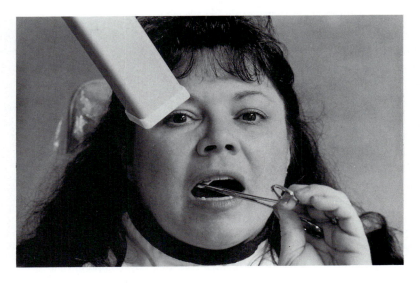

FIGURE 9-46 The hemostat is placed against the tooth with patient stabilizing the handle. Horizontal, vertical, and cone centering for the hemostat is shown using the bisecting angle technique.

Step 1   Grasp the edge or corner of the film with the needle end of the hemostat and lock the handle closed (Figure 9-45b).

Step 2   Place the film against the tooth being radiographed with the film edge slightly lower than the occlusal or incisal edge and instruct the patient to stabilize the hemostat with the hand (Figure 9-46).

Step 3   Visualize the angle formed by the film and long axis of the tooth. Bisect the angle and position the beam at right angles to the bisecting line (Figure 9-46).

SNAP-A-RAY

The snap-a-ray is also a film holding device used with the bisecting angle technique. The advantages of this device are its lightweight quality and ease of maneuverability. It is also autoclavable. Disadvantages are the need for the patient to stabilize the device and absence of an extension arm for alignment of the beam.

Film Technique

The technique is similar to the other devices discussed in that the film is placed in the holder and then stabilized by the patient once it is placed in the mouth. The film is placed at the end of the device in a vertical orientation for the anterior projections (Figure 9-47a) and in a

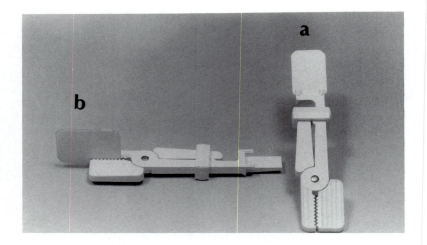

FIGURE 9-47 (a) Snap-a-ray showing the film placement for an anterior projection. (b) Snap-a-ray showing the film placement for a posterior projection.

horizontal position for posterior projections (Figure 9-47b). The bisecting angle technique is used primarily with this device, although the mandibular posterior projections closely resemble film placement using the paralleling technique.

Step 1 Place the film in the holder according to the area of the mouth to be imaged.

Step 2 Place the film against the tooth being radiographed with the film edge slightly lower than the occlusal or incisal edge and instruct the patient to stabilize the film holder with the hand (Figure 9-48).

Step 3 Visualize the angle formed by the film and long axis of the tooth. Bisect the angle and position the beam at right angles to the bisecting line (Figure 9-48).

SUMMARY

This chapter presented a variety of intraoral radiographic techniques that are acceptable alternatives if an area can not be radiographed using the paralleling technique with a rectangular collimated position-indicating device. Each technique has specific advantages and disadvantages that should be applied to the individual clinical situation. When making these clinical decisions, the primary concern of the dental radiographer is to produce a diagnostically acceptable radiograph while

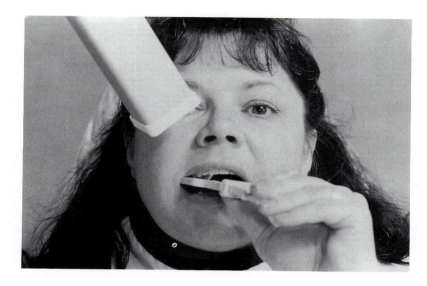

FIGURE 9-48 Placement of the snap-a-ray in the mouth with the patient stabilizing the film. Horizontal, vertical, and cone centering for the snap-a-ray device is shown using the bisecting angle technique.

keeping the radiation dose to the patient as low as reasonably achievable.

BIBLIOGRAPHY

COUNCIL ON DENTAL MATERIALS, INSTRUMENTS AND EQUIPMENT. Recommendations in Radiographic Practices: An Update, 1988. *JADA* 1989; 118(1): 115–117.

MATTESON SR, WHALEY C, SECRIST VC. *Dental Radiography,* 4th ed. Chapel Hill, NC: University of North Carolina Press, 1988.

REVIEW QUESTIONS

1. The major disadvantages for using the bisecting angle technique include all *except*

a. superimposition of the zygomatic arch on molar apices.
b. close film-to-object distance.
c. tooth distortion.
d. guesswork used to bisect angle.

2. Film-holding device(s) that can be used with the bisecting angle technique is (are)

a. styrofoam bite block.
b. hemostat.
c. snap-a-ray.
d. all of the above
e. none of the above

3. The advantages of using a styrofoam bite block and rectangular collimator include all *except*

a. good imaging principles.
b. patient comfort.
c. stabilization of holder by biting.
d. beam alignment.
e. all of the above

4. The steps that should be used with all intraoral radiographic procedures that do not use a beam alignment device are

a. packet placement, beam alignment.
b. packet placement, vertical, horizontal, cone centering.
c. packet placement, horizontal, Cone centering.
d. packet placement, vertical, horizontal.

5. When using the bisecting angle technique, the beam is directed perpendicular to

a. the long axis of the tooth.
b. the long axis of the film.
c. the line bisecting the angle formed by the film and occlusal plane.
d. the line bisecting the angle formed by the film and tooth.
e. none of the above

Radiographic Imaging for the Dental Team, by Sally Mauriello. J.B. Lippincott Company, Philadelphia © 1995.

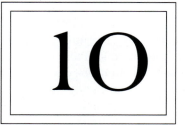

Supplemental Radiographic Procedures

Upon the completion of this chapter, the student should be able to:

1. Identify the types of supplemental radiographic procedures used in dentistry.

2. Discuss the rationale for using supplemental radiographic procedures in dentistry.

3. Apply the principles for taking supplemental radiographs.

INTRODUCTION

Often the standard intraoral or extraoral radiographic procedures will not reveal the necessary structures for certain dental procedures. In addition, certain patient conditions, such as a fractured mandible, impacted third molars, location of cyst or foreign object, or a very small mouth, will require special radiographic procedures.

The supplemental radiographs discussed in this chapter include occlusal radiographs, disto-oblique radiographs, localization techniques, edentulous and partially edentulous surveys, and endodontic and pediatric projections. Some of these projections require specific types of film, as well as unique packet placement and adjustment of technique factors (machine settings).

OCCLUSAL RADIOGRAPHS

Occlusal radiographs are taken to obtain a wider view of either the maxilla or mandible—typically the palate or the floor of the mouth and their surrounding structures. The film that is used for occlusal radiography (size 4) is a relatively large film, measuring approximately 3 in. × 2¼ in. (57 mm × 76 mm) (Figure 10-1). The film is placed between the arches; the X-ray beam is directed toward either the maxillary or mandibular arch, depending on which you are radiographing.

Occlusal radiographs are particularly useful in the following cases

1. To locate pathology in the palate or the floor of the mouth, such as cysts and malignancies.

2. To take radiographs on patients, who have a limited ability to open their mouths.

3. To locate fractures of the maxilla or mandible.

4. To locate foreign bodies.

5. To locate impacted or supernumerary teeth.

6. To take radiographs on small children who cannot tolerate the standard placement of intraoral film packets.

Two basic types of occlusal radiographs can be exposed. The topographical occlusal radiograph demonstrates the anterior area of the arch. This view can be taken on either the maxilla or mandible. The cross-sectional occlusal radiograph is a view of the mandible that allows us to study the floor of the mouth. This view is similar to looking at the mandible from below. Each type of occlusal radiograph can be placed so to achieve a standard anterior or lateral view of the arch.

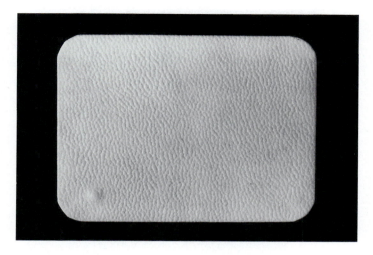

FIGURE 10-1 Occlusal film packet.

Topographic Views

A standard topographical occlusal view of the maxilla shows the palate, the nasal septum, the zygomatic processes, and the teeth from second molar to second molar (Figure 10-2). This projection is accom-

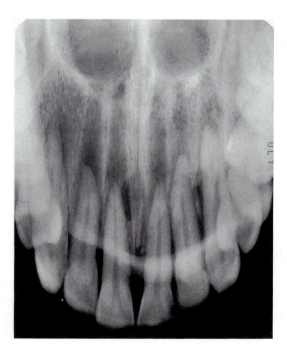

FIGURE 10-2 Standard maxillary topographical occlusal radiograph.

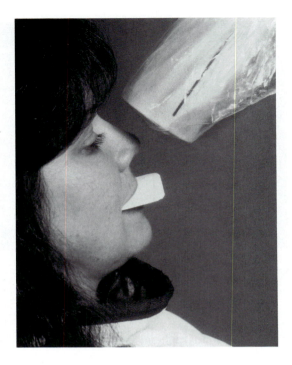

FIGURE 10-3 Proper patient, film, and PID positioning for the standard maxillary topographical occlusal radiograph.

plished by placing the occlusal film between the patient's teeth with the tube side (stippled) of the film toward the maxilla. The patient is seated so that occlusal plane is parallel to the floor. The film is placed crosswise in the mouth and pushed back as far as possible. The patient closes gently on the film to stabilize it. The beam is directed so that the central ray is a vertical angulation of +65 degrees and a horizontal angulation toward the middle of the film. The central ray typically enters the patient's face at the bridge of the nose (Figure 10-3).

The anterior topographical occlusal view of the maxilla shows the anterior portion of the maxilla and the canine to canine teeth. This view is taken with the same patient positioning, vertical angulation, and horizontal angulation as the standard view. The only differences are that the packet is placed anteriorly, and the central ray is directed to enter the patient at the tip of the nose (Figures 10-4 and 10-5).

The lateral topographical occlusal view of the maxilla is used to view half of the maxilla, with its surrounding structures and teeth. The film is placed with the long axis directed toward the posterior of the mouth and on the side of the mouth being studied. The patient is seated so that the occlusal plane is parallel to the floor. The beam is directed at +60 degrees vertical angulation at a point approximately 2 cm below the canthus of the eye (Figures 10-6 and 10-7).

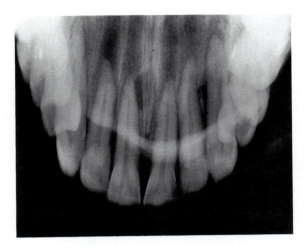

FIGURE 10-4 Anterior maxillary topographical occlusal radiograph.

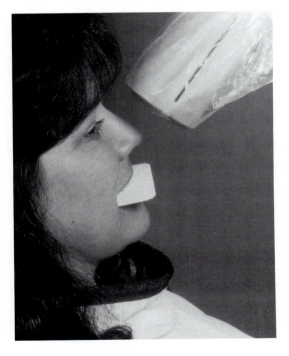

FIGURE 10-5 Proper patient, film, and PID positioning for the anterior maxillary topographical occlusal radiograph.

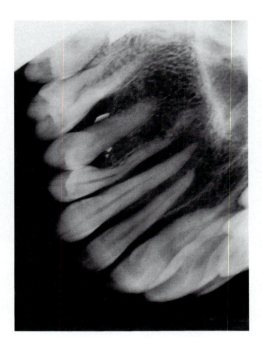

FIGURE 10-6 Lateral maxillary topographical occlusal radiograph.

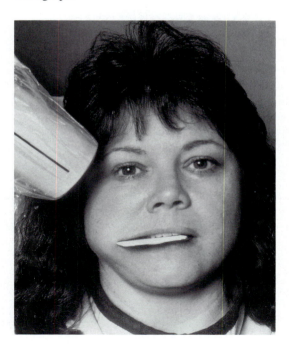

FIGURE 10-7 Proper patient, film, and PID positioning for the lateral maxillary topographical occlusal radiograph.

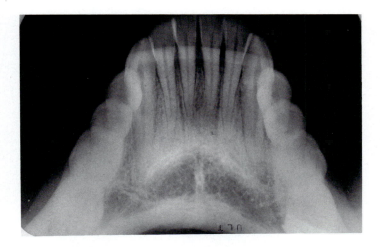

FIGURE 10-8 Anterior mandibular topographical occlusal radiograph.

The anterior topographical occlusal view of the mandible is used to view the mandibular anterior teeth and their surrounding structures. The film is placed crosswise in the patient's mouth and the patient's head is tilted back so that the occlusal plane is approximately 45 degrees to the floor. The film is placed so the tube side is directed toward the mandibular teeth, and the patient bites gently on the film to stabilize it. The beam is directed towards the center of the film with a −55 degrees vertical angulation. The beam is centered on the tip of the chin (Figures 10-8 and 10-9).

Cross-Sectional Views

Cross-sectional views are exposed on the mandibular arch mainly to view the floor of the mouth. A standard cross-sectional view is accomplished by placing the film crosswise in the patient's mouth and as far back as possible. The tube side of the film faces the mandible, and the patient bites down gently on the film to stabilize it. The patient's head is tilted back (often it is necessary to have the patient in a reclining position), so that the occlusal plane is almost perpendicular to the floor. The beam is directed so that it is at a right angle (90 degrees) to the plane of the film and toward the center of the film (Figures 10-10 and 10-11).

The lateral cross-sectional view covers the floor of one-half of the mouth. The film is placed lengthwise on the side of the mouth to be studied. The patient and beam placement is the same as with the standard and anterior views (Figures 10-12 and 10-13).

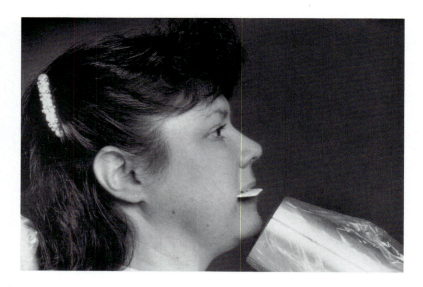

FIGURE 10-9 Proper patient, film, and PID positioning for the anterior mandibular topographical occlusal radiograph.

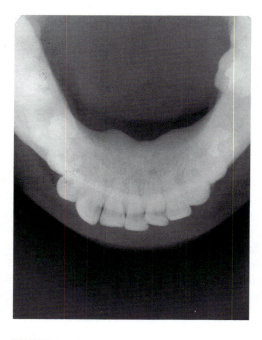

FIGURE 10-10 Standard mandibular cross-sectional occlusal radiograph.

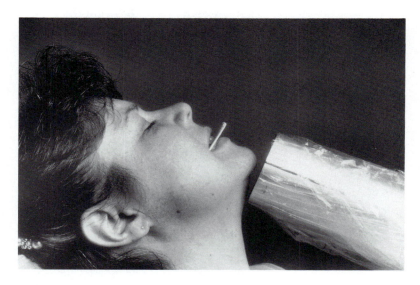

FIGURE 10-11 Proper patient, film, and PID positioning for the standard mandibular cross sectional occlusal radiograph.

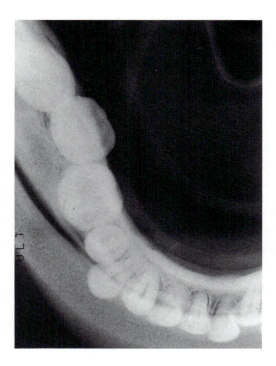

FIGURE 10-12 Lateral mandibular cross-sectional occlusal radiograph.

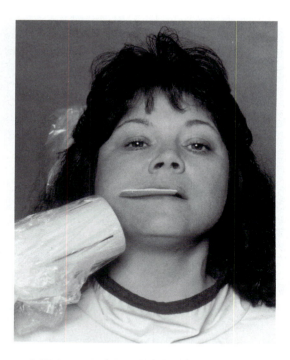

FIGURE 10-13 Proper patient, film, and PID positioning for the mandibular lateral cross sectional occlusal radiograph.

DISTO-OBLIQUE RADIOGRAPHS

Disto-oblique radiographs are useful to view the most posterior areas of the mouth, such as impacted third molars. Often, patients are unable to tolerate intraoral film packets so far back in their mouths. Therefore, these projections are used to project the images of the third molars onto the film without having to place them as far back as the third molars extend. One drawback to this projection is the increased interproximal overlapping that will occur in the image because of the excessive horizontal angulation needed to project the third molar onto the film.

Maxillary

For the maxillary third molars, the film packet is placed as far back as the patient can tolerate. The tubehead is aligned as it would normally be for a molar projection and then shifted to increase the vertical angulation by 10 degrees. The horizontal angulation is then also shifted so the beam is 5 to 10 degrees further from the distal (Figures 10-14, 10-15, and 10-16).

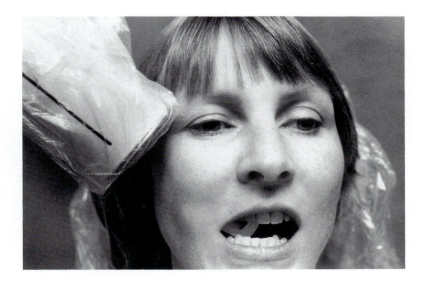

FIGURE 10-14   Proper vertical positioning of the PID for the maxillary disto-oblique radiograph.

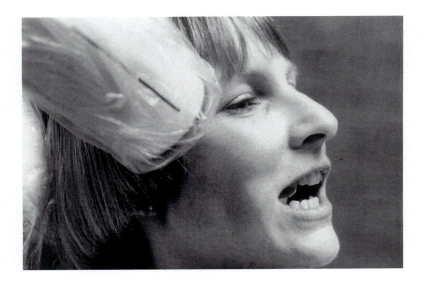

FIGURE 10-15   Proper horizontal positioning of the PID for the maxillary disto-oblique radiograph.

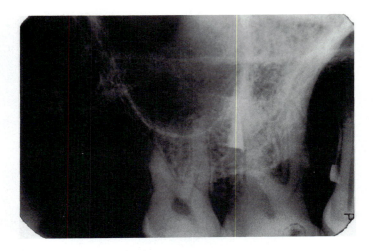

FIGURE 10-16   Maxillary disto-oblique radiograph.

Mandibular

The mandibular third molars can be imaged by placing the film packet as it would be placed for a molar projection. The tubehead is then aligned for the standard projection. After this alignment, the tubehead is shifted 10 degrees horizontally from the distal. No change is made in the vertical angulation (Figures 10-17, 10-18, and 10-19).

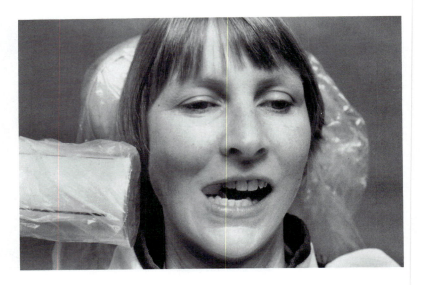

FIGURE 10-17   Proper vertical positioning of the PID for the mandibular disto-oblique radiograph.

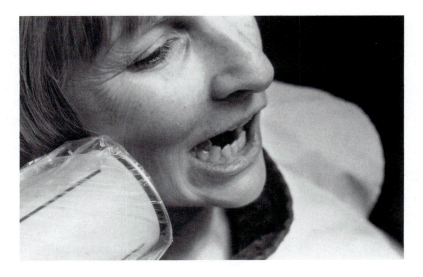

FIGURE 10-18 Proper horizontal positioning of the PID for the mandibular disto-oblique radiograph.

LOCALIZATION

Often it is necessary to locate a foreign object, supernumerary, or impacted tooth in the mouth. Before these objects can be dealt with surgically, one must determine if the object being viewed is facial or

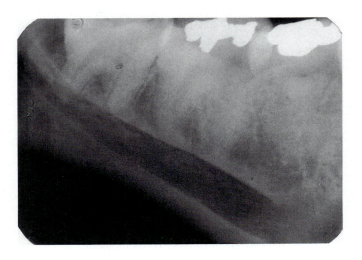

FIGURE 10-19 Mandibular disto-oblique radiograph.

lingual to the adjacent teeth. Since radiographs are simply a two-dimensional representation of a three-dimensional area, objects facial or lingual appear to be superimposed over the teeth. Therefore, their exact location cannot be determined. There are generally two methods for locating these objects. The first—the right angle technique—uses two films exposed at right angles to one another. The second—the tube shift technique—follows the concepts revealed in the buccal object rule, or Clarke's rule.

Right Angle Technique

This technique takes a standard periapical radiograph of the area of interest and then exposes an occlusal radiograph of that arch. This provides two projections at right angles to one another. For example, if a mandibular molar projection shows radiopacity below the apex of the second molar, then a standard cross-sectional occlusal radiograph can be taken of the mandible to determine if the radiopacity is facial or lingual to the second molar (Figures 10-20 and 10-21).

Tube Shift Technique

This technique is based on the concept that images will shift in position as the projection angle changes. For example, a standard periapical

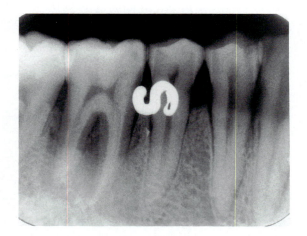

FIGURE 10-20   A foreign object is represented by a lead letter in this radiograph. It is impossible to determine from this radiograph if the foreign object lies facial or lingual to the teeth.

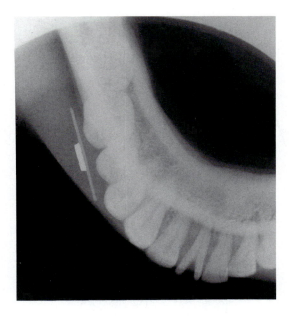

FIGURE 10-21 This occlusal radiograph shows that the foreign object represented by the lead letter is facial to the teeth.

radiograph of the mandibular premolar area shows a radiolucency below the mandibular second premolar. Another projection of the same area is taken, but this time the tubehead is shifted mesially beyond the standard horizontal angulation. In comparing the two radiographs, the second one shows the radiolucency to be below the area between the first and second premolar. The object seems to have shifted mesially with the tube shift. This indicates that the object in question is lingual to the teeth. If the object had appeared to move distally, the object would be lying facially. These results follow a concept known as the SLOB rule: *s*ame *l*ingual, *o*pposite *b*uccal. This states that as the tube is shifted mesially, a lingual object will move in the same direction. If the object moves distally, it is considered to lie buccal or facial (opposite direction) (Figures 10-22 and 10-23). This concept can also be seen in a panoramic radiograph with a split image. The anterior area is imaged twice in the radiograph. Any foreign object imaged in this area will shift following the SLOB concept.

This concept can also be described using the buccal object rule (also known as **Clarke's rule**). This rule states that a buccal (or facial) object will move in the same direction as the beam is directed. For example, as the beam is directed mesially, the buccal object appears to shift mesially.

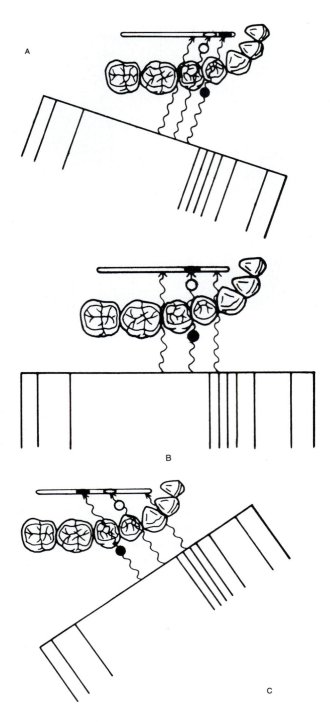

FIGURE 10-22 This drawing depicts how the image on the radiograph shifts position as the beam is directed either distally or mesially.

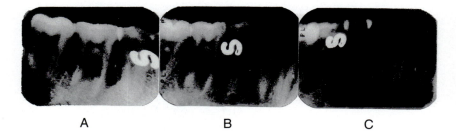

FIGURE 10-23 Radiograph B is the standard projection. In Radiograph A, as the tube is shifted distally (beam directed mesially), the foreign object moves mesially. In Radiograph C, as the tube is shifted mesially (beam directed distally), the foreign object moves distally. This indicates that the foreign object is located facial to the teeth.

EDENTULOUS AND PARTIALLY EDENTULOUS RADIOGRAPHIC SURVEYS

Radiographic examination of edentulous and partially edentulous patients should not be neglected solely because there are no teeth present. Areas that do not have teeth present may contain root tips, cysts, residual infection, or malignancies that can adversely affect the patient's health or compromise their ability to tolerate such prosthetic appliances as partial and full dentures.

With partially edentulous patients, film packet placement may be difficult in the areas of missing teeth. For example, a patient may be missing the two mandibular right premolars and the second molar. When placing the film packet for the molar projection, it may tilt forward in the premolar area. To stabilize the film packet, it may be necessary to fill the edentulous area with cotton gauze or a cotton roll upon which the film holder can rest.

When taking radiographs on fully edentulous patients, it is recommended to take as few exposures as necessary to cover the entire edentulous areas. Usually a full radiographic survey of an edentulous patient can be accomplished with approximately 14 periapical projections (seven maxillary, seven mandibular). Film packet placement and stabilization can pose a particular problem in these patients. It is recommended that cotton rolls be attached to the film holder bite block in order to stabilize the film and provide the necessary vertical spacing on the radiograph (Figure 10-24). However, the patient may keep the opposing denture in place in order to aid in biting on the bite block. The denture covering the area to be radiographed must be removed.

Another consideration when radiographing the edentulous patient is the exposure factors. Without the teeth, the alveolar ridge attenuation

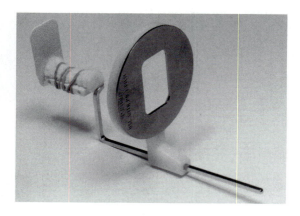

FIGURE 10-24 Cotton roll attached to a biteblock on the film holder will aid in radiographing edentulous areas.

factor is much less. Therefore, using the same exposure factors on edentulous patients as is used on dentate patients would result in radiographs that are much too dark. It is therefore necessary to decrease the exposure factors when radiographing edentulous ridges by approximately 25 percent.

If possible, panoramic radiographs of the edentulous patients can serve the purpose for studying the alveolar ridges. If there are specific areas of concern, periapical projections can supplement the panoramic radiograph.

ENDODONTIC RADIOGRAPHIC PROJECTIONS

Radiographs are required in all phases of endodontic therapy, including diagnosis, treatment planning, preparation and restoration of the tooth, and monitoring the healing process. Radiographs must be taken to estimate canal length before the procedure begins and also during the root canal procedure to affirm instrument placement. In addition, radiographs are recommended before the final filling of the canal.

Endodontic radiographs taken during treatment must be exposed under difficult conditions. The rubber dam, clamp, and root canal instruments and fillings projecting from the tooth create less than ideal radiographic conditions. Because the root length estimates should be as precise as possible, the paralleling radiographic technique should be employed. This technique provides the truest image. The bisecting the angle technique in contrast, could possibly result in a distortion in root length.

Because the patients cannot close their mouths or bite on standard film holders, altered or specialized film holders must be used that allow patients to bite and not interfere with the endodontic instruments. A

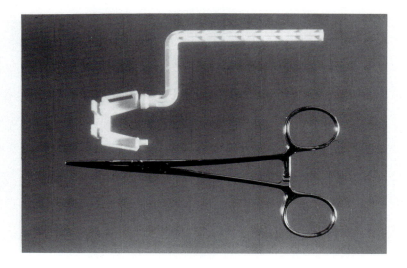

FIGURE 10-25 Film holders used in endodontic procedures.

straight hemostat or Endo-Ray™ film holder (Figure 10-25) are two such film holders available.

No special machine setting modifications are used to expose endodontic radiographs. Although many practitioners choose to overexpose these radiographs in order to speed the developing process (they are assuming that greater density will shorten the developing time that is required to view the image), this unacceptable procedure results in a poor image. The more acceptable procedure is to use rapid processing chemistry after using standard exposure factors. These chemicals allow the developing and fixing process to be completed in a few minutes. The films should still be returned to the fixer and final wash for the standard times after the initial viewing of the films.

PEDIATRIC RADIOGRAPHIC SURVEYS

Because of children's sensitivity to ionizing radiation, caution should be exercised when taking radiographs on the pediatric patient. Consideration should be given to the patient's caries history and teeth present. These patients can also pose special management problems because of age, apprehension, and size of the mouth. The number of projections required depends on the teeth present in the child's mouth. In addition, exposure factors should be modified to ensure the proper density. Because the pediatric patient is smaller than the adult patient and the bone is less dense, the exposure factors (mAs) should be reduced by 50 percent for children under 10 years of age and by 25 percent for children between 10 and 15.

For the patient with a total primary dentition, the typical survey consists of a maxillary and a mandibular occlusal radiograph (using

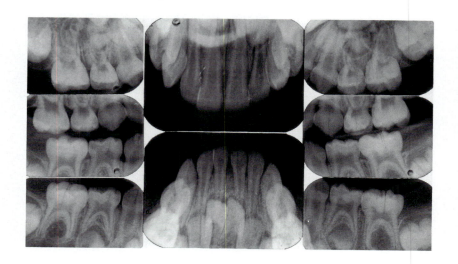

FIGURE 10-26 Full-mouth radiographic series of primary dentition.

size 2 film), 4 molar projections (one in each quadrant, using size 0 film), and 2 bitewings (one on each side, using size 0 film). The patient with a mixed dentition usually requires anterior periapicals to replace the occlusal radiographs. This includes maxillary and mandibular central projections, 4 lateral-canine projections (one in each quadrant), 4 molar projections (one in each quadrant), and 2 or 4 bitewing radiographs (depending on the presence of the permanent premolars and second molars). The film size used with a patient with a mixed dentition depends on the size of the patient's mouth. Size 1 and 2 film should be used when possible (Figures 10-26 and 10-27).

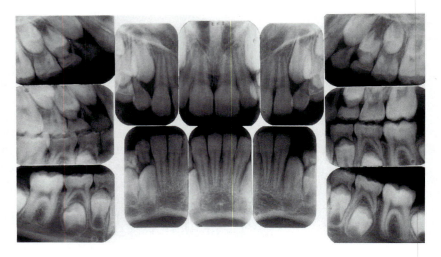

FIGURE 10-27 Full-mouth radiographic series of a mixed dentition.

SUMMARY

For maximum flexibility in handling all radiographic situations, the operator should be able to use the supplemental techniques that complement the standard radiographic procedures. This includes assessing the need to use a supplemental procedure as an alternative to the standard technique. These techniques include occlusal, disto-obliques, localization, edentulous and partially edentulous techniques, and endodontic and pediatric techniques. With the skill to apply these techniques, the operator should be able to deal with most radiographic requirements of the patient.

BIBLIOGRAPHY

GOAZ PW, WHITE SC. *Oral Radiology: Principles and Interpretation,* 2nd ed. St. Louis: CV Mosby, 1987.

LANGLAIS RP, LANGLAND OE, MORRIS CR. Radiographic Localization Technics. *Dental Radiography and Photography* 1979; 52(4): 69–77.

RICHARDS AG. *The Buccal Object Rule.* Dental Radiography and Photography 1980; 53(3): 37–56.

REVIEW QUESTIONS

1. In what situations are occlusal radiographs useful?

   a. _____
   b. _____
   c. _____
   d. _____
   e. _____
   f. _____

2. The cross-sectional occlusal radiograph is a view of the maxilla which demonstrates the anterior area of the arch.

   a. True
   b. False

3. Disto-oblique radiographs are used to view what structures?

   a. Third molars
   b. Salivary glands
   c. Sinuses
   d. Anterior teeth

4. The two techniques used for localization are known as

a. _____

b. _____

5. It is not necessary to take radiographs on a fully edentulous patient.

a. True
b. False

Radiographic Imaging for the Dental Team,
by Sally Mauriello. J.B. Lippincott Company,
Philadelphia © 1995.

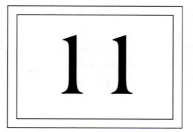

Patient Management in Dental Radiology

Upon the completion of this chapter, the student should be able to:

1. Discuss management problems due to oral anatomical constraints and various ways to manipulate the radiographic technique.

2. Describe technique modifications that can be used with physically or mentally disabled patients.

3. Discuss management techniques that can be used with phobic or apprehensive dental radiography patients.

Patients come in a variety of sizes, physical and mental abilities, dentitions, and personalities. Management of radiology patients will be dictated by these factors and govern the way the radiology appointment is handled. For example, a pediatric radiology patient will dictate the number and type of radiographic films needed, in addition to the way the radiographer speaks to and handles the patient. The ability to make the necessary adjustments in technique and management will increase the likelihood of obtaining the diagnostic information desired on the radiograph. Therefore, this chapter will address some of the more common situations a radiographer may encounter.

ORAL ANATOMICAL CONSTRAINTS

Palate

The hard palate comes in all shapes and sizes. If a patient has a palate that is shaped very narrow with a deep vault, the standard film size and placement become a problem. What does one do when the size 2 film used for the maxillary central projection does not fit? The easiest modification is to use a size 1 film. The result will be a radiograph with centrals imaged on the film and minimal or nonexistent appearance of the laterals (Figure 11-1). This is not a major concern, because the laterals can be imaged on the lateral/canine projection.

The hard palate can also have a wide shallow vault. This shape poses a problem because the radiographer is unable to place the film parallel to the long axis of the tooth. What does one do? Obviously, the radiographer must resort to one of the alternative techniques discussed in Chapter 9. Ideally, use of another film-holding device using the paralleling technique would be the first choice. If one is still unable to position the film without excessive bending of the film, then a film holder using the bisecting angle technique would be the second choice.

The anterior extent of the palate can present constraints in film placement for the premolar projection. Sometimes, it is impossible to place the premolar film forward (mesial) enough in the palate to image the entire first premolar onto the film. This may be due to the shape of the palate or mesial drifting of the premolar. In either case, the radiographic technique must be modified. This can be best accomplished by using the projection geometry principles discussed in Chapter 7. By placing the film as far forward (mesial) in the mouth as possible, with the anterior film edge turned toward the opposite canine area, (Figure 11-2) and adjusting the horizontal angulation so that the beam is directed towards the distal, the image of the first premolar will be projected on the film (Figure 11-3). This will occur even though the film is

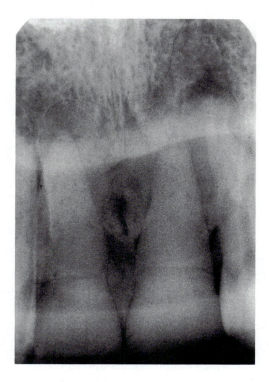

FIGURE 11-1 This figure demonstrates the appearance of a maxillary central projection exposed on a size 1 film.

not directly behind the entire tooth. It should be noted that horizontal overlap will occur with this modification because of the change in horizontal angulation. The horizontal overlap will not be a problem since this area can be viewed on the bitewing projection.

Floor of the Mouth

The floor of the mouth can also present special challenges to the radiographer. Most often during the mandibular central and lateral/canine projections, the patient will complain of the film cutting the floor of the mouth or the gingiva. This usually occurs because the radiographer is trying to force the film into the floor of the mouth, while the patient has his/her mouth wide open. In this open position, the muscles in the floor of the mouth are tight. This makes it difficult to accommodate the film. To correct this, place the film in a bisecting angle position with the edge of the film as far under the tongue as possible (Figure 11-4). As the patient is instructed to close, the muscles in the floor of the mouth will become flexible, and the radiographer will be able to upright the film in the floor of the mouth without

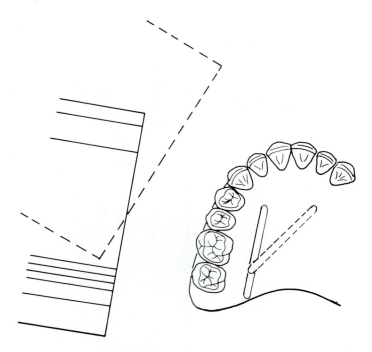

FIGURE 11-2 Positioning the film behind the opposite canine area enables the mesial of the first premolar to be projected onto the film.

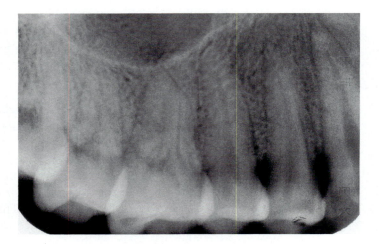

FIGURE 11-3 Modification of the horizontal beam angulation allows the first premolar to be projected onto the film.

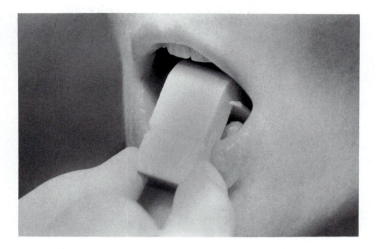

FIGURE 11-4 Placement of the film packet prior to positioning as the patient closes.

causing undue discomfort to the patient (Figure 11-5). The film will then be parallel to the long axis of the tooth.

Another possible cause for discomfort in this area may be due to the edge of the film cutting into the tissue. Dental products can be applied to the film to soften the edge (e.g., Edge-Ease X-ray Comfort Cushion*) or more easily, the film can be repositioned away from the teeth toward the midline of the mouth with the patient biting on the end of the biteblock. Another method would be to wrap the sharp edges of the film with a 2 × 2 gauze to cushion it in the mouth. Any of these methods will usually alleviate the cutting or jabbing feeling of the film.

As with the maxillary premolar, the mandibular premolar can also be difficult to image depending on the shape of the mandibular arch, musculature of the floor of the mouth, and position of the premolar. By using the same technique as with the maxillary arch, position the film as far forward in the floor of the mouth as possible and angle the film behind the canine of the opposite side (Figure 11-6). Adjust the horizontal angulation of the beam by directing it towards the distal, thereby projecting the premolar image onto the film.

Lingual Frenum

When the lingual frenum is attached high, towards the tip of the tongue (ankyloglossia), it can create a difficult environment for exposing radiographs on the mandibular arch. The mandibular central and lateral/canine radiographs would be the ones most likely affected. In this

---

*Strong Dental Products, Saratoga, CA

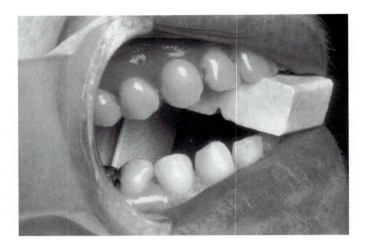

FIGURE 11-5   Correct film positioning for the mandibular central projection.

circumstance, you are often unable to get the radiograph parallel to the tooth because you are unable to slide it under the tongue. The only alternative is to place the film on top of the tongue and have the patient bite on the free end of the bite block (Figure 11-7). Usually, the film will be placed in a parallel relationship to the tooth. If it is not, then position the film holder and x-ray beam form a bisecting angle technique. A cotton roll may be necessary between the biteblock and opposing arch to keep the film holder straight. Consideration should be given to increasing the technique factors by 5 kVp or increasing expo-

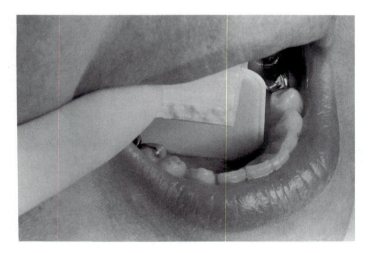

FIGURE 11-6   Positioning of the film packet in the mandibular arch to image the mesial of the premolar.

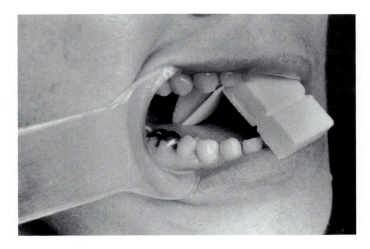

FIGURE 11-7 Placement of the film packet for a mandibular projection in a patient with ankyloglossia.

sure time if the film is placed on top of the tongue. This will allow for adequate density on the film since the tongue will absorb some of the x-ray beam. Note that during radiographic interpretation, the soft tissue image of the tongue will be present if this technique modification is used.

Maxillary and Mandibular Tori

Tori (bony growths) are commonly found in the midline of the palate and lingual surfaces along the premolar area in the mandibular area. Usually, the tori are small and do not interfere with the radiographic technique. Occasionally, the growths are very large and thus present problems in positioning the film.

When exposing a film with a large torus palatinus present, the radiographer will often have to place the film on the opposite side of the torus (Figure 11-8). More than likely, one of the alternative film-holding devices will have to be used. Therefore, the beam alignment for vertical angulation should be as close to 90 degrees as possible. The technique factors should be increased by 5 to 10 kVp to maintain the proper film density.

In the mandibular arch, a unilateral tori would be handled similarly to the torus palatinus. The film packet should be placed away from the tooth and the kVp increased. The vertical and horizontal angulation should not be effected. Bilateral tori present a different problem. Often, the tori have grown so large that they meet at the midline under the tongue, and it is impossible to insert a film between them. In this situation, place the film as far forward as possible and adjust the horizontal angulation to image the teeth onto the film (Figure 11-9).

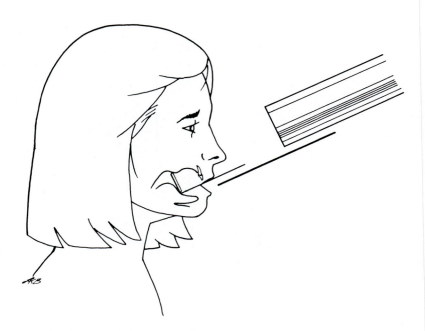

FIGURE 11-8 Placement of the film packet for a patient with a large torus palatinus.

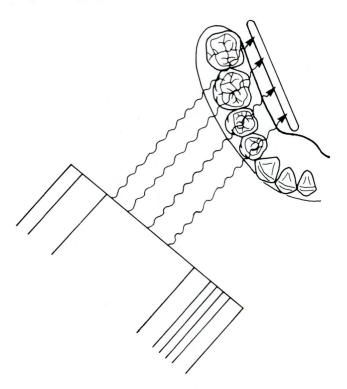

FIGURE 11-9 Placement of the tubehead to allow imaging of the first premolar on the film.

This will compensate for the inability to position the film directly behind the premolars. Again, the kVp must be increased in order to maintain film density.

Gag Reflex

Some people are unable to tolerate foreign objects in their mouth without gagging. This **gag reflex** presents a real challenge for the radiographer. The basis for the gagging can be mental or physical. Regardless, the radiographer must deal with a situation that is unpleasant for both the patient and the radiographer.

Once you realize you have a "gagger," first expose the films that will not trigger the gag reflex; leave the difficult films until last. When it is time to expose the difficult films, remember to have everything set prior to placing the film in the mouth. That includes chair adjustments, technique factors, and tube angulation. Speak calmly to the patient and explain everything that is being done. No Surprises!

There are various "remedies" that may help the situation, although they will not work for everyone. Some of the techniques that may be tried are listed as follows.

1. Special antigag film (cold film from the refrigerator). Tell the patient you are going to get some special antigag film that is kept in the refrigerator. Leave the operatory to get the film and use the cold film upon return. Take the difficult projections with this film.

2. Having the patient concentrate on something else, such as breathing through the nose, lifting a finger, and so on.

3. Let the patient place the film holder with your guidance and assistance.

4. Use of a topical anesthetic sprayed in the soft palate may be indicated in extreme cases, but should be used cautiously. A mouthwash with a mild anesthetic can be swished in the mouth and produce a numbing effect.

5. The temporal tap, which involves tapping firmly three times in the temporal area (in front of the ears), has been acclaimed as an effective antigagging technique. Tap three times with the fingertips and tell the patient that he/she will not gag. To increase the effectiveness of this technique, the taps should be done before the patient experiences a gag response.

6. Sucking on ice or swallowing ice water between exposures can help control gagging. Do not use this technique if the patient reports having cold-sensitive teeth.

7. Placing salt on the tongue or rinsing with salt water is sometimes effective. Do not use this technique if the patient is on a salt-restricted diet.

These techniques often seem to aid the patient, even though there is no scientific data to support them. Remember that if you are unable to position the film to get the information you want, then do not expose the radiograph. Supplemental radiographs may be an alternative.

Trismus

Trismus is a condition that limits or prevents the patient from opening the mouth. It often occurs following radiation therapy to the oral cavity, fixation of a broken mandible, or infection/inflammation of the temporomandibular joint (TMJ). Therefore, if it is necessary to take a radiograph, normal procedures should be modified. The easiest film holder to use for a periapical projection would be the hemostat (see Chapter 9). The film can be placed properly without opening the mouth wider than a couple of millimeters (Figure 11-10). Other appropriate techniques to consider would be an extraoral projection (see Chapter 13) or an occlusal projection (see Chapter 10). In circumstances where trismus has been caused by edema, it may be necessary to adjust the exposure factors to maintain an adequate film density.

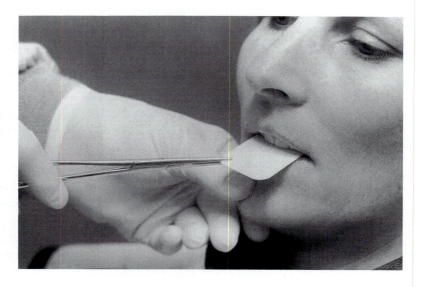

FIGURE 11-10   Insertion of the film on a patient unable to open the mouth.

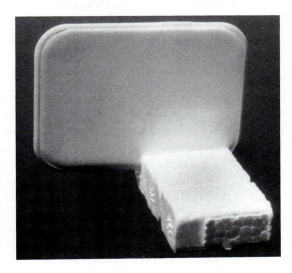

FIGURE 11-11 Off-centering the film in the holder will allow imaging of an edentulous area.

MODIFIED DENTITION

Missing or Broken Teeth

Some patients will present with a single or multiple missing or broken teeth. This situation may present a challenge in taking a particular radiograph when there are no teeth present for the patient to occlude against. In such cases, a few alternatives can be considered. First, determine if it is possible to off-center the film in the film holder and have the adjacent teeth stabilize the film holder. For example, the mandibular premolars are missing. In order to expose this area, off-center the film in the film holder toward the distal (Figure 11-11). Then, place the film holder so that the canines occlude on the film holder and the film is positioned distally. When off-centering the film in the holder, remember to align the x-ray beam with the film and not the film holder. If the beam is aligned to the film holder, then a cone cut on the film will result. Another alternative would be to use cotton rolls in the edentulous area.

Supererupted Teeth

If a tooth does not have an opposing tooth against which to occlude, then often the tooth will continue to erupt and be out of alignment with the occlusal surface. In these situations, it is difficult to keep the film holder from tipping when the patient bites. To steady the film holder, try using cotton rolls or centering the supererupted tooth in the middle of the film holder.

Severely Overlapped Teeth

Severely overlapped teeth can present a special challenge to the radiographer. Often, one will try to adjust the horizontal angulation so that the interproximal space appears open. The result is a film that does not have the correct teeth displayed, because the exaggerated horizontal angulation projects the tooth off of the film. When it is necessary to use an extreme horizontal angulation, compensate by moving the film packet in the direction in which the beam is directed (See Chapter 7, especially Figure 7-14).

PHYSICAL AND MENTAL DISABILITIES

Patients may present with physical and/or mental disabilities. The radiographer must determine the extent of the patient's limitation(s) and make a judgment as to the appropriate radiographic technique that should be used. Every attempt should be made to help the patient understand the procedure that will be performed. The caregiver can often be a valuable asset in communication and should be asked the words and actions to which the patient best responds. Speed is of the utmost importance and every attempt should be made to minimize the amount of time the film packet is in the mouth (e.g., fast-speed film, short exposure times, and so on).

Some patients require a wheelchair. If possible, the patient should be transferred to the dental chair. If not, a portable headrest that attaches to the wheelchair or a mechanism to stabilize the head is imperative (Figure 11-12). Some situations will not allow for intraoral radiographs. In this case, an extraoral projection may be the radiograph of choice. Sedation may be a final solution if patient coordination or lack of cooperation makes it impossible to expose intraoral or extraoral radiographs.

TRAUMA PATIENTS

A trauma patient may have extreme difficulty in tolerating a film packet in the oral cavity. Therefore, the extraoral projection will probably be the radiographic technique of choice. In some cases, the patient may be bedbound, which would make it impossible to expose an extraoral film. Alternative solutions would be the occlusal technique or hemostat film-holding device.

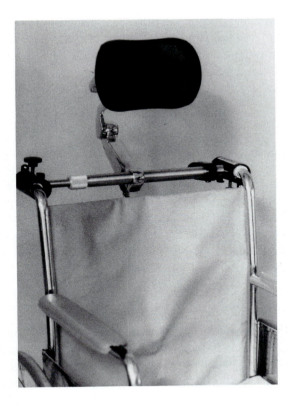

FIGURE 11-12 A portable headrest attached to the hand grips on the wheelchair.

As with the disabled patient, move quickly in order to minimize the pain to the patient. Using modified exposure techniques (e.g., increased kVp or time) and fast-speed film. In addition, the patient may not be able to tolerate a heavy film-holding device. Therefore, another type of film holding device, such as a stabe, may be indicated.

PERSONALITY TRAITS

Apprehension and Fear

Apprehension due to the unknown or fear of pain are two very real emotions experienced by some dental patients. These emotions can escalate until they interfere with the radiographer's ability to expose a projection. It is important to explain the procedure to the patient before exposing the radiographs. Alert the patient to the senses that will be stimulated during the procedure, such as the weight of the film-holding device, the sound of the exposure, and any discomfort. Try to determine the cause of the apprehension or fear and reassure the patient. Placing and removing the film as quickly as possible will help alleviate any apprehension and fear.

Pregnancy

During pregnancy, the fetus is undergoing continual growth and change. As discussed in Chapter 3, cells are most sensitive during the mitosis stage of cell development. Therefore, exposure of a pregnant woman during the first three months could potentially be harmful to the fetus. Although new technology has greatly reduced the possibility of danger to the fetus, elective radiographs are not recommended during this time. If possible, radiographs of the mother should be delayed until after the birth of the child.

Concern for Radiation Exposure

Public awareness of the harmful effects of ionizing radiation has increased and made dental radiologists accountable for their actions. Often a patient will question the necessity of having routine radiographs exposed because of the possible harmful effects. The dental professional should be able to explain to the patient the amount of risk that is associated with dental radiographs. Risk estimates have been discussed in Chapter 3. It is helpful to have this information posted in the radiology clinical area, with brochures available to help answer patient questions. Radiographs should never be exposed on a patient unless the patient understands the need for the radiographs, and the dental practitioner has received the consent of the patient. To receive this consent, it is essential that the patient gain a thorough and complete understanding of the rationale for radiographs prior to the clinical experience.

SUMMARY

This chapter reviewed various management situations that the dental radiographer may encounter during the radiographic clinical examination. The radiographer should be knowledgeable about radiation exposure and its harmful effects, as well as competent in performing various radiographic techniques. As discussed, there are many anatomical constraints, dentition limitations, and physical and mental barriers that can impact on the appropriate treatment to be rendered.

BIBLIOGRAPHY

CURRY III TS, DOWDY JE, MURRY JR RC. *Christensen's Physics of Diagnostic Radiology,* 3d ed. Philadelphia: Lea and Febiger, 1990.

GOAZ PW, WHITE SW. *Oral Radiology: Principles and Interpretation,* 3d ed. St. Louis: CV Mosby, 1994.

MANSON-HING, LR. *Fundamentals of Dental Radiography,* 3d ed. Philadelphia: Lea and Febiger, 1990.

MATTESON SR, WHALEY C, AND SECRIST V. *Dental Radiology,* 4th ed. Chapel Hill, NC: University of North Carolina Press, 1988.

REVIEW QUESTIONS

1. An acceptable technique modification that can be used to image central incisors with a narrow palate is to use

   a. size 0 film.
   b. size 1 film.
   c. size 3 film.
   d. size 4 film.
   e. none of the above

2. Film placement for the lateral/canine projection in a patient with ankyloglossia would involve

   a. moving the film distal.
   b. directing the beam mesial.
   c. directing the beam distal.
   d. placing the film on top of the tongue.

3. Technique adjustments for mandibular tori may include

   I. increasing kVp.
   II. decreasing kVp.
   III. distal movement of the film.
   IV. decreasing Ma.
   V. directing the beam distal.

   a. I, III, and V only
   b. II, III, and V only
   c. I, III, IV, and V only
   d. II, III, IV, and V only
   e. I, IV, and V only

4. A patient experiencing trismus may require the use of a

   a. styrofoam bite block.
   b. Rinn BAI instruments.
   c. Rinn XCP instruments.
   d. Precision instruments.
   e. hemostat.

5. "Remedies" that can be used with a "gagger" are

   a. antigag film (cold film).
   b. temporal tap.
   c. topical anesthetic.
   d. all of the above
   e. b and c only

Radiographic Imaging for the Dental Team,
by Sally Mauriello. J.B. Lippincott Company,
Philadelphia © 1995.

12

Exposure Factors and Image Production

Upon the completion of this chapter, the student should be able to:

1. Discuss image quality and identify the main factors affecting it.

2. Explain density and contrast, and their relationship to the exposure factor.

3. Explain the basis for the selection of exposure factors.

4. Demonstrate the use of the 15 percent rule.

5. Formulate interchangeable exposure factors.

6. Discuss the importance of collimation.

7. Distinguish among the different types of exposure controls.

8. Select alternative exposure factors given different image detectors.

IMAGE QUALITY

Although image quality is difficult to define, most agree that a quality image is one that faithfully displays anatomical objects and furnishes the appropriate information needed to diagnose a patient's condition or monitor a therapeutic procedure. For example, a periapical film demonstrating proper placement of an endodontic file may have an acceptable image quality. However, if this same film was used to determine periapical pathology, its image quality may not be adequate. The tolerances for acceptable quality in this regard depend on the diagnostic task. In the clinical setting, image quality is subjectively ranked from high to low. This rating is derived mostly from experience, personal taste, and perception. A working knowledge of the major factors involved in image production and a comprehensive understanding of how these factors interact with each other is required to accurately control image production. Figure 12-1 depicts factors known to influence image production. These factors work synergistically to affect the final image.

Factors Affecting Image Quality

The factors affecting image quality depicted in Figure 12-1 can be broken down into the following components:

1. Illuminator (Chapter 17)

   a. view box condition
   b. view box light
   c. extraneous light
   d. room light

2. Motion artifacts (Chapter 18)

   a. tube head motion
   b. film and cassette movement
   c. patient movement

3. Processing and darkroom (Chapter 6)

   a. chemistry conditions, such as concentration and age of solutions
   b. temperature of chemical agents and water
   c. time length at each processing step
   d. condition of processor
   e. lighting conditions
   f. safelighting conditions
   g. cleanliness of area

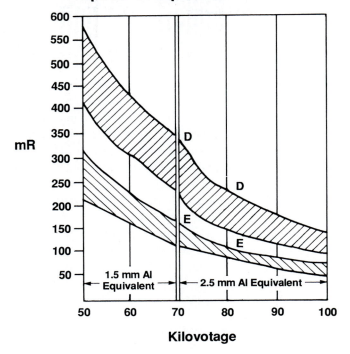

FIGURE 12-2 Acceptable x-ray exposure ranges for speed group D and E films. (Department of Health and Human Services.)

impulses (mAi) is the primary factor used in controlling film density. mAs is calculated by multiplying the milliamperes by the exposure time (mA × s). Likewise the mAi is calculated by multiplying the milliamperes by the number of impulses (mA × i). For example, if 10 mA is applied to the x-ray tube for .30 seconds, the mAs is 3; if 15 mA is applied to the x-ray tube for 24 impulses, the mAi is 360. Kilovoltage can also be used to regulate density, but not without affecting image contrast. Although source-to-film distance, processing conditions, and the amount of filtration affect density, these factors are not recommended as methods to control density. However, film speed may be used to control density and reduce patient exposure. For example, E-speed film may be substituted for D-speed film. Since E-speed film is more sensitive to radiation than D-speed film, it produces approximately the same amount of density as the D-speed film with about half the radiation exposure. This results in a reduction of radiation exposure to the patient. The minimum adjustment necessary to cause a visible change in density is 30 percent of the mAs or mAi or the equivalent.

Contrast

Contrast may be defined as the difference between radiographic densities. Contrast results from the density variations in the anatomical objects being radiographed. More radiopaque areas attenuate (stop) more x-rays than less radiopaque areas. Thus, by the time the x-ray beam reaches the film, it will have been altered by the different radiopacities in the object. Anatomical variations produce different degrees of tonal shades on the film. These tonal shades can range from clear to black with grays in between. The tonal grays are called contrast shades and can be further described as being short scale in contrast and long scale in contrast. A film with short scale contrast produces a major difference in density between two adjacent areas. A film with short-scale contrast is sometimes referred to as a high-contrast film. A film with long-scale contrast on the other hand provides less differences in density and could be referred to as a low contrast film (Figure 12-3). Contrast scales are primarily controlled by kilovoltage, even though other factors, such as processing conditions, size, and shape of the anatomical objects being radiographed, filtration, and film used also have an effect. As the kilovoltage increases, the amount of contrast decreases; as the kilovoltage decreases, the amount of contrast increases. As a general rule, radiographic examinations intended for the evaluation of dental decay require high-contrast images, whereas examinations of the soft tissue, such as cephalometric radiography and

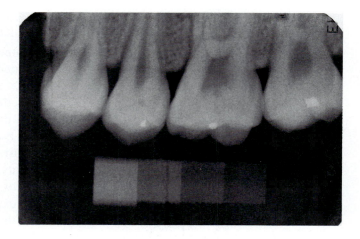

FIGURE 12-3 Low-contrast film.

examinations for evaluation of periodontal disease, require low-contrast images.

Selection of Exposure Factors

The selection of **exposure** factors is somewhat dependent on the radiographic unit itself. A great number of units allow only the selection of exposure times, since their milliampere and kilovoltage values are fixed. Others units may give the operator a choice of two kilovoltage values and different exposure times; these units usually have fixed milliampere values. A third type may offer a selection of a range of kilovoltages, exposure times, and milliampere values. In the first case, the operator is limited to the selection of exposure time values as a means of controlling density, because the milliampere and kilovoltage values are fixed. This limits the operator's ability to control exposure factors if the patient is larger or smaller than average. In the second case, the operator may choose from one of two kilovoltages and a range of exposure times. Two kilovoltages allow the operator some control over image contrast. Figure 12-4 displays two images of the same area obtained with two different kilovoltage settings. In the third case, a variable kilovoltage, a range of exposure times, and a choice of at least two milliampere selections allows the operator to exercise more control over image contrast and x-ray penetration and to limit the effects of patient movement. For example, techniques A and B theoretically should produce identical images, but technique B would be better for controlling patient motion because the exposure time is shorter.

Technique A
10mA, 30i, (300mAi) 70kVp

Technique B
15mA, 20i, (300mAi) 70kVp

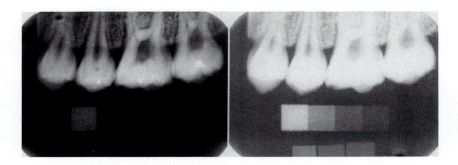

FIGURE 12-4 Images with different tonal values. The image on the left is higher in contrast than the image on the right.

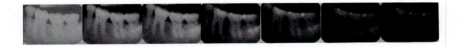

FIGURE 12-5 Images exposed with different kilovoltage values.

Selection of Kilovoltage

The kilovoltage is the potential difference applied to the x-ray tube needed to produce the desired exposure. Kilovoltage provides the force necessary to drive the electrons from the cathode to the anode. The greater the kilovoltage, the greater the speed of the electrons and the greater the energy of the x-rays produced. As the kilovoltage increases so does quality and penetrating power of the beam. Kilovoltage should be selected to insure adequate penetration of the object being radiographed. Each anatomical part has an effective and a maximum **kilovoltage** value. The effective kilovoltage is the lowest kilovoltage required to penetrate an object to produce an image. The maximum kilovoltage is the greatest kilovoltage that can be applied to an object before over penetrating it and producing an image too dark to see. Figure 12-5 illustrates images of a dental phantom exposed at different kilovoltage values. The exposure times were adjusted to compensate for the increase in the kilovoltage value. In this example, it is apparent that even though the time has been adjusted to compensate for the increase or decrease in kilovoltage, the images with the highest and lowest kilovoltages have fallen outside the effective and maximum kilovoltage values. As mentioned earlier, kilovoltage is the primary factor responsible for controlling contrast. As a general rule contrast decreases as kilovoltage increases. This is because as the kilovoltage increases, a greater portion of scatter and secondary x-rays are emitted in the forward direction, thus reaching the film.

15 Percent Rule

Kilovoltage not only controls contrast, but also affects film density. As the kilovoltage is increased, film density is also increased. Sometimes it is necessary to increase kilovoltage and yet maintain the same radiographic density. This can be achieved by the use of the 15 percent rule, which states that increasing the kilovoltage by 15 percent is the equivalent of doubling the milliamperage or the exposure time. If the kilovoltage is increased by 15 percent, a 50 percent reduction in the milliampere or exposure time is required to maintain the same radiographic density. For example, with a periapical film exposed at 10mA, 15i, and 70kVp, a reduction in exposure time to 50 percent of the original value and an increase in the kilovoltage by 15 percent will maintain approximately the same radiographic density. The new factors will be as follows: 10mA, 7.5i (50 percent of 15, or 7.5), 80.5kVp (70 + 15 percent of 70, or 10.5). In addition, with the 15 percent rule, the operator may exercise control of contrast by increasing or decreasing the kilovoltage to obtain the desired results. The examples below using the 15 percent rule will produce films of approximately the same density but different contrasts.

10 mA	30 i	70 kVp	(High Contrast)
5 mA	30 i	80.5 kVp	(Lower Contrast)

Selection of Milliamperage

The milliamperage controls the amount of electrons available for x-ray production, and therefore the quantity of x-rays produced. There is a direct relationship between milliamperage and radiation exposure. If the milliamperage is doubled, the radiation exposure is also doubled. Milliamperage is the primary factor used in controlling density provided there is sufficient kilovoltage to penetrate the object. In dental radiography, milliamperage values usually range from 7 to 15 milliamps. Selecting the highest milliamperage available permits the use of the lowest exposure time. For example, the techniques listed below should theoretically produce films with identical densities and contrasts, while using different exposure times.

10 mA	45 i (450mAi)	70 kVp
15 mA	30 i (450mAi)	70 kVp

Selection of Exposure Time (Impulses)

Time controls of the duration of the exposure and therefore the quantity x-rays produced. There is also a direct relationship between time (impulses) and radiation exposure. That is, if the time (impulses) is doubled, the radiation exposure is also doubled. Dental x-ray units may have either time selectors or impulse selectors. Timers allow the selection of a time fraction needed for a particular exposure, while impulse counters allow the selection of impulses. On this basis, when 30 impulses are selected for an exposure, the machine delivers 30 distinct impulses of electricity. If the current is half-wave or self-rectified, the delivery of 30 impulses will take ½ of a second (30/60). If the current is full-wave rectified, the delivery of 30 impulses will take ¼ of a second (30/120). Machines that use full-wave rectification or direct current usually use electronic timers instead of impulse counters. Most older dental x-ray machines, however, are half-wave rectified and use impulse counters, while newer units use constant potential (or direct current).

Selection of Distance

In dental radiography the distance between the x-ray source and the object is determined in part by the length of the position indicating device (PID). Generally, short PIDs are used with the bisecting angle technique and long PIDs with the paralleling technique. PIDs may range from 8 in. to 16 in. in length. The length is important because it affects image detail and magnification. The longer the PID, the better the detail and the lesser the magnification. Long PIDs are recommended with the paralleling technique and whenever possible. Operators should insure that the end of the PID is consistently placed at the same distance from the skin, so that film density is not affected.

Focal Spot Size

The size of the focal spot is fixed and can not be changed by the operator. The size of the **focal spot** affects image detail. Dental x-ray units are equipped with focal spots ranging from about .6 mm to .8 mm in size. Larger focal spots are employed in medical x-ray units for general purpose radiography.

Collimation

Collimation refers to the restriction of the x-ray beam. Collimation is important because it affects image contrast and radiation exposure to the patient. Restricting the size of the beam improves the visibility of image details by confining the primary beam to an area no larger than the field of interest. Restriction of the primary beam decreases the amount of scatter and secondary radiation produced. Scatter and secondary radiation cause image "fog" that reduces contrast and decreases the visibility of detail. In dental radiography, lead-lined circular cylinders are most often used to collimate the x-ray beam. The diameter of the cylinder determines the amount of tissue radiated. However, the amount of tissue radiated can be further reduced by the use of such beam-restricting devices as the Precision Instrument and the XCP snap-on ring collimator shown in Figure 10-8. Rectangular PIDs are also available. Restricting the size of the beam to conform to the size of the film improves image contrast, reduces a patient's radiation exposure, and allows use of the most sensitive image receptors. One of the major complaints from practitioners who have attempted to convert from D-speed film to E-speed film is that the images obtained with E-speed film are not as "crisp." This can be improved by restricting the size of

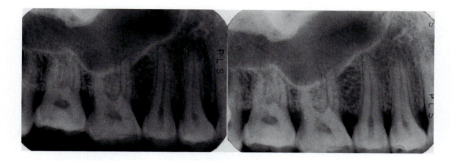

FIGURE 12-6 The image on the left was exposed without collimation and the image on the right with a precision instrument. Notice the difference in contrast.

the beam to the size of the film and by keeping processing conditions at an optimum level. Compare the E-speed films shown in Figure 12-6, exposed with and without collimation.

Icon-Driven Selection Controls

Icon-driven selection controls are consoles with a technique management system (see Figure 12-7). Each icon selection is preset for a particular exposure time. The operator makes the technique selections by simply depressing the appropriate icon. In most cases the operator may select from two kilovoltage values (60kVp or 70kVp) and various anatomic areas. In addition, the operator may compensate for different patient sizes by depressing the preprogrammed density compensator. The preset exposures can be overridden manually. The use of icon-driven selection controls simplifies machine operation, promotes consistent quality radiographs, and reduces errors due to improper technique selection.

Technique Charts

Technique charts should be placed next to every x-ray console. The purpose of the chart is to guide the operator in the selection of the appropriate technical factors that are necessary for the production of high-quality images. Generally, technique charts are organized to show the projection, exposure time, milliamperage, kilovoltage, and type of film used. Before a technique chart is formulated, the following should be accomplished:

1. Have a processor quality control program in place (see Chapter 17).

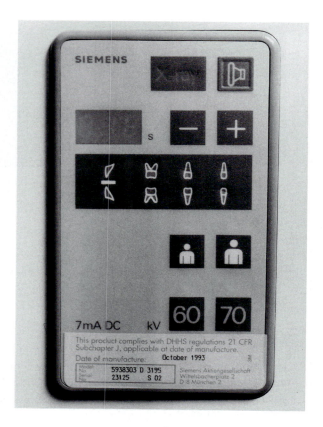

FIGURE 12-7 Icon-driven controls.

2. Be certain that the radiographic unit has been properly calibrated and a preventive maintenance program is in place (see Chapter 17).

3. Factors should be selected to promote the lowest radiation dosage possible to both patients and operators. The use of E-speed film should be strongly considered.

4. Include the projection, the milliamperage, the kilovoltage, the exposure time, and the type of film used. Provide guidelines for large and small patients (see Figure 12-8 for example).

Key Factors in Technique Selection

Kilovoltage

Kilovoltage selection may be limited to machine type. If the unit has a fixed kilovoltage value, the operator does not have control of the kilovoltage. When machines have variable kilovoltages, the operator has a

TECHNICS CHART: GENDEX (GE) 1000

PROJECTION	mA	kVp	TIME in SECONDS	FILM TYPE
ANTERIOR	15	70	21/60	E
PREMOLAR	15	70	24/60	E
MOLAR	15	75	24/60	E
BITEWING	15	75	30/60	D
OCCLUSAL	15	75	30/60	D

For **Large** Patients Add 5 Killovolts (kVP.)
For Small Patients Reduce 5 Killovolts (kVP)

FIGURE 12-8 Sample of a technique chart.

range of kilovoltages available for selection. As mentioned earlier, high kilovoltage techniques produce longer gray images (low contrast) and improve soft tissue and dense bone visualization. In addition, high kilovoltage techniques permit the use of shorter exposure times, which help reduce radiation dose to patients. High kilovoltages are desirable for periodontic and cephalometric radiography. Low kilovoltages generally produce short-scale (high-contrast) images and are well suited for caries detection and endodontic radiography. For example, 70kVp may be more appropriate for caries detection than 90kVp. 90kVp would be more useful when performing radiography to detect periodontal disease and image calculus deposits.

Milliamperage

Milliamperage selection may be limited by machine type. Some units have fixed milliamperage values, while others may offer a choice of two values. Most intraoral systems are available in milliamperage values ranging from 7 to 15 milliamps. The advantage of having more than one mA value is flexibility. The operator may select different milliamperages and exposure times while maintaining the same exposure value. For example, techniques A and B have different mA values and different exposure times but the same exposure value.

Technique A	15mA	30i (450mAi)	70kVp
Technique B	10mA	45i (450mAi)	70kVp

The advantage of technique A is that it uses a lower impulse value and reduces the chances of the production of motion artifacts.

Exposure Time

When selecting exposure times, possible unwanted patient movement should be taken into consideration. For example, if the patient is a child who has difficulty remaining still or if the patient suffers from a condition warranting a speedy procedure, a short exposure time is desired. This is only possible, of course, if the unit has more than one mA value or more than one kilovoltage selection. Consider techniques A and B in our previous example. Also consider techniques C and D below, when more than one kilovoltage is available.

Technique C	10mA	30i	60kVp
Technique D	10mA	15i	70kVp

Clearly, technique D uses a faster time, but the kilovoltage had to be increased by 15 percent to compensate for the loss in density that would have resulted from a reduction in time. If, additionally, we change the mA we can further decrease the time, as shown below with techniques D and E.

Technique D	10mA	15i (150mAi)	70kVp
Technique E	15mA	10i (150mAi)	70kVp

Technique E employs a higher mA and a lower exposure time. Therefore it is more suitable for controlling patient motion. The major differences between technique C and the others is that technique C will produce the image with the highest contrast. Theoretically, techniques D and E should produce radiographs with the same density and contrast.

Film Speed

The use of E-speed film should be strongly considered for intraoral radiography. The use of E-speed film with a beam-restricting image holder, or a rectangular PID, has been shown to produce images of excellent radiographic quality. In addition to reducing radiation exposure, the use of E-speed film allows the use of a shorter exposure time when compared to D-speed film. As previously discussed, the use of a lower exposure time reduce the chance of producing motion artifacts. Consider techniques F and G:

Technique F	15mA	30i	70kVp	D-speed film
Technique G	15mA	15i	70kVp	E-speed film

Since Technique G uses E-speed film (approximately twice as fast as D-speed film), it only requires half the time to produce an image with the same radiographic density.

Radiographic Exposure Conversions

When the dental radiographer is able to control the technical factors, adjustments can be made to satisfy the particular needs of the exam.

For example, an increase in the kilovoltage may better penetrate an object, change image contrast, and allow the use of a shorter exposure time to reduce motion. Altering exposure factors necessitates the understanding of the interrelationship between the factors themselves. Radiographic units with fixed kilovoltage and mA systems do not provide any flexibility for changing exposure factors since the only variable is the time of exposure.

Relation of Exposure Factors to Film Speeds

In dental radiography, two film speeds are presently being used, D-speed film and E-speed film. E-speed film is approximately twice as fast, or twice as sensitive, as D-speed film. It requires only about half the x-ray energy to produce a film of comparable density. For example, if for a periapical examination of molars, 15mA, 30i, 75kVp, and D-speed film is used, changing to E-speed film presents several options. All options assume the use of a unit with two mA settings and variable kilovoltage.

Option 1: Reduce time in half to deliver half the energy.

Original Factors	15mA	30i	75kVp	D-speed
New Factors	15mA	15i	75kVp	E-speed

Option 2: Reduce the mA to 10 and use the appropriate exposure time to maintain the same mAs or mAi.

Original Factors	15mA	30i	75kVp	D-speed
New Factors	10mA	23i*	75kVp	E-speed

*The way to arrive at 23i is as follows:

$$15\text{mA} \times 30\text{i} = 450\text{mAi}$$
$$10\text{mA} \times \quad \text{i} = 450\text{mAi}$$
$$\text{i} = 450\text{mAi}/10\text{mA}$$
$$\text{i} = 45$$

Since the faster film requires half the exposure, we divide 45i by 2 and obtain 22.5. Rounded to the nearest tenth = 23.

Option 3: Reduce the kilovoltage.

Original Factors	15mA	30i	75kVp	D-speed
New Factors	15mA	30i	64kVp	E-speed

The new kilovoltage was obtained using the 15 percent rule, therefore 15 percent of 75 = 11.25, 75 − 11.25 = 63.75, rounded off to 64.

RELATION OF EXPOSURE FACTORS WITH DIFFERENT INTENSIFYING SCREEN AND FILM COMBINATIONS

Intensifying screens are used mainly for extraoral radiography. The speed of the screen and the speed of the film make up the relative speed factor. On this basis, a screen/film with a relative speed of 400 is two times as fast as one with a relative speed of 200 or four times as fast as one with a relative speed of 100. For example, changing from a panoramic 200 screen/film system to a 400 system, provides options that assume utilization of a specific unit (Siemens Orthopantomograph 10S). This unit has variable kilovoltage, 57-90, and variable mA, 5-12. The exposure time is preset at 15 seconds.

Option 1:

Original Factors	12mA	85kVp	200 screen/film system
New Factors	6mA	85kVp	400 screen/film system

Option 2:

Original Factors	12mA	85kVp	200 screen/film system
New Factors	12mA	72kVp	400 screen/film system

The 72kVp was obtained using the 15 percent rule. 15 percent of 85 = 12.75, 85 − 12.7 = 72.

Option 3:

This option reduces the kilovoltage and the mA half way each, as follows.

Original Factor	12mA	85kVp	200 screen/film system
New Factor	9mA	79kVp	400 screen/film system

Changing the time is not an option since panoramic units have a fixed exposure time.

PATHOLOGIES REQUIRING EXPOSURE CHANGES

Some pathological conditions may require either an increase or decrease of technical factors. This is due to disease processes causing additive pathology (bone density increases) or destructive pathology (bone density decreases). Additive pathology is hard to penetrate and destructive pathology is easy to penetrate. Since penetration is controlled mainly by kilovoltage, changes in exposure factors should be made primarily by altering the kVp. Table 12-1 illustrates some common pathological conditions requiring exposure changes.

TABLE 12-1
Common pathological conditions requiring exposure changes

Hard to Penetrate	Easy to Penetrate
Torus	Multiple Myeloma
Exostosis	Fibrosis
Hydrocephalus	Osteolytic Metastasis
Osteosclerotic Metastasis	Osteoporosis
Osteoma	Radiation Necrosis
Paget's Disease	Emaciation
Sclerosis	Apical Rarefying Osteitis
Edema	Cysts
Apical sclerosing Osteitis	

SUMMARY

The diagnostic information provided by a radiographic image is proportional to its quality. That is, the higher the quality of the image, the greater the information gained and the greater the chance of obtaining a more accurate diagnosis. A comprehensive understanding of exposure factors and the role they play in image production will enhance the operator's ability to better serve the patient and the doctor.

BIBLIOGRAPHY

BUSHONG SC. *Radiologic Science for Technologists: Physics, Biology, and Protection,* 3d ed. St. Louis: CV Mosby, 1984.

CARLTON RR, MCKENNA ADLER A. *Principles of Radiographic Imaging: An Art and a Science,* Albany: Delmar, 1992.

CULLINAN AM. *Producing Quality Radiographs.* Philadelphia: J.B. Lippincott, 1987.

GOAZ PW, WHITE SW. *Oral Radiology: Principles and Interpretation,* 3d ed. St. Louis: CV Mosby, 1994.

THOMPSON TT. *Cahoon's Formulating X-ray Techniques,* 9th ed. Durham: Duke University Press, 1979.

REVIEW QUESTIONS

1. When changing exposure factors to alter image contrast, which factor will have the most noticeable effect?

   a. Milliamperage
   b. Exposure time
   c. Kilovoltage
   d. Processing

2. Which combination of exposure values will produce the highest image contrast?

   I.   10 mA, 15 impulses, 70 kilovolts
   II. 15 mA, 10 impulses, 70 kilovolts
   III. 5 mA, 30 impulses, 70 kilovolts
   IV. 30 mA, 5 impulses, 70 kilovolts

   a. I, II, and III only
   b. I, III, and IV only
   c. II, III, and IV only
   d. I, II, III, and IV will produce the same contrast

3. Using the 15 percent rule, select equivalent exposure factors.

   I.   15 mA, 10 impulses, 70 kilovolts
   II. 15 mA, 5 impulses, 60 kilovolts
   III. 15 mA, 20 impulses, 80 kilovolts
   IV. 15 mA, 20 impulses, 60 kilovolts

   a. I and II only
   b. I and III only
   c. I and IV only
   d. II and III only

4. All of the following are considered advantages of collimation except:

   a. reduced exposure to the patient.
   b. a decrease in exposure time.
   c. simple to use.
   d. increased image contrast.

5. A periapical of the premolar region requires the use of 15 mA, 30 impulses, 75 kilovolts, and D-speed film. Select the equivalent factors when using E-speed film.

   I.   15 mA, 15 impulses, 75 kilovolts
   II. 15 mA, 30 impulses, 64 kilovolts
   III. 10 mA, 30 impulses, 64 kilovolts
   IV. 15 mA, 60 impulses, 75 kilovolts

   a. I and II only
   b. I and III only
   c. II and IV only
   d. III and IV only

6. When changing from a 200 to a 400 screen/film system, it is necessary to do one of the following:

    I.   Decrease the mA in half

    II. Decrease the kilovoltage by 15 percent

    III. Decrease the mA by 15 percent

    IV. Double the mA to compensate for increase in speed

a. I or II only

b. II or III only

c. II or IV only

d. I only

Radiographic Imaging for the Dental Team,
by Sally Mauriello. J.B. Lippincott Company,
Philadelphia © 1995.

13

Extraoral Radiography

Upon the completion of this chapter, the student should be able to:

1. Differentiate between intraoral and extraoral radiography.

2. Describe equipment needed to perform extraoral radiography.

3. Discuss specific extraoral projections and their application to dentistry.

4. Define tomography and explain the principles of tomographic operation.

5. Discuss tomography and its clinical applications to dentistry.

6. Define panoramic radiography and explain the principles of panoramic operation.

7. Discuss panoramic radiography and its basic application to dentistry.

8. Recognize various extraoral projections.

Extraoral radiography is the production of radiographic images when the film and x-ray source are placed outside of the patient's mouth.

EQUIPMENT

The equipment required to produce extraoral radiographs varies according to the objectives of the exam. For example, an intraoral unit and a film cassette is all that is needed for producing an oblique view of a mandible. However, a specialized unit is required for the production of a panoramic image. The equipment most relevant to dentistry will be discussed in this chapter.

Cassette

Basic to all extraoral radiography image production is the use of a film cassette. The cassette is a light-tight container slightly larger than the film. In most cases, the front of the **cassette** is made of a radiolucent material, such as bakelite, that allows the transmission of the radiation with little or no interference. The back of the cassette uses a light-weight metal, such as magnesium, that is dense enough to absorb x-rays and prevent back scatter radiation production. Some panoramic units use flexible cassettes that wrap around a drum that rotates during the exposure. These cassettes are usually made of a vinyl material (see Figure 13-1 for examples).

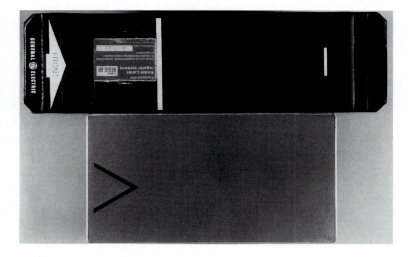

FIGURE 13-1 Photographs of flexible and rigid cassettes.

Film Size and Screen/Film Systems

The most common extraoral film sizes used in dentistry are 5 × 7 inches, 8 × 10 inches, 5 × 12 inches, and 6 × 12 inches. Often, 5 × 7 inch films are used for temporomandibular joint radiography, 8 × 10 inches for facial bones, and 5 × 12 and 6 × 12 inches for panoramic radiography. Most extraoral film is classified as indirect exposure film, because the film is exposed by the light emitted from the **intensifying screen,** a device used to convert x-ray energy to light energy, rather than by the x-rays emitted from the tube. As discussed in Chapter 5, speed is a characteristic of intensifying screens and extraoral films. Their combined speed determines the total speed of the screen/film system. Screen/film systems may be designed for specific applications. For example, a Kodak T-Mat L film combined with Kodak Lanex regular screens provides good soft-tissue visualization and a wide range of densities (low contrast), while a Kodak T-Mat G film with the same screens results in higher-contrast images. It is advantageous to use high-speed screen/film systems because they reduce the radiation dose to patients. In addition, high-speed screen/film systems require shorter exposure times, which reduce the chance of patient motion and potentially extending the life of the x-ray tube.

Grid

A **grid** is a device placed between the patient and the film for the purpose of reducing the amount of scattered and **secondary radiation** reaching the film. Grids are normally used during radiographic examinations of large anatomical parts, such as the skull and facial bones.

The use of a grid should be considered for anatomical objects measuring more than 12 cm in thickness. Grids are constructed of lead strips that alternate with strips of a radiolucent material (Figure 13-2). The lead strips are oriented to allow the passage of the primary x-ray beam between them. The lead strips absorb most of the scattered and secondary radiation before it reaches the film. In short, grids act as "cleaning devices" that improve image contrast. Grids are characterized by the way they are constructed as linear or focused. Linear grids have the lead strips parallel to each other in the longitudinal dimension and focused grids have the lead strips angled with the primary beam. Grids are rated by their **grid ratio,** which is the ratio of the height of the lead strips to the width of the space between them. The higher the grid ratio, the greater the "cleanup" of scattered and secondary radiation. Some grids remain stationary during the time of exposure, others move. Images produced with stationary grids often show grid lines (Figure 13-3), while the motion applied to moving grids

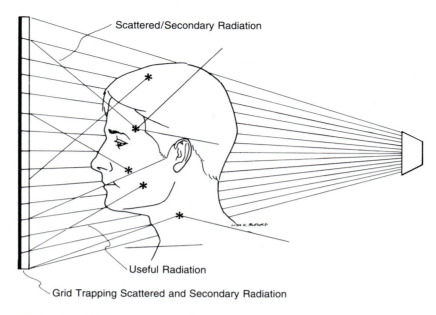

Scattered/Secondary Radiation

Useful Radiation

Grid Trapping Scattered and Secondary Radiation

FIGURE 13-2 An example of a radiographic grid.

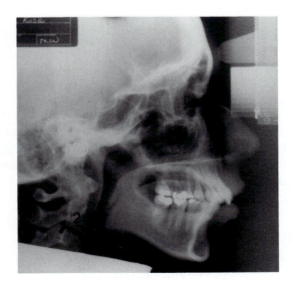

FIGURE 13-3 Grid lines characteristically present in images exposed with stationary grids.

causes the grid lines to blur out. For radiographic studies of the maxillofacial complex, a minimum of an 8:1 grid ratio should be used.

Radiographic Units

The three main types of radiographic units used for extraoral radiography are intraoral, panoramic, and "medical." Intraoral units feature a fixed anode and are used widely for cephalometric and temporomandibular joint radiography. Panoramic units also feature a fixed anode and are used mainly for imaging the maxilla and mandible. "Medical" units feature rotating anodes and are more frequently used for imaging skulls and facial bones. Although intraoral units may be adequate for most dental applications, their limitation lies in the amount of energy that they produce. "Medical" units are found more frequently in dental schools, large maxillofacial surgery practices, and maxillofacial radiology laboratories.

Specific Projections Applicable to Dentistry

Cranial and maxillofacial radiography employ a series of specific projections and protocols designed to demonstrate certain anatomical structures from different perspectives. For example, a skull series may consist of five specific views, while a paranasal sinus series may consist of four. Sometimes the same projection utilizing different technical factors is used to demonstrate a specific anatomical object.

PROJECTIONS OF THE CRANIUM, PARANASAL SINUSES, MANDIBLE, AND FACIAL BONES

Posterior Anterior (PA) Skull

This view is used as a general survey examination of the cranium. The forehead and nose rest on the cassette, with the midsagittal plane of the skull perpendicular to the cassette. The **central ray** is directed to the nasion from behind the head and aimed at right angles to the cassette (see Figure 13-4).

Lateral Skull (Cephalometric)

This view is used as a general survey examination of the cranium and facial bones from the lateral aspect. The **lateral skull projection** is used in orthodontics to study the contact relationship of the occlusal surfaces of the teeth, as well as the morphology and correlation of skull, facial bones, and soft tissue. The patient's head rests on the

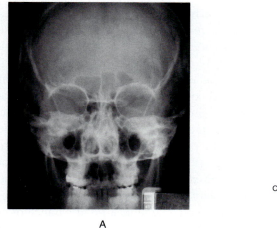

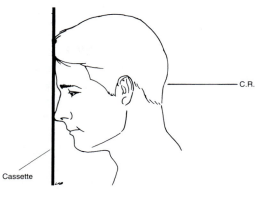

A   B

FIGURE 13-4 Posterior anterior (PA) skull. (A) Radiograph.
(B0) Projection.

cassette, with the midsagittal plane parallel to the cassette plane. A
cephalostat—a device that holds the head in place during cephalometric radiography—is used to ensure accurate positioning, magnification, and image reproducibility (Figure 13-5). The x-ray source is
located 5 feet from the center of the head holder, and the sagittal plane
to film distance is 11.5 cm. To attenuate more x-rays and enhance the
soft tissue area in the anterior of the face, wedge filters are often used.
The filters can either be placed on the cassette or at the point where the

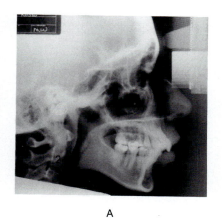

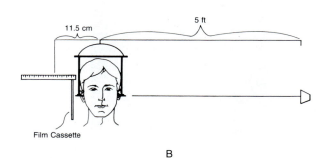

A   B

FIGURE 13-5 Lateral cephalogram. (A) Radiograph. (B) Projection.

x-rays exit the tube. The most efficient method is to filter the beam where it exits the tube before it reaches the patient. This reduces the radiation dose to the anterior region of the face. Successful production of cephalometric images is highly dependent on operator skill, proper positioning, and manipulation of exposure parameters. The operator should give the patient clear and concise instructions during the exam. Instructions include, but are not limited to, assuming the natural head position, not moving, and occluding or biting together properly. These instructions are determined by the person requesting the images. Errors related to cephalometric radiography fall in the category of too dark, too light, not enough soft tissue shown, faulty processing, and poor handling. Refer to Chapters 6 and 12 for tips on exposure manipulation, processing, and film-handling. To achieve a good balance of soft and hard tissue in the anterior of the face, use a low-contrast film and place the wedge filter at a level where the thickest portion of the filter attenuates more radiation in the anterior portion of the face.

Posterior Anterior (PA) Mandible

This view is used to visualize the anterior aspect of the mandible and the mandibular rami. The patient is seated facing the film. The head is adjusted so that the midsagittal plane is perpendicular and centered on the film. The patient's chin and nose are resting on the film and the central ray is directed between 20 and 30 degrees so that it exits at the acanthion (Figure 13-6).

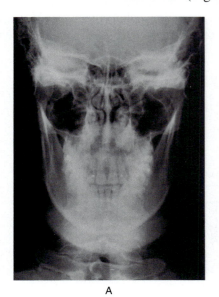

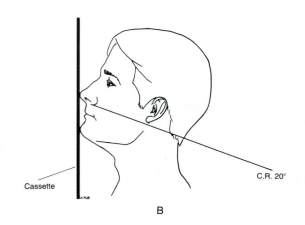

A

B

FIGURE 13-6 Posterior/anterior (PA) mandible. (A) Radiograph. (B) Projection.

Lateral Oblique Mandible

The **lateral oblique of the mandible** is used to visualize the mandibular body and ramus from the side. Usually the body is seen from the angle to the region of the canine. To obtain this projection, the patient is seated and the head is adjusted so that the long axis of the mandibular body is parallel with the transverse axis of the film. Adjust the rotation of the head so that the broad surface of the mandibular body is parallel with the plane of the film. Direct the central ray approximately 25 degrees cephalad aimed at the first molar region (Figure 13-7).

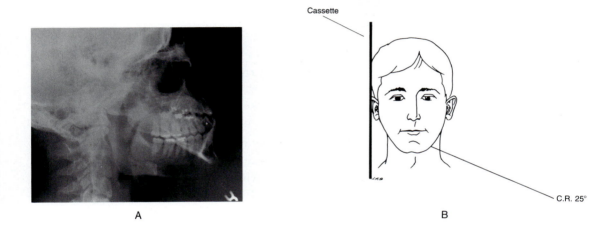

A   B

FIGURE 13-7   Oblique Mandible. (A) Radiograph. (B) Projection.

Towne Projection

The **Towne** projection demonstrates the occipital bone, petrous pyramids, and condyles of the mandible. The patient's head is positioned so that the midsagittal plane and the orbitomeatal line are perpendicular to the film. The central ray is directed at 35 degrees caudally (toward the feet) through the condyles. The projection may be performed in open and closed mouth positions. In the open mouth position the condyles are brought down and are more easily seen (Figure 13-8).

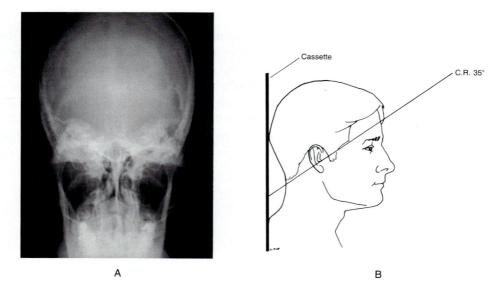

A   B

FIGURE 13-8   Towne Projection. (A) Radiograph.
(B) Projection.

Waters Projection

This projection demonstrates the maxillary sinuses and facial bones.
The patient is positioned with the chin extended so that the orbitomeatal line forms a 37 degree angle with the film. The midsagittal plane is
perpendicular to the plane of the film and the central ray is directed at
right angles to the film, and to the acanthion (Figure 13-9).

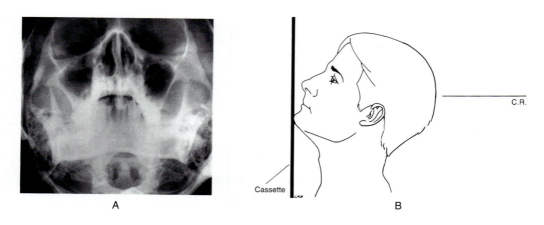

A   B

FIGURE 13-9   Waters Projection. (A) Radiograph. (B) Projection.

Submentovertical (SMV) Projection

This projection demonstrates an axial projection of the mandibular
body, showing the coronoid and condyloid processes of the rami. It is

used for angle corrected tomography in which the angle of the condyle is measured to determine the correct amount of head rotation needed when performing lateral tomograms of the temporomandibular joints (Figure 13-10).

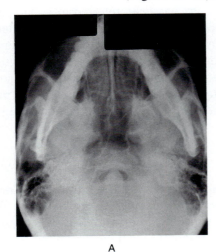

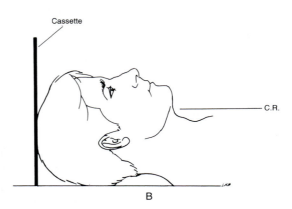

A

B

FIGURE 13-10 Submentovertical (SMV) Projection. (A) Radiograph. (B) Projection.

Transcranial Projection

This projection is used to visualize the temporomandibular joints in the open and closed positions. The patient is positioned with the side of interest closest to the film. The midsagittal plane is parallel to the film and the central ray is angled 25 degrees entering the upper parietal region and passing through the temporomandibular joint being studied (Figure 13-11).

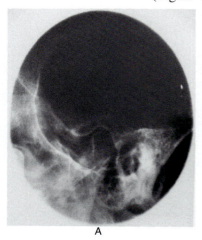

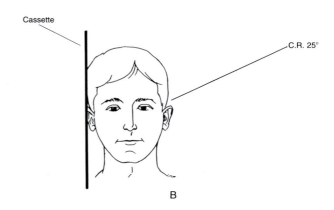

A

B

FIGURE 13-11 Transcranial Projection. (A) Radiograph. (B) Projection.

TOMOGRAPHY

Tomography, or body section radiography, is a radiographic technique that uses motion to blur out unwanted structures while the region of interest remains clear. Tomography has been referred to as bloodless dissection, since selected sections of the body can be individually imaged one at a time. If the human body was a loaf of bread, an image of the entire loaf would be equivalent to a conventional radiograph. However, an image of an individual slice of the bread would be equivalent to a tomogram. Tomography allows the study of structures in more detail since structures above and below them are blurred out during the exposure.

Principle of Operation

To accomplish body section radiography, the tube and the film move synchronously and opposite to each other during the exposure. The tube moves in one direction, while the film moves in the opposite direction about a pivot point or fulcrum. Anything not in the plane of focus determined by the level of the fulcrum is displaced relative to it and is deliberately obscured by the blurring motion of the tube and film. In Figure 13-12 the fulcrum has been placed at the level of the circle and the triangle and cube have moved relative to the circle. Consequently, their images are blurred out while the image of the circle remains relatively sharp.

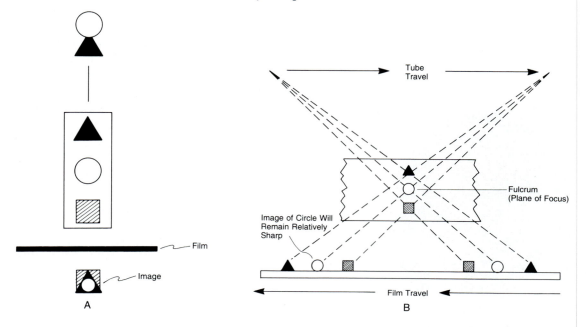

FIGURE 13-12 Diagrams depicting the set-up for producing image of circle using tomography.

There are many types of tomography—linear, circular, elliptical, hypocycloidal, spiral, and computed. Linear tomography is the simplest and least complicated. In linear tomography, the tube and film move in opposite directions to each other by means of a lever attached to the x-ray tube and the bucky tray (film-holding device). In more modern units, the linkage is electronic. The pivot point, or fulcrum, about which the lever rotates is adjustable, so that different layers within the body can be selected for imaging. Circular, elliptical, hypocycloidal, and spiral tomography all require specialized equipment. The advantage of these more complicated motions is their ability to produce very thin tomographic layers, or slices. Recently, several multidirectional tomography units designed specifically for dentomaxillofacial imaging have been introduced into the market (Figure 13-13 a–b). Computed tomography will be discussed in Chapter 14.

Dental Applications

Tomography is used in dentistry for the radiographic examination of the temporomandibular joint and implant sites. It can also be used to evaluate fractures of the maxillofacial complex. Figure 13-14 displays a linear tomogram of the temporomandibular joint depicting osseous structures. It can demonstrate congenital abnormalities, posttraumatic deformities, and changes secondary to infection and arthritis. It can also demonstrate sclerosis of the condyle and osteophyte formation associated with degenerative joint disease. Figure 13-15 demonstrates a

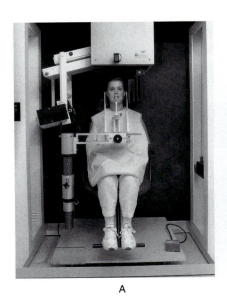

A

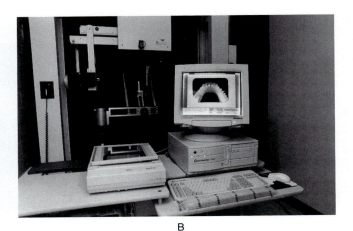

B

FIGURE 13-13 Components of the IS2000 tomographic unit used mainly for dental applications.

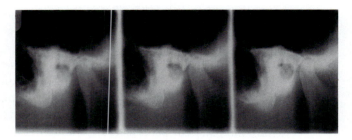

FIGURE 13-14 Linear tomogram of the temporomandibular joint.

series of radiographs obtained using linear tomography to evaluate anatomical sites for dental implants. This technique shows the location of the mandibular canal relative to the lingual and buccal dimensions.

Panoramic Radiography

This special radiographic technique is used for imaging the mandible, maxilla, temporomandibular joints, and dental arches. In panoramic radiography, the radiation source and the film holder are rotated around the patient's head, while the film inside the holder moves in the opposite direction to the beam. Unlike conventional tomography, the image layer is fixed and cannot be changed. The image layer, or focal trough as it is most commonly known, is dependent on the speed at which the film travels relative to the x-ray source. The size and shape of the focal trough is determined by the machine manufacturer. During the exam, the patient is positioned so that the dental arches are placed in the zone corresponding to the focal trough. The x-ray tube and film holder both rotate during the exposure and only the structures in or near the focal

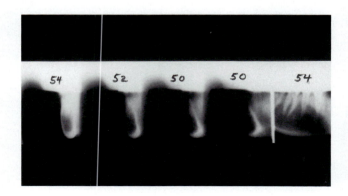

FIGURE 13-15 Radiographic images of cross-sections of the mandible being evaluated for implants.

trough are defined in the image. Figure 13-16 displays a panoramic radiograph of an adult patient. Notice the anatomical structures shown. The panoramic radiograph is widely used in dentistry as a screening tool to provide a broad view of the anatomic regions of the maxillofacial complex. It is useful for patients who are unable to open their mouths or cannot tolerate intraoral radiographs. It is also useful in the evaluation of trauma, tooth development, and developmental anomalies. However, panoramic radiographs should not be used as a substitute for examinations requiring high image resolution such as when evaluating a patient for caries.

Positioning

Accurate and correct positioning of the head is one of the key elements for producing high quality panoramic radiographs. Before positioning takes place, all artifact-producing devices should be removed from the patient. These include earrings, eyeglasses, neck chains, dentures, and partials. These items usually produce unwanted images that may overlap important anatomical details. It is also helpful to tell the patient how the machine is going to move and what type of instructions you are going to give them before the exposure is made.

Procedure

1. Bring the patient into the examining area and make sure they have removed any artifact-producing devices.

2. Drape a lead apron to protect patient from any scatter and secondary radiation.

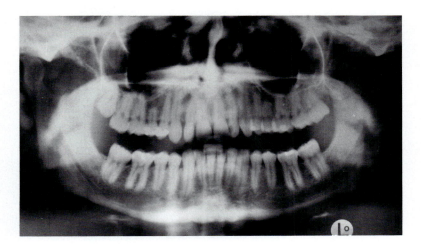

FIGURE 13-16 Panoramic image of adult patient.

3. Instruct the patient to bite on the biteblock. When biting correctly, the biteblock will place the average patient's upper and lower arches in the focal trough or zone of sharpness.

4. Adjust the patient's head so that the infraorbital meatal line, or **Frankfort horizontal plane,** is parallel to the horizon.

5. Keep the patient's head completely straight and the shoulders relaxed so that they do not interfere with machine movement.

6. Before making the exposure, instruct the patient to swallow while keeping the tongue on the roof of the mouth. This will prevent the apices of the maxillary teeth from becoming obscured by a radiolucency created from the air in between the palate and tongue.

Figures 13-17 through 13-22 display some of the most common errors associated with panoramic radiography. Tips on how to correct them are also included.

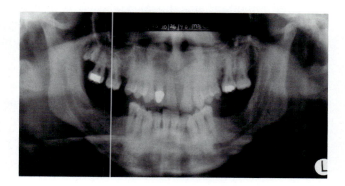

FIGURE 13-17 Exaggerated "smile" resulting from the chin being tipped too low. Adjust the Frankfort plane so that it is parallel to the horizon.

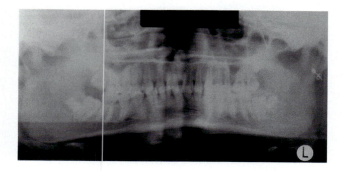

FIGURE 13-18 "Frown" resulting from the chin being tipped too high. Adjust the Frankfort plane so that it is parallel to the horizon.

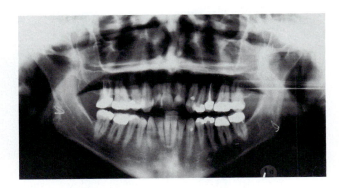

FIGURE 13-19 Apacies of maxillary teeth are obscured by air space. Instruct patient to swallow while keeping the tongue on the roof of the mouth.

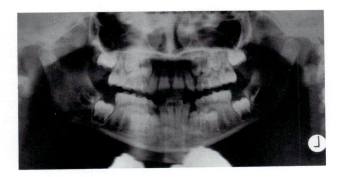

FIGURE 13-20 Radiopacity representing the image of the lead apron. Adjust the lead apron so that it is not in the path of the beam.

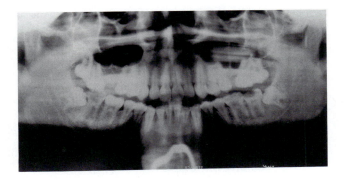

FIGURE 13-21 Lighter density at the center of the image caused by the cervical spine being in the path of the beam. Ask patient to stand or sit erect and stretch the neck to prevent spine from being in the path of the beam.

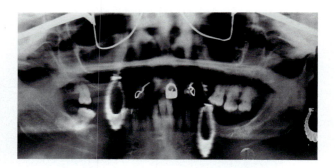

FIGURE 13-22 Multiple ghost shadows resulting
from items left on the patient during the exposure.
Have the patient remove all jewelry, glasses, and so on.

SUMMARY

Although the majority of extraoral radiographs produced in dental offices are panoramic, an increasing number of dental professionals are using additional extraoral radiographic exams as part of their diagnostic work-up. Knowledge and understanding of the extraoral procedures outlined in this chapter will enable the radiographer not only to perform a wider spectrum of imaging services, but increases his/her ability to better serve the patient and doctor.

BIBLIOGRAPHY

BALLINGER PW. *Radiographic Positions and Radiologic Procedures.* St. Louis: CV Mosby, 1986.

CARLTON RR, MCKENNA ADLER A. *Principles of Radiographic Imaging.* Albany: Delmar, 1992.

UNGER JM. *Head and Neck Imaging.* New York: Churchill, Livingstone, 1987.

REVIEW QUESTIONS

1. When film/screen systems are used, image production can be mainly attributed to

   a. blue light energy.
   b. x-ray energy.
   c. light energy.
   d. x-ray and light energy.

2. Grids are devices that are used to

    a. improve image contrast.
    b. improve image quality.
    c. clean up scatter and secondary radiation.
    d. all of the above

3. In tomography, the image layer is selected by the

    a. fulcrum adjustment.
    b. blurring motion.
    c. lever.
    d. bucky tray.

4. In most panoramic machines, the image layer is

    a. determined by its elliptical motion.
    b. cannot be changed.
    c. adjusted by the fulcrum.
    d. none of the above

5. A panoramic image resembling a frown was probably caused by the patient's chin being tipped

    a. too flat.
    b. too high.
    c. too low.
    d. to one side more than the other.

6. The presence of air in the apacies of the maxillary teeth may be eliminated by instructing the patient to

    a. take a deep breath.
    b. place tip of tongue on palate.
    c. swallow while keeping the tongue on the roof of the mouth.
    d. exhale slowly.

Radiographic Imaging for the Dental Team,
by Sally Mauriello. J.B. Lippincott Company,
Philadelphia © 1995.

14

Specialized Imaging

Upon the completion of this chapter, the student should be able to:

1. Define magnetic resonance imaging, computed tomography, nuclear medicine imaging, ultrasound imaging, computerized radiography, and digital subtraction radiography.

2. Explain the clinical applications in dentistry of the modalities mentioned above.

3. Explain the use of contrast media in radiography.

4. Differentiate among the different types of radiation used in ultrasound, nuclear medicine, magnetic resonance, and computed tomographic imaging.

5. Recognize magnetic resonance, computer tomography, nuclear medicine, and ultrasound images.

This chapter introduces the reader to advanced imaging techniques and describes some of their clinical applications in dentistry. Because the theories of operation for each modality are beyond the scope of this text, the interested reader should consult the references at the end of the chapter.

In the past twenty-five years, medical radiology has been affected by technological changes. These changes have gradually filtered down to influence dental radiology and its practice. It is not uncommon to come across the words **magnetic resonance imaging** (MRI), **computed tomography** (CT), **ultrasound,** digital **subtraction radiography,** or **nuclear medicine** when evaluating a patient's medical history. Understanding these procedures, and the roles they play in diagnosis, not only enhances the dental auxiliaries ability to communicate with patients, but also improves the delivery of patient care services. For example, if a patient is referred by a dentist or dental specialist for a nuclear medicine exam, the auxiliary may be a resource if the patient is seeking information or has concerns.

MAGNETIC RESONANCE IMAGING (MRI)

Magnetic resonance imaging is probably one of the most revolutionary imaging tools available for diagnostic purposes. Unlike radiographs, which use ionizing radiation, MRI uses a magnetic field, a radio frequency, and the natural magnetism of the atoms of the body to produce diagnostic images. The image is reconstructed using a powerful computer that displays the results on a monitor. Pictures of the images are usually printed on film and are known as hard copies. As of today, MRI is considered to be a safe procedure with no known detrimental effects on humans.

MRI allows diagnosticians to view the soft tissues of internal organs in great detail. For example, patients suspected of having disc problems in the temporomandibular joint (TMJ) can benefit from MRI. The technique can show noninvasively (without the painful injection of dyes) the position of the disc, the presence of joint fluid, and the osseous anatomy. Figure 14-1 shows an MRI study of the TMJ. MRI images are usually displayed in cross-sectional or sagittal form, with anatomical details shown free of superimposition. The exam does not require any type of preparation. However, patients who have had metal implants such as pacemakers, aneurysm clips, or inner ear implants should not have the exam. These objects, secured only by soft tissue, may be pulled by the strong magnetic force and cause internal bleeding. Implants that are fixed to bone, permanent appliances, and amalgam restorations have not been known to pose a health threat. Encour-

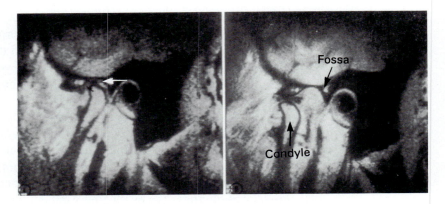

FIGURE 14-1   Sagittal magnetic resonance study of the TMJ.

age patients to discuss these issues with the physician or technologist performing the exam. MRI units are usually found in large medical centers or large medical radiology practices.

COMPUTED TOMOGRAPHY (CT)

Computed **tomography** is the radiographic examination of body structures in cross-sectional form. This technique allows the operator to selectively "cut" the body in slices, thereby producing an unobstructed view of the inner structures. In conventional radiography, structures are usually hidden by bone or other organs. In CT, because the images are cross-sectional, they are free from superimposition. On a lateral cephalogram, for example, all of the bones of the skull and face are superimposed on one another, but on a CT they can be seen in three-dimensions rather than two.

Information can also be acquired and displayed in different planes. For example, Figure 14-2 shows a coronal view of the temporomandibular joint, while Figure 14-3 shows a sagittal view of the temporomandibular joint. CT makes it possible to diagnose certain diseases and conditions that previously were not able to be seen on radiographs, such as pancreatic disease or disc problems. CT has the ability to distinguish minor differences between body tissues. The technique uses x-ray energy and a computer to acquire and display the images. The images are displayed on a monitor and can be printed on film as hard copies. One of the benefits of CT is that the images can be manipulated by changing the contrast to highlight or accentuate areas of interest. In comparison with other diagnostic tools, such as exploratory surgery, CT involves less risk and discomfort to the patient. Preparation for the procedure varies according to the examination to be performed. The examination is carried out while the patient lies on a "couch." The

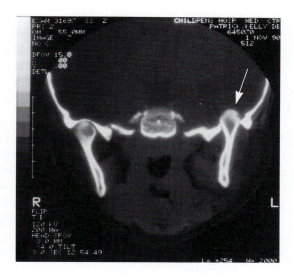

FIGURE 14-2 Coronal computed tomographic view of the temporomandibular joint demonstrating left condyle perforation through the mid-cranial fossa.

couch can be moved into the gantry (the round opening) which houses the x-ray source and data acquisition equipment. Special programs have been designed for dental needs. One such program is the Dentascan, which is marketed by General Electric (GE) Medical Systems. With this program, CT scans can show axial, cross-sectional, and sagit-

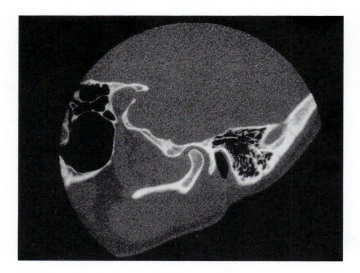

FIGURE 14-3 Sagittal computed tomographic view of the temporomandibular joint.

tal views of both the mandible and maxilla. The images produced can identify patients who have insufficient bone for an implant as well as help diagnose pathosis in and around the oral region.

NUCLEAR MEDICINE

Nuclear medicine is the branch of medicine that uses radioactive materials or radioisotopes for diagnostic and therapeutic purposes. The materials that are used in nuclear medicine follow the same basic laws of physiology that nonradioactive materials do. For example, iodine is selectively removed from circulation by the thyroid gland as is radioactive iodine. The quantities of radioactive materials used in the clinical studies are so small that the physiological balance is not altered. Radioactive materials used in clinical studies are also known as tracers. Tracers concentrate differently in healthy tissue and diseased tissue. This makes nuclear medicine very precise in identifying the location of the disease. Many conditions become visible in nuclear scans before they are recognized in conventional radiography. Examples of such conditions are metastases of cancer to the skeleton, stress fractures, and osteomyelitis. Nuclear medicine scans are considered safe. The most widely used radioactive isotope in nuclear medicine is Technetium-99m, which has a very short physical **half-life** (6 hours). The physical half-life of radioactive materials is the length of time it takes for the original number of atoms in a given sample to disintegrate or decay to one-half the original number. Depending on the exam, Technetium-99m is added to a compound that physiologically goes to the appropriate organ. Then the organ can be studied for size, shape, and function. There is no set of instructions for nuclear medicine exams, but the patient may be asked to avoid certain foods that could interfere with the accuracy of the test. For example, if a patient is having a thyroid scan, he/she might be asked to avoid foods or medicines containing iodine, because the iodine in these substances can affect the accuracy of the test. Figure 14-4 shows a nuclear exam displaying an ossifying fibroma. Notice that the diseased region detects the isotope in greater concentrations than the normal tissue surrounding it. This is due to the high metabolic activity found in the disease site. Nuclear medicine scans of the salivary gland and bones may be performed to assess dentally related conditions.

ULTRASOUND

Unlike CT scanning or nuclear medicine, ultrasound uses high-frequency sound waves to create a picture of the interior of the body.

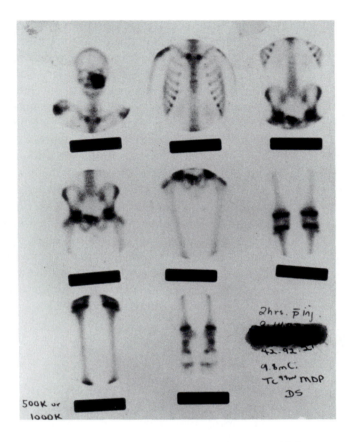

FIGURE 14-4 Bone scan demonstrating an ossifying fibroma on the left side of the patient's face. The dark density is indicative of more activity in the tumor site.

Ultrasound uses the pulse–echo principle. The pulse is generated in a device called a transducer. The transducer sends and receives these pulses, which are converted into visual signals and displayed on a monitor. For example, a pulse of ultrasound is generated and discharged into the body. The pulse travels through tissue, encounters a reflecting surface, and is reflected back toward the source of the pulse. Photographs of the images can be made on paper or film. Ultrasound examinations can portray the internal organs in motion or still. Only structures capable of reflecting sound can be examined using ultrasound. Reflection is the redirection of a portion of the ultrasound beam back toward its source. When the sound waves pass through different tissues, some of the sound waves are reflected back and the reminder continue. Water, blood cells, fat, liver cells, and blood vessel walls all have sufficiently different densities to create interfaces or cause some of the sound to be reflected. Since bone is so dense, about 70 percent of the sound is reflected, therefore, the sound is exhausted very quickly. This explains why it is not possible to perform ultrasound on bone. As far as it is known, there are no risks associated with the use of diagnostic ultrasound. Most of the energy that is absorbed by the tissue is converted into heat, which is the basis for ultrasound diathermy. However, at the low energy levels used in diagnostic ultrasound, the biologic effects have been found to be negligible. Ultrasound is used to diagnose many types of diseases and abnormalities of the heart, various tumors, and cysts, as well as monitoring progress during pregnancy. It is also used to evaluate diseases of the parotid and submandibular glands. Ultrasound may be used to investigate neck masses as well. Preparation for ultrasound may vary. Patients may be asked to avoid foods and beverages that produce gas; they may be asked to drink lots of liquid because, in some cases, a full bladder is required for the exam. A mineral oil or gel is applied to the body part being examined and the sonographer moves the transducer over the area being examined. Images are then displayed on a video monitor and permanent copies can be made for further study (Figure 14-5).

DIGITAL RADIOGRAPHY

Digital radiography is a system of electronic elements that allows images to be displayed in digitized form. In conventional radiography, images are displayed as signals recorded on film or on a television monitor. In digital radiography these signals are converted into binary

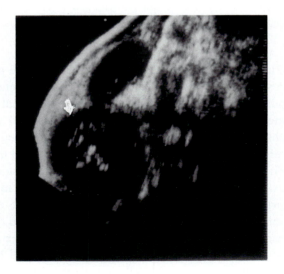

FIGURE 14-5 Ultrasound image of a parotid gland, notice the tumor demarcated by the arrow.

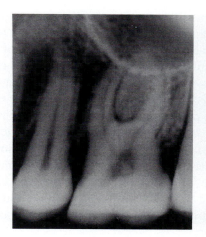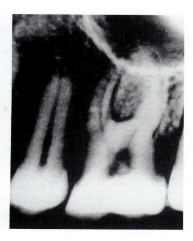

FIGURE 14-6 The image on the right was altered with the contrast enhancement feature of the imaging system.

numbers (digitized) and stored in a digital memory. The digital numbers are assigned a gray level (shades of gray) and displayed on a monitor. Images that have been digitized can be manipulated—that is, the contrast of the images can be changed by altering certain parameters on the system being used. Figure 14-6 shows an image that was digitally manipulated. One of the most useful applications of digital radiography in dentistry is that it allows the performance of digital subtraction. There are many types of digital subtraction, such as mask subtraction, dual energy subtraction, time interval differencing, and temporal filtering. Temporal image subtraction is being investigated in dentistry to assess tooth structure and bone loss or growth. In temporal image subtraction, two images are exposed at different times (e.g., 6 months, 1 year, etc.) and then subtracted from each other. The resultant image is a record of changes that took place between the time the two images were exposed. Reproducibility of positioning is key for performing temporal subtraction radiography. The difference between digital and analog signals can be best explained by observing how two watches provide time. One actually displays the time in numbers (for example, 10:45); the other by the hands pointing to numbers. The watch that provides the actual numbers is a digital device, and the watch that uses hands is an analog device.

RADIOGRAPHIC EXAMINATIONS USING CONTRAST MEDIA

Some radiographic examinations require the use of **contrast media** to visualize the appropriate anatomical details. Examples of exams that use contrast media are **arthrography** and **sialography.** Arthrography is the radiographic examination of soft tissue. "Dyes," for example, are substances that, when introduced into the site of interest, render certain anatomic details more visible. Contrast agents can be radiopaque (that is, they can stop or slow x-ray beams as they travel) or radiolucent (that is, they allow x-ray beams to travel with little or no interference). An example of a radiopaque contrast agent is Ethiodol, which is used for sialography—a radiographic examination of the salivary glands, ducts, and associated structures. An example of a radiolucent contrast agent is carbon dioxide or gas, used in radiography of the stomach or in arthrography of the TMJ. Arthrography allows the visualization of osseous abnormalities and disc position. It can demonstrate disc size, shape, integrity, and presence of disc perforations and tears.

SUMMARY

Profound technological changes in the field of oral and maxillofacial radiology are quickly filtering into general and specialty practices. The use of MRI to diagnose TMJ abnormalities and the use of CT, as well as specialized tomography, to image implant sites is rapidly increasing. It will not be long before digital radiography is used in dental offices as commonly as conventional radiography. A basic understanding of the uses of the technology not only increases the radiographer's understanding of his/her environment, but provides the information needed to better communicate with patients and peers.

BIBLIOGRAPHY

BALLINGER PW. *Radiographic Positions and Procedures*. St. Louis: CV Mosby, 1986.

DELBALSO AM. *Maxillofacial Imaging*. Philadelphia: WB Saunders, 1990.

UNGER JM. *Head and Neck Imaging*. New York: Churchill Livingstone, 1987.

REVIEW QUESTIONS

1. Which of the following imaging techniques does not use ionizing radiation?

a. Nuclear medicine
b. CT
c. MRI
d. Digital radiography

2. Computed tomography

   a. has the ability to distinguish minor differences between body tissues.
   b. allows manipulation of image contrast.
   c. uses a computer to reconstruct images.
   d. All of the above
   e. Only two of the above

3. Radioactive materials used in clinical studies are known as

   a. tracers.
   b. Technetium-99m.
   c. radioisotopes.
   d. Two of the above
   e. None of the above

4. From the items listed below, please choose the one that causes sound to reflect the most.

   a. Blood cells
   b. Fat
   c. Water
   d. Bone

5. Digital subtraction radiography shows potential applications in the assessment of

   a. cysts.
   b. caries.
   c. bone loss.
   d. hard tissue masses.

6. Select the technique that best demonstrates the presence of disc perforations and tears in the temporomandibular joint?

   a. Arthrogram
   b. CT scan
   c. Nuclear medicine
   d. Ultrasound

Radiographic Imaging for the Dental Team,
by Sally Mauriello. J.B. Lippincott Company,
Philadelphia © 1995.

15

Normal Radiographic Anatomy

Upon the completion of this chapter, the student should be able to:

1. Discuss the rationale for a knowledge of normal radiographic anatomy.

2. Identify the radiographic appearance of the teeth and their surrounding structures.

3. Identify the normal radiographic structures in both periapical and panoramic radiographs.

4. Apply the knowledge of radiographic anatomy in exposing and mounting intraoral radiographs.

Knowledge of normal radiographic anatomy is essential in the practice of dentistry for several reasons. First, correct film mounting requires a good knowledge of normal radiographic anatomy. In addition, to be able to detect abnormal findings, the radiographer must be able to identify what is considered normal anatomy in the radiograph. This chapter will discuss the most common anatomical landmarks seen in both periapical and panoramic radiographs. Often the landmarks may be seen in more than one projection. But they may appear different depending on the angulation of the radiograph. The landmarks discussed will be identified on both radiographs and a skull.

APPEARANCE OF THE TEETH AND SURROUNDING STRUCTURES

The teeth seen in a radiograph are made up of several structures that are of varying density and thus attenuate (absorb) the x-ray beam at different levels. Therefore, each structure will appear to have a different density or contrast in the radiograph. The enamel, which is the tissue that surrounds the crown of the tooth, is one of the hardest tissues in the body. Therefore, the enamel appears more radiopaque on the radiograph. The dentin and cementum are less hard and have a gray appearance on the radiograph. The junction between the enamel and the dentin on the tooth can be easily distinguished by this difference in appearance. This area is known as the dentinoenamel junction (DEJ). The cementum is the tissue that covers the root of the tooth and has similar density to that of the dentin. Therefore, it cannot be distinguished on the radiograph from the dentin. The pulp of the tooth contains the nerve and blood tissue. Therefore, this tissue is very soft and appears radiolucent on the radiograph because it absorbs very little of the x-ray beam (Figure 15-1).

The surrounding structures of the teeth include the bone and the periodontal ligament spaces. There are two types of bone seen in dental radiographs: cortical and cancellous. The **cortical bone** is very dense and contains no marrow spaces. This bone is seen surrounding the tooth (also known as the lamina dura) and carried over the aveolar crest. Because this bone is very dense, it appears radiopaque, similar to the appearance of enamel. The **cancellous bone** has a "spider web" appearance because of the fact that it surrounds the marrow spaces. It varies in shades of gray and white. This pattern is referred to as a trabecular pattern or trabeculae. This type of bone makes up the majority of the bony structure in the maxilla and mandible. The periodontal ligament surrounds the root of the tooth and is similar in density to the

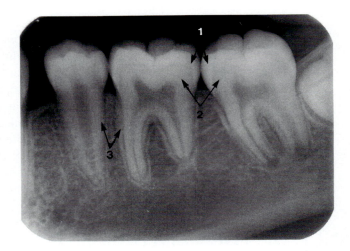

FIGURE 15-1 This radiograph depicts the (1) enamel; (2) dentin; and (3) cementum.

pulp of the tooth. Therefore, it appears as a thin black line surrounding the root of the tooth. In a healthy mouth, the periodontal ligament space is thin and continuous around the root of the tooth (Figure 15-2).

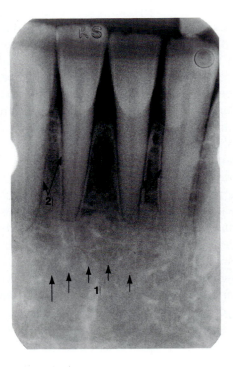

FIGURE 15-2 This radiograph depicts the (1) bone; (2) the periodontal ligament spaces.

SKULL OSTEOLOGY

Figures 15-3 through 15-5 illustrate the landmarks found in the maxillary and mandibular radiographs as they are seen in a human skull.

PERIAPICAL ANATOMY

Maxillary Anterior Landmarks

There are several anatomic landmarks that are found in the maxillary anterior region (see Figures 15-6 and 15-7).

1. **Nasal fossa:** This is the air-filled radiolucent area inside the nasal cavity.

2. **Nasal septum:** This is the thin line of bone that separates the right and left nasal cavities. In the radiograph, the nasal septum appears as a radiopaque line.

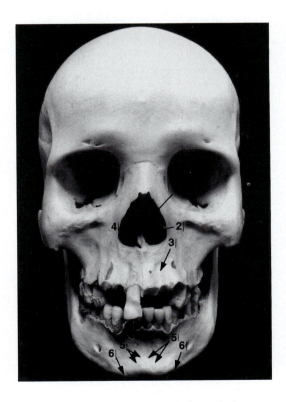

FIGURE 15-3 Human skull, frontal view: (1) nasal cavity; (2) nasal septum; (3) lateral or canine fossa; (4) anterior nasal spine; (5) mental ridge; (6) inferior border of the mandible.

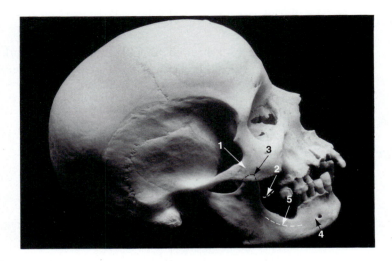

FIGURE 15-4   Human skull, side view: (1) zygomatic arch (malar process); (2) maxillary tuberosity; (3) coronoid process; (4) mental foramen; (5) external oblique ridge.

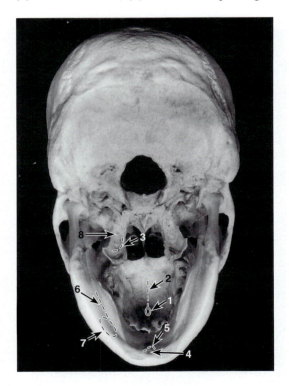

FIGURE 15-5   Human skull, inferior view: (1) incisive foramen; (2) mid palatine suture; (3) hamulus; (4) lingual foramen; (5) genial tubercles; (6) mylohyoid ridge; (7) submandibular fossa; (8) lateral pterygoid plate.

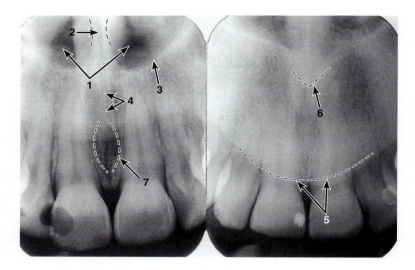

FIGURE 15-6 Maxillary central incisor projection: (1) nasal fossa; (2) nasal septum; (3) floor of the nasal cavity; (4) mid palatine suture; (5) shadow of the nose; (6) anterior nasal spine; (7) incisive foramen.

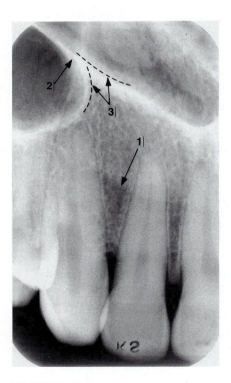

FIGURE 15-7 Maxillary lateral/ canine projection: (1) lateral or canine fossa; (2) anterior wall of the maxillary sinus; (3) typical inverted "Y" formation.

3. **Floor of the nasal cavity:** This is a thin line of bone that forms the lower boundaries of the nasal fossae. This structure appears as a curved, radiopaque line.

4. **Midpalatine suture:** This structure appears as a thin, radiolucent line between the central incisors. This line represents the area where the bony plates come together to form the palate.

5. **Shadow of the nose:** The nose can be seen as a soft tissue shadow, usually radiopaque, along the roots of the maxillary incisors.

6. **Anterior nasal spine:** This structure appears as a radiopaque area at the base of the nasal septum. It represents a bony protuberance to which the nasal cartilage is attached.

7. **Incisive foramen:** This structure is an opening through which the nasopalatine nerves and artery pass. This area appears as a radiolucent, oval-shaped structure between the central incisors.

8. **Lateral Fossa:** This appears as a radiolucent area between the lateral incisor and the canine. This structure represents a depression in the surface of the maxilla in that area.

9. **Anterior wall of the maxillary sinus:** This is a radiopaque line separating the nasal fossa and the maxillary sinus that appears around the maxillary canine region.

10. **Canine fossa:** This fossa may be seen in the canine region because of an indentation in the surface of the maxilla in that area (this is also known as the lateral fossa).

11. **Typical inverted "Y" formation** (Y of Ennis): This is a "Y"-shaped, radiopaque line that represents the intersection of the nasal cavity and the maxillary sinus.

Maxillary Posterior Landmarks

The following landmarks demonstrated in the maxillary posterior region (see Figures 15-8 and 15-9).

1. **Inferior border of the maxillary sinus:** This structure is seen as a thin, radiopaque line that represents the front wall of the maxillary sinus.

2. **Maxillary sinus:** This is an air-filled space above the maxillary premolars and molars and appears radiolucent.

3. **Malar process** of the zygomatic arch (Typical "U" or "J" shape): This radiopaque shape appears superimposed over the maxillary molars and represents the bony structure that joins the maxilla, frontal, and temporal bones.

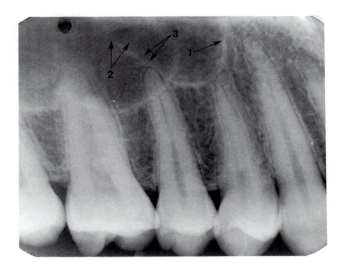

FIGURE 15-8 Maxillary premolar projection:
(1) inferior border of the maxillary sinus; (2) maxillary
sinus; (3) sinus septum.

4. **Maxillary tuberosity:** This bony structure appears as a bulge distal
   to the maxillary molars and at the end of the maxillary aveolar
   ridges.

5. **Hamulus:** This bony projection, which appears radiopaque and
   extends downward from the medial pterygoid plate, is located behind the maxillary tuberosity region.

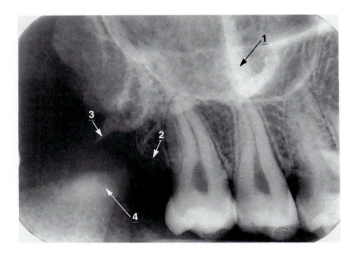

FIGURE 15-9 Maxillary molar projection: (1) malar
process of the zygomatic arch; (2) maxillary tuberosity;
(3) hamulus; (4) coronoid process of the mandible.

6. **Floor of the nasal fossa:** This thin, radiopaque line is often seen over the maxillary premolar area and represents the floor of the nasal fossa.

7. **Coronoid process** of the mandible: This structure may be seen in a molar projection that is placed extremely to the distal. It appears as finger-shaped projection extending upward from the mandible distal to the maxillary molars.

8. **Sinus septum:** These thin, radiopaque lines appear within the sinuses and represent bony walls that form the compartments of the sinuses.

Mandibular Anterior Landmarks

The following landmarks can be demonstrated in the anterior region of the mandible on periapical radiographs (see Figures 15-10 and 15-11).

1. **Inferior border of the mandible:** If mandibular radiograph is exposed using an extreme negative angulation, the inferior border of the mandible can be seen as a radiopaque ridge below the anterior teeth.

2. **Lingual foramen:** This structure appears as a tiny, radiopaque hole below the roots of the mandibular central incisors. This foramen provides an opening through which a small blood vessel is able to pass.

3. **Genial tubercles:** These bony projections surround the lingual foramen and appear as a radiopaque ring around it.

4. **Mental ridge:** The mental ridge is a bony prominence on the external portion of the mandible which extends in a sloping fashion from the premolar area to the central incisors. It appears as a radiopaque, curved ridge below the mandibular anterior teeth.

5. **Nutrient canals:** These can be seen as radiolucent lines extending downward from the mandibular anterior teeth. These canals provide a mean for the blood vessels and nerves to reach the teeth.

6. **Lip line:** Often the soft tissue of the lip can be seen as a radiopaque, curved line that appears below the crowns of the mandibular teeth.

7. **Mandibular tori:** Tori are bony protuberences often seen as small, rounded, radiopaque areas superimposed on the roots of the teeth in the canine and premolar regions of the mandible.

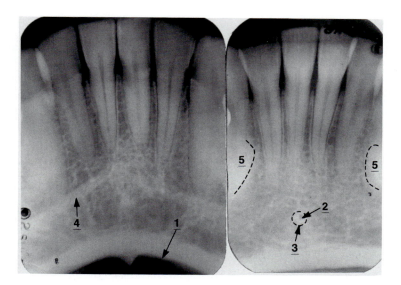

FIGURE 15-10 Mandibular central incisor projection:
(1) inferior border of the mandible; (2) lingual foramen;
(3) genial tubercles; (4) mental ridge; (5) mandibular tori.

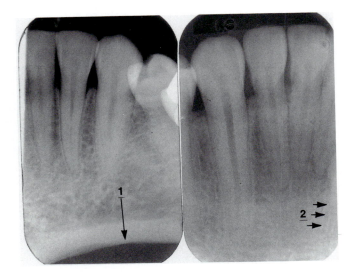

FIGURE 15-11 Mandibular lateral/canine projection:
(1) inferior border of the mandible; (2) nutrient canals.

Mandibular Posterior Landmarks

The following landmarks can be seen in the mandibular posterior areas (see Figures 15-12 and 15-13).

1. **Mental foramen:** This structure provides a means for the blood vessels and nerves to supply the lower lip. It appears as a radiolucent, round- or oval-shaped area located near the apices of the mandibular premolars. This structure is often misinterpreted as some type of periapical lesion.

2. **Mandibular canal:** This canal extends the length of the mandible and provides a passageway for blood vessels and nerves. It appears as a radiolucent band following the roots of the mandibular posterior teeth.

3. **Internal oblique ridge** (Mylohyoid Ridge): This ridge is a bony prominence that provides an attachment site for the mylohyoid muscle to the internal surface of the mandible. It is seen as a wide, curved, radiopaque line extending downward and anteriorly in the molar region. It is often superimposed over the roots of the molar teeth.

4. **External oblique ridge:** This ridge provides an attachment site for the buccinator muscle. It appears as a wide, curved, radiopaque line that travels near the CEJs of the molar teeth.

5. **Submandibular fossa:** This is a depressed area on the lingual side of the mandible. It appears radiographically as a radiolucent area below the internal oblique ridge.

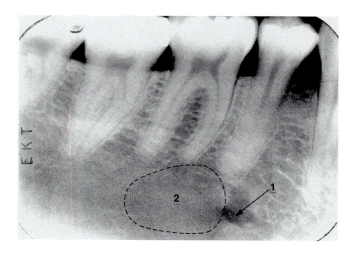

FIGURE 15-12 Mandibular premolar projection: (1) mental foramen; (2) submandibular fossa.

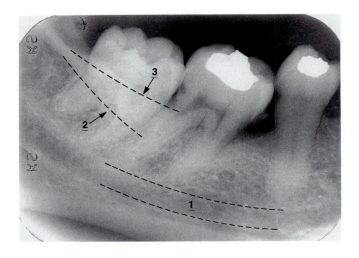

FIGURE 15-13 Mandibular molar projection: (1) mandibular canal; (2) internal oblique ridge (mylohyoid); (3) external oblique ridge.

PANORAMIC ANATOMY

Panoramic Landmarks

The following diagram and panoramic radiograph illustrate common landmarks found in panoramic radiographs (Figures 15-14 and 15-15). Many of these landmarks are the same as appear in the periapical radiographs previously discussed.

1. Lateral pterygoid plate
2. Incisive foramen
3. Mastoid process
4. Styloid process
5. External auditory meatus
6. Hamulus
7. Zygomatic process
8. Malar bone

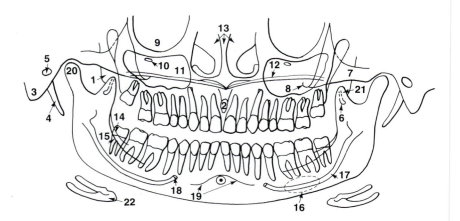

FIGURE 15-14 Panoramic Anatomy: (1) lateral pterygoid plate; (2) incisive foramen; (3) mastoid process; (4) styloid process; (5) external auditory meatus; (6) hamulus; (7) zygomatic process; (8) malar process; (9) orbit; (10) infraorbital foramen; (11) maxillary sinuses; (12) hard palate; (13) nasal fossae and septum; (14) external oblique ridge; (15) internal oblique ridge; (16) submandibular fossa; (17) mandibular canal; (18) mental foramen; (19) mental ridge; (20) mandibular condyle; (21) coronoid process; (22) hyoid bone.

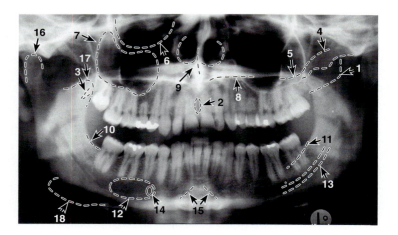

FIGURE 15-15 Panoramic Anatomy: (1) lateral pterygoid plate; (2) incisive foramen; (3) hamulus; (4) zygomatic process; (5) malar process; (6) orbit; (7) maxillary sinuses; (8) hard palate; (9) nasal fossae and septum; (10) external oblique ridge; (11) internal oblique ridge; (12) submandibular fossa; (13) mandibular canal; (14) mental foramen; (15) mental ridge; (16) mandibular condyle; (17) coronoid process; (18) hyoid bone.

9. Orbit

10. Infraorbital foramen

11. Maxillary sinuses

12. Hard palate

13. Nasal fossae and septum

14. External oblique ridge

15. Internal oblique ridge

16. Submandibular fossa

17. Mandibular canal

18. Mental foramen

19. Mental ridge

20. Mandibular condyle

21. Coronoid process

22. Hyoid bone

Panoramic Artifacts and Shadows

In panoramic radiographs, shadows and artifacts often appear superimposed over the normal radiographic structures even though correct technique has been followed. These shadows are due to air spaces in the skull, soft tissues, and such panoramic machine structures as the chin rest. The following diagrams and radiographs demonstrate these artifacts and shadows.

Shadows (Figures 15-16 and 15-17)

1. Vertebral column

2. Submandibular shadow

3. Ghost shadow of the opposite mandible

4. Bite block

5. Chin rest

6. Ghost shadow of the opposite chin rest

7. Pancentric head positioning device

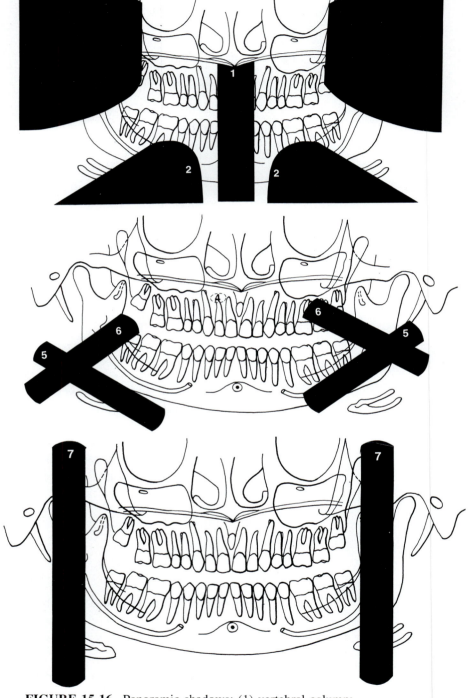

FIGURE 15-16 Panoramic shadows: (1) vertebral column;
(2) submandibular shadow; (3) ghost shadow of the opposite mandible;
(4) bite block; (5) chin rest; (6) ghost shadow of the opposite chin rest;
(7) pancentric head position device.

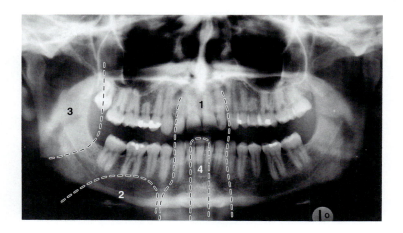

FIGURE 15-17 Panoramic shadows: (1) vertebral column; (2) submandibular shadow; (3) ghost shadow of the opposite mandible; (4) bite block.

Soft tissues images (Figures 15-18 and 15-19)

8. Tongue

9. Ear

10. Soft palate and uvula

11. Lip line

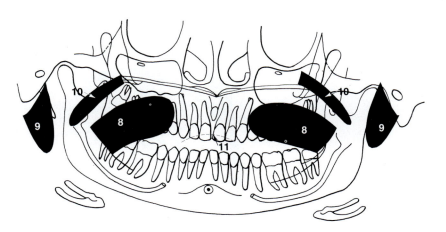

FIGURE 15-18 Panoramic soft tissue images: (8) tongue; (9) ear; (10) soft palate and uvula; (11) lip line.

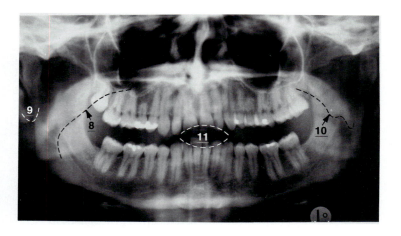

FIGURE 15-19 Panoramic soft tissue images: (8) tongue; (9) ear; (10) soft palate and uvula; (11) lip line.

Air spaces: (Figures 15-20 and 15-21)

12. Palatoglossal air space

13. Nasopharyngeal air space

14. Glossopharyngeal air space

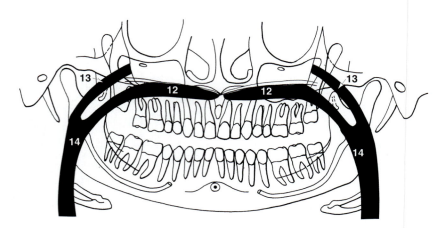

FIGURE 15-20 Panoramic air spaces: (12) palatoglossal air space;(13) nasopharyngeal air space; (14) glosspharyngeal air space.

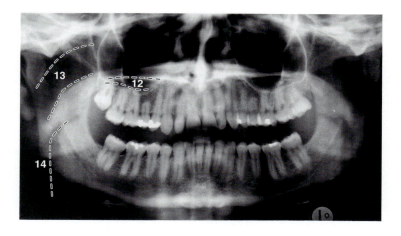

FIGURE 15-21 Panoramic air spaces: (12) palatoglossal air space; (13) nasopharyngeal air space; (14) glosspharyngeal air space.

SUMMARY

This chapter identified the normal radiographic appearance of intraoral and some extraoral structures seen in both periapical and panoramic radiographs. With the knowledge of these structures, the radiographer should be able to properly mount dental radiographs (this is discussed step by step in Chapter 19) and identify normal structures. This can aid in the ultimate identification of abnormal structures or disease processes through the use of radiographs.

BIBLIOGRAPHY

DAE PROJECT. *Normal Radiographic Landmarks.* New York: Teachers College Press, 1982.

GOAZ PW, WHITE SC. *Oral Radiology: Principles and Interpretation,* 2d ed. St. Louis: CV Mosby, 1987.

HARING JI, LIND LJ. *Radiographic Interpretation for the Dental Hygienist.* Philadelphia: WB Saunders, 1993.

MATTESON SR, WHALEY C, SECRIST VC. *Dental Radiology,* 4th ed. Chapel Hill: University of North Carolina Press, 1988.

REVIEW QUESTIONS

1. The pulp of the tooth appears radiographically as

  a. radiopaque.
  b. radiolucent.
  c. clear.
  d. undistinguishable.

2. Cancellous bone has a "spider web" appearance.

  a. True
  b. False

3. The "U"- or "J"-shaped radiopaque structure found in the maxillary molar projection is the

  a. hamulus.
  b. maxillary sinus.
  c. sinus septum.
  d. malar process.

4. The small, bony, radiopaque structure that encircles the lingual foramen in the mandibular central incisor radiograph is the

  a. genial tubercles.
  b. mental ridge.
  c. inferior border of the mandible.
  d. tori.

5. The radiopaque band that extends along the roots of the mandibular molars is known as the

  a. submandibular fossa.
  b. internal oblique ridge.
  c. external oblique ridge.
  d. mental ridge.

6. The small radiolucent round structure seen between the mandibular premolar and is often mistaken for pathology is known as the

  a. mental foramen.
  b. lingual foramen.
  c. mandibular canal.
  d. genial tubercles.

Radiographic Imaging for the Dental Team,
by Sally Mauriello. J.B. Lippincott Company,
Philadelphia © 1995.

16

Principles of Radiographic Interpretation

Upon the completion of this chapter, the student should be able to:

1. Discuss the basic principles of radiographic interpretation.

2. Define the terminology used in radiographic interpretation.

3. Identify radiographically the appearance of restorative materials.

4. Distinguish between normal anatomy and pathological processes.

5. Identify radiographically, the signs of caries, periodontal lesions, developmental abnormalities, trauma, and benign and malignant lesions.

6. Apply radiographic interpretation to dental hygiene services.

Interpretation of radiographs can be defined as reading what is seen on the radiograph. Often, the terms interpretation and diagnosis are used interchangeably, but there are distinct differences between the two terms. Diagnosis involves using the information found on the radiograph, along with the medical and dental history and clinical examination, to distinguish disease processes from normal findings. Only the dentist is legally qualified to diagnose. But the interpretation of radiographs can be accomplished by both the dentist and dental hygienist. The dental hygienist can play a vital role in the preliminary interpretation of the radiographs in order to direct the dentist to areas of concern. But primarily, the dental hygienist uses the radiographs to plan and implement dental hygiene treatment. This can include such things as identifying clinically periodontal pockets that appear radiographically, identifying calculus deposits, and educating the patient through the use of radiographs.

This chapter will aid the dental hygienist in the use of radiographs to identify the appearance of abnormal radiographic signs and pathological processes. In addition, it will help to establish the terminology and basic principles needed to interpret dental radiographs.

BASIC PRINCIPLES
OF RADIOGRAPHIC INTERPRETATION

In addition to analyzing information displayed in the radiograph, radiographic interpretation involves the use of high-quality radiographs and technique, proper processing procedures, proper film mounting and viewing techniques, a systematic approach in viewing the radiographs, and communication and documentation of accurate descriptions of radiographic findings. The dental hygienist can play an important role in providing this information to the dentist and patient.

As discussed in previous chapters, the radiographic technique can obscure important clinical information through distortion, horizontal overlap, and failure to project information on the radiograph. Improper exposure settings and processing techniques can influence the contrast, density, and appearance of the object on the radiograph. Therefore, measures should be taken to insure that radiographs of good diagnostic quality are rendered prior to displaying the films for radiographic interpretation.

When preparing the radiographs for interpretation, they should be mounted properly according to the American Dental Association guidelines (discussed in Chapter 19). The use of proper viewing conditions is also essential for the detection of subtle information present on the radiograph. This would include the following (see Figure 16-1):

1. Masked **viewbox** to omit extraneous light.

2. Film mount that omits extraneous light.

3. Viewbox with an even intensity of light.

4. Viewbox with an adjustable light level.

5. Viewing room should be dimly lit.

Masking or covering the unused portion of the viewbox will help reduce glare and enable the observer to adapt to the brightness of the displayed radiographs. This effect will also be enhanced by room dimness and opaque film mounts. The viewbox light can optimize the radiographic image, while evenly lighting the entire image. Dark or light radiographic films can be maximized by increasing or decreasing the viewbox light with a variable intensity light source. This will enhance the radiographs and enable the observer to maximize information gained from the illuminated image.

Once the radiographs are properly displayed, they are ready for a preliminary interpretation. This should include both a global and local viewing. The global viewing should assess symmetry of form and density, cortical symmetries, and the number of teeth present. Locally, one should assess the periodontal ligament space and lamina dura, evaluate the root form, and assess the tooth crowns for caries and abnormalities. Most importantly, a systematic approach should be used when interpreting radiographs.

Much of radiographic interpretation involves the differentiation of normal versus abnormal conditions. This emphasizes the need for a

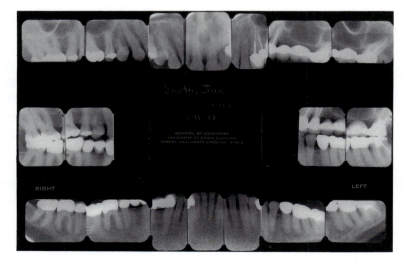

FIGURE 16-1 Radiographs mounted and prepared for interpretation.

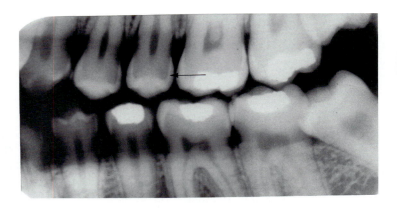

FIGURE 16-2 An example of Mach banding mimicking a carious lesion.

good understanding of normal radiographic anatomy and patterns in the oral cavity. Knowledge of artifacts, such as Mach banding and cervical burnout, is also essential. The **Mach band effect** occurs when a dark coloring is next to a light coloring. Due to the receptors in the eye, the dark color appears even darker and the light color appears lighter as they approach their joining (Figure 16-2). An example of this would be the joining of the dentin and enamel, which may mimic the appearance of a carious lesion because of the Mach banding. One method for differentiating between Mach bands and caries is to place an index card or paper over the darker density. If it is an illusion caused by the Mach band, then it will disappear. Another artifact that can mimic cervical caries is **cervical burnout.** (Figure 16-3) As the name denotes, it occurs in the cervical region of the tooth and will be discussed later in this chapter.

A major point to remember when evaluating radiographs for interpretation is to integrate clinical data and information provided by the patient with the radiographic data. Radiographs provide a two-dimensional picture of a three-dimensional object. Radiographic limitations that occur in the detection of periodontal disease include the inability to differentiate between buccal and lingual bone height, the inability to visualize bony defects because overlying bone, and the density of the root superimposed over the defect. Therefore, both clinical and radiographic data is necessary in helping the dentist render an accurate diagnosis.

VOCABULARY OF INTERPRETATION

Just as descriptive terms are applied to clinical findings in order to describe the appearance of lesions, the same applies to radiographic

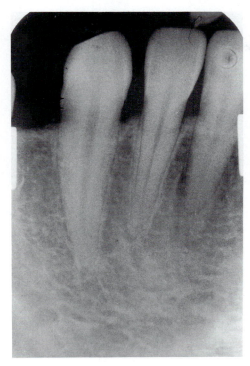

FIGURE 16-3 The radiographic appearance of cervical burnout mimics cervical caries.

findings. It is imperative to provide accurate documentation that describes all conditions found radiographically.

Density

The terms used to describe density are **radiolucent** and **radiopaque.** Radiolucent objects appear black, or dark, on the radiograph. This occurs because few photons are attenuated by the object. Thus, many photons interact with the film emulsion. Examples of low-density structures or lesions that would appear radiolucent on a radiograph are **pulp, caries, sinus, and foramen.** Radiopaque structures appear white, or light, on the radiograph because of the attenuation of most photons by the object. Examples of radiopaque structures are enamel, bone, dentin, and amalgam or gold restorations. When interpreting radiographs, a statement should be made based on the overall degree of radiolucency or **radiopacity** of the object/structure being described (Figure 16-4).

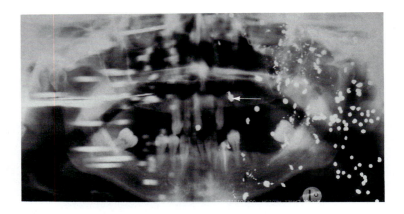

FIGURE 16-4 The foreign object noted by the arrow is an example of a radiopaque object.

Location

It is important to note the location of the object/structure. Terms that can be used to describe location are maxilla or mandible, unilateral (one side) or bilateral (both sides), and symmetrical or asymmetrical.

Size, Shape, and Number

The size of the lesion should be documented for two reasons. First, treatment plan options may be dictated by the size of the lesion. Second, comparisons can be made by monitoring the size of the lesion over time. Lesions will vary in size. Often the diameter will measure from millimeters to centimeters.

The shape and number of lesions can also vary. Some of the different shapes that can occur are circular, oval, pear-shaped, heart-shaped, or irregular (Figure 16-5). Lesions can occur singularly or in multiples (Figure 16-6). Documentation of the size, shape, and number of lesions is paramount in determining growth, monitoring change, and diagnosis.

Borders

Borders of lesions can also be indicative of a particular type of lesion; therefore, they are important in identification of the lesion type. Terms that can be used to describe various borders are distinct or poorly-defined (Figure 16-7), corticated or uncorticated (Figure 16-8), smooth or ragged (Figure 16-9), and scalloped.

Internal Architecture

The cortex can reveal much about the nature of the lesion. It can be termed **unilocular** (having one compartment) (Figure 16-10) or **multi-locular** (having more than one compartment) (Figure 16-11). Some

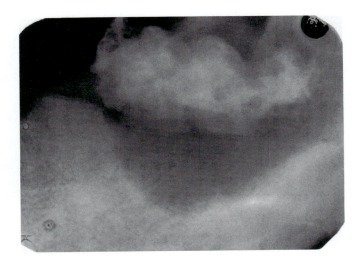

FIGURE 16-5   This is an example of an irregular lesion.

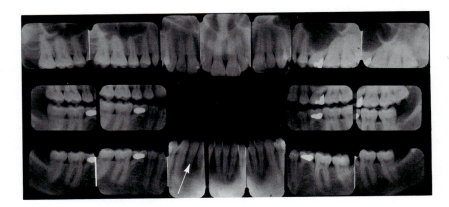

FIGURE 16-6   This is an example of a singular lesion.

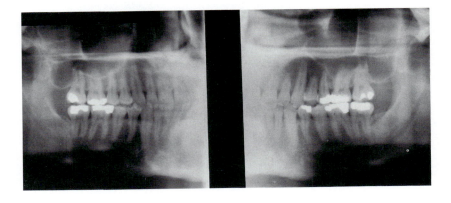

FIGURE 16-7   The borders of the lesion are distinct.

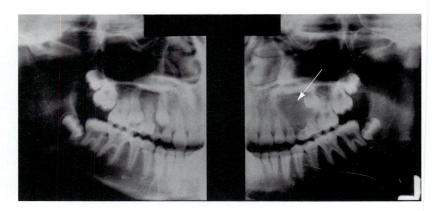

FIGURE 16-8 The borders of the lesion are corticated.

lesions are radiolucent, have radiopaque flecks, or may be of a mixed density.

Effect on Adjacent Structure

A lesion can often affect adjacent structures. It can be through movement of roots, displacement of teeth, or resorption of roots. In addition, bone swelling paresthesia, and pulp death can occur.

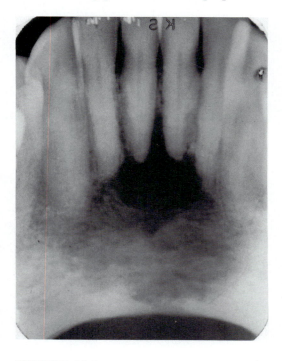

FIGURE 16-9 The borders of the lesion are ragged.

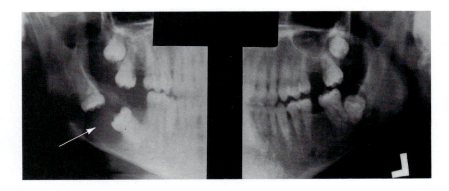

FIGURE 16-10 The cortex of this lesion is described as being unilocular.

RADIOGRAPHIC APPEARANCE OF RESTORATIVE MATERIALS

Metallic Restorations

Metallic restorations used in dentistry include such materials as amalgam, gold, and stainless steel. Amalgam is the most common restorative material used in dentistry. Its radiographic appearance is completely radiopaque because it is a very dense material and absorbs x-ray beams. Absorption prevents x-rays from reaching the film. Amalgams vary in size and shape and can cover very little to almost all of the tooth surface (Figure 16-12).

Gold restorations, such as crowns, bridges, and onlays, have approximately the same density as amalgam. Thus, they appear totally radiopaque. It may be difficult to distinguish gold from amalgam on the radiograph. Gold restorations may only be distinguished by their contour and smooth borders. A clinical examination would be required in order to verify what type of metallic restoration has been used.

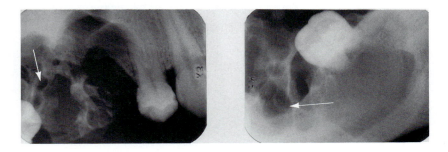

FIGURE 16-11 The cortex of this lesion is described as being multilocular.

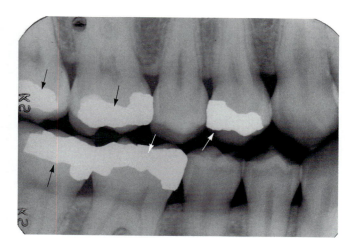

FIGURE 16-12 Amalgam restoration

Stainless steel and chrome crowns are often used as temporary restorations and are prefabricated. Therefore, their contour and shape may not follow the tooth anatomy as closely as gold or amalgam. In addition, a stainless steel or chrome crown is thinner than a cast restoration or amalgam, allowing more of the x-ray beam to pass through. As such, these restorations appear radiopaque, but less radiopaque than amalgam or gold (Figure 16-13).

Nonmetallic Restorative Materials

Nonmetallic restorative materials include composites and acrylic resins (Figure 16-14). These restorations can vary in appearance from slightly

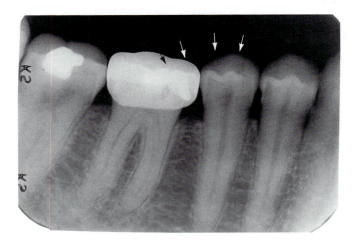

FIGURE 16-13 Stainless steel crown

radiopaque to radiolucent, depending upon their density. Acrylic resins are the least dense and often appear radiolucent. This makes it difficult to distinguish in the radiograph if any restorative material is present at all. A clinical examination would be required to verify the presence of a resin material.

Manufacturers often incorporate radiopaque particles in composite restorations to make them more distinguishable on the radiographs. Still a clinical examination may be required to distinguish this restorative material from dental caries.

OTHER CAST RESTORATIONS

In addition to gold restorations, porcelain, porcelain fused to metal, and post and core restorations can be distinguished on dental radiographs. Porcelain restorations are seen as slightly radiopaque with a thin outline of the tooth preparation apparent through the restoration. This radiopaque line outlining of the tooth preparation represents the cement used in securing the restoration (Figure 16-15).

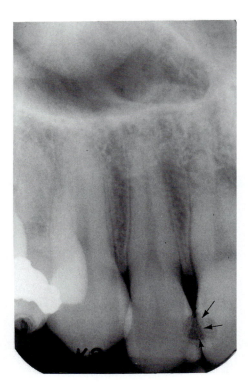

FIGURE 16-14 Composite restorations

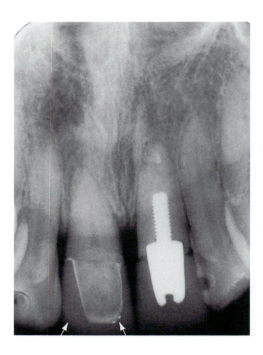

FIGURE 16-15   Porcelain crown

Porcelain fused to metal restorations (Figure 16-16) have a similar appearance to the all-porcelain restorations, except that the metallic component in the center appears totally radiopaque.

Post and core restorations are seen on endodontically treated teeth. The total restoration is radiopaque and has an extension (the post) into the pulp canal (Figure 16-17).

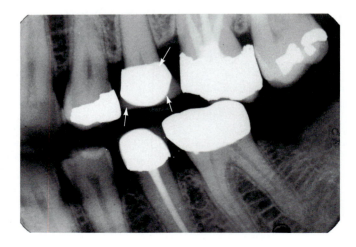

FIGURE 16-16   Porcelain fused to metal crown

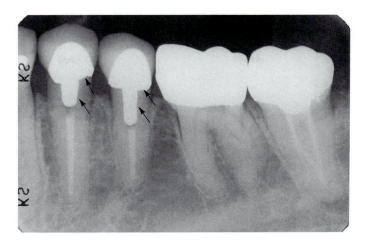

FIGURE 16-17 Post and core restoration

Other Materials Used in Dentistry

Several materials used in restorative, orthodontic, and surgical procedures can be identified radiographically. These include metallic pins, base materials, gutta percha, silver points, suture wires, splints, implants, plates, and orthodontic wires, bands, and brackets.

Metallic pins can be identified in large amalgam or composite restorations. They are used to help retain the restoration and can be seen as radiopaque projections at the base of the restoration (Figure 16-18).

Gutta percha and silver points can be seen in endodontically treated teeth as radiopaque material filling the root canal. Gutta percha appears less radiopaque than silver points because the gutta percha is a soft material and silver points are a metallic material (Figure 16-19).

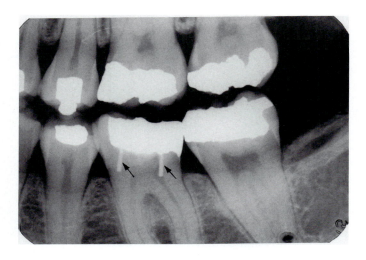

FIGURE 16-18 Restorations supported by metallic pins

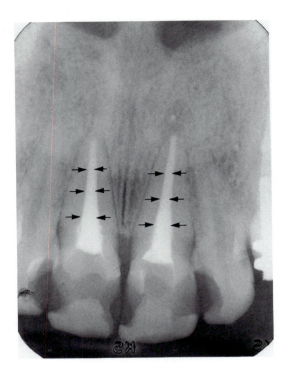

FIGURE 16-19   Gutta percha

Base materials are often used under restorations to protect the pulp of the tooth. These materials are placed on the floor of the cavity preparation and appear as a thin radiopaque line. These materials include zinc phosphate, and zinc oxide and eugenol (Figure 16-20).

Oral surgery may require the use of wires, stabilizing plates or splints, and, more recently, implants. All of these materials appear radiopaque and can vary in size, shape, and location (Figure 16-21).

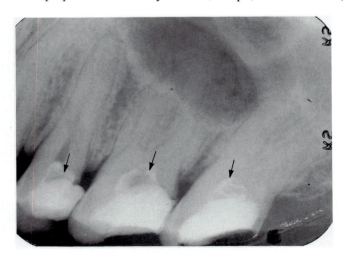

FIGURE 16-20   Zinc phosphate cement

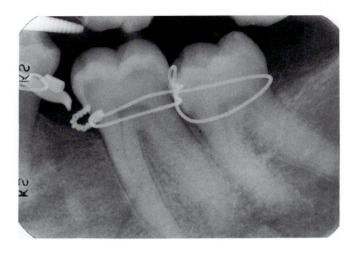

FIGURE 16-21 Stabilizing wires

Orthodontic bands, brackets, and wires can be seen radiographically. These all appear radiopaque and usually can be identified without much trouble as orthodontic appliances (Figure 16-22).

Materials Used in Prosthodontics

Complete and partial dentures can be identified in a dental radiograph if they are left in during radiographic exposure. Since the teeth of the dentures are typically acrylic, they are slightly radiopaque. But any metallic framework on the partial denture or retention pins in the full denture appear totally radiopaque (Figure 16-23).

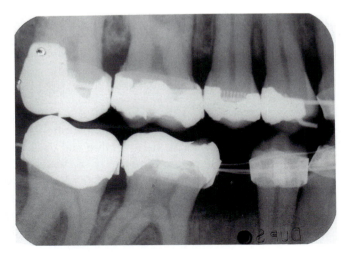

FIGURE 16-22 Orthodontic bands

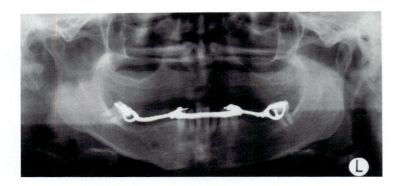

FIGURE 16-23 Partial denture left in during a panoramic exposure

Relation of Identification to Dental Hygiene Services

In order for dental hygienists to distinguish signs of pathological processes, they must be able to identify common restorative materials. This aids in planning dental hygiene treatment for the patient. Identification of such things as overhangs on amalgam restorations and their implications on tissue and bone health in the patient's mouth can effect scaling procedures. In addition, the contour and shape of the margins and borders of cast restorations can have an effect on the buildup of calculus deposits and subsequent scaling and root planing appointments. Therefore, knowledge of the types and integrity of the patient's restorations can play a vital role in dental hygiene treatment.

RADIOGRAPHIC APPEARANCE OF NORMAL ANATOMY MIMICKING PATHOLOGICAL PROCESSES

The location and appearance of normal anatomy sometimes mimics a pathological process.

Mandible

The mental foramen, which is most often seen about halfway between the lower border of the mandible and the crest of the alveolar process usually in the region of the apex of the second premolar, may simulate periapical pathosis. In Figure 16-24 the image of the mental foramen at the level of the apex of the second premolar simulates a periapical lesion, but continuity of the lamina dura around the apex indicates the absence of periapical disease. The image on the right displays a radiograph containing a tooth with a periapical lesion.

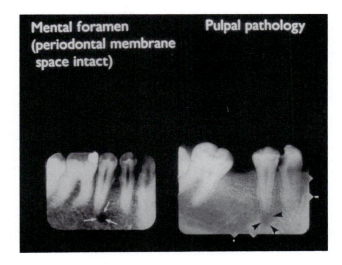

FIGURE 16-24 The radiograph on the left demonstrates the mental foramen at the level of the apex of the second premolar. The radiograph on the right demonstrates pulpal pathology. Courtesy of Dr. Donald A. Tyndall, UNC School of Dentistry.

Maxilla

In the maxillary region, the maxillary sinus may pneumatize into dentate and/or edentulous spaces. **Pneumatization** is the formation of pneumatic cells or cavities in tissue. Radiographically, a pneumatized region is seen as a large radiolucency resembling pathology. Figure 16-25 shows a large radiolucency between the first premolar and the

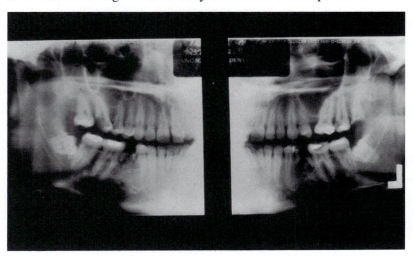

FIGURE 16-25 Radiolucency between the second premolar and the first molar on the right maxilla represents an example of pneumatization.

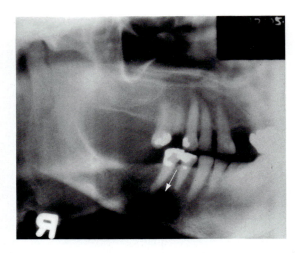

FIGURE 16-26 Radiolucency caused by the sub-mandibular salivary gland pressing against the lingual surface of the mandible.

first molar. Close examination reveals that the radiolucency is part of the maxillary sinus. Another example in which a large radiolucency is frequently seen is in the posterior aspect between the apices of the teeth and the inferior border of the mandible. This radiolucency is caused by the submandibular salivary gland pressing against the lingual surface of the mandible known as the submandibular gland depression. Figure 16-26 shows an image displaying the radiographic appearance of the submandibular salivary gland depression. The incisive foramen between the maxillary centrals is sometimes displayed as a large ovoid radiolucency; The canine fossa, which can appear as a depression in the bone around the canine, can present radiographically as an ill-defined radiolucency. It is important for the radiographer to be able to recognize and identify normal radiographic anatomy and be familiar with the range of common variations. Knowledge of radiographic anatomy makes the radiographer a more valuable member of the dental team.

RADIOGRAPHIC SIGNS OF CONGENITAL AND DEVELOPMENTAL ANOMALIES

The term **anomaly** implies a marked deviation from the normal or a departure from the regular order of things. Developmental anomalies may be hereditary or result from environmental insults. The effects of anomalies may or may not cause problems to the patient or the dentist in the formulation of treatment. Dental anomalies generally reflect either a change in the number of teeth, their size, their form, or their position.

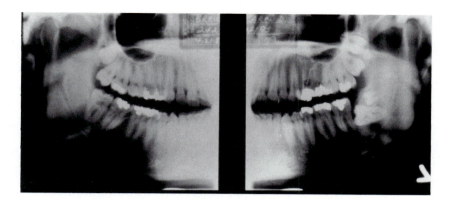

FIGURE 16-27 This image demonstrates an example of hyperdontia in the right and left maxillary region and the left mandibular region. Notice the presence of 4th molars.

Anomaly of Number

An example of anomaly in the number of teeth is hyperdontia or supernumerary teeth expressed by an increased number of teeth over that which is normal. The panoramic radiograph shown in Figure 16-27 shows an example of a case where hyperdontia is present. The most common areas for supernumeraries are between the upper central incisors, below the mandibular premolars, and behind the third molars.

Anomaly of Size

In the case of anomaly of size, conditions range from macrodontia, in which the teeth are larger than normal, to microdontia, in which the teeth are smaller than normal. Figure 16-28 shows an example of microdontia. Maxillary third molars are the most common microdont teeth.

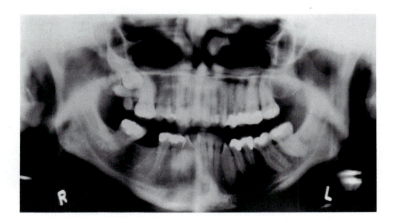

FIGURE 16-28 Image displaying a microdont supernumery tooth in the right side of the patient.

Anomaly of Form

Anomaly of form may be manifested in the following (see Figures 16-29 and 16-30):

1. Fusion, in which there is union of two or more teeth and the dentin of these structures become confluent.

2. Gemination, in which there is formation of a bifid crown.

3. Concrescence, in which only the cementum of two or more teeth become united.

4. Dens-in-Dente, produced by an infolding of the outer surface of a tooth into the interior.

5. Taurodontia, characterized by a tooth having a long body and short roots.

6. Dilaceration, in which the root is curved or bent.

7. Dentin dysplasia or "rootless teeth."

8. Amelogenesis imperfecta or defective development of enamel formation.

Anomaly of Tooth Position

In anomalies of tooth position, impaction, transposition of teeth, rotations, and hypereruptions may occur. Figure 16-31 shows an example of anomalies of tooth position.

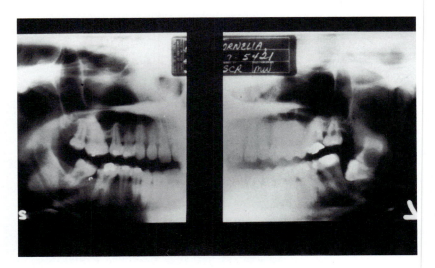

FIGURE 16-29 This panoramic radiograph shows an example of taurodontia. Notice the long bodies and short roots of the mandibular molars.

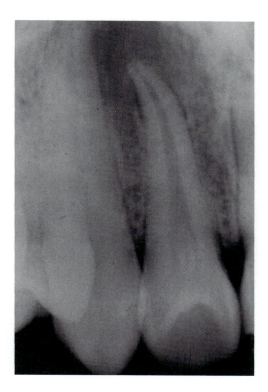

FIGURE 16-30 This periapical view of the lateral incisor shows an example of dens en dente.

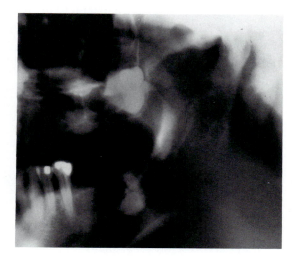

FIGURE 16-31 This panoramic radiograph reveals tooth #16 to be impacted vertically. This is an example of an anomaly of tooth position.

RADIOGRAPHIC SIGNS OF CARIOUS LESIONS

Accurate detection of carious lesions can be accomplished with a thorough clinical examination and the use of radiographs to view areas that cannot be seen clinically. The bitewing radiograph is the most appropriate projection to use for caries detection because it gives a view of both the maxillary and mandibular crowns of the posterior teeth. Caries that are apparent in dental radiographs are clinically further advanced than seen on the radiograph. This occurs because demineralization does not effect the density of the tooth structure and therefore cannot be detected on the radiograph. As the lesion progresses and tooth structure is altered in density, it begins to become detectable in the radiograph.

Dental caries appear as radiolucent areas within the tooth structure and can be mimicked by such other things as restorative materials, attrition, abrasion, and radiographic artifacts. Therefore a systematic approach must be used in evaluating radiographs for dental caries and the hygienist should be knowledgeable about the appearance of different types of carious lesions.

Carious lesions can be classified by their extent—mild (or incipient), moderate, advanced, and severe, and by their location—interproximal, occlusal, buccal or lingual, cemental, and recurrent. Depending on their extent and location, carious lesions can have different appearances.

Interproximal Caries

Incipient, or mild, carious lesions appear between teeth as small radiolucent notches in the enamel. These lesions are just present in the enamel and do not appear to extend to the dentoenamel junction (DEJ) (Figure 16-32).

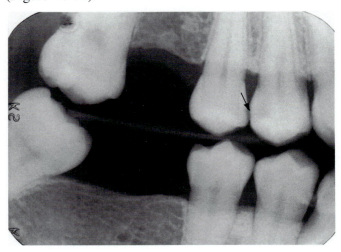

FIGURE 16-32   Mild interproximal caries

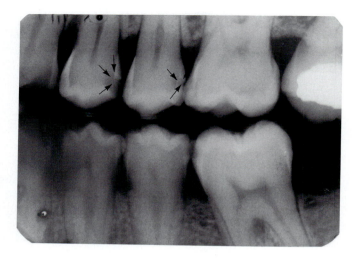

FIGURE 16-33 Moderate interproximal caries

Moderate interproximal caries appear as triangular notches in the enamel and may extend just to the DEJ. This triangular radiolucent area does not involve the DEJ (Figure 16-33).

Severe interproximal caries also appear as a triangular shaped radiolucent area in the enamel extending all the way to the DEJ. In addition, the lesion invades the dentin. This is seen as a radiolucent "half-moon" shape extending into the dentin from the lesion area at the DEJ, but not reaching more than half way to the pulp (Figure 16-34).

Advance interproximal caries have the same appearance as severe caries but they often extend into the dentin more than half way to the pulp. These lesions usually appear clinically as a large hole in the tooth (Figure 16-35).

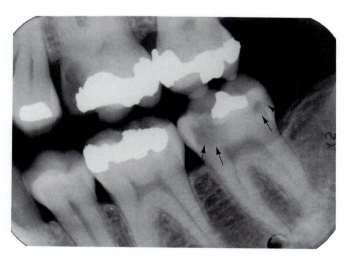

FIGURE 16-34 Severe interproximal caries

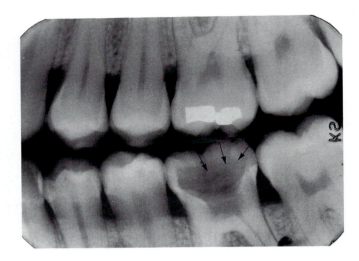

FIGURE 16-35   Advanced interproximal caries

Occlusal Caries

Occlusal caries are difficult to visualize on the radiograph until they are in an advanced stage because the enamel in occlusal areas is dense and the cusps are superimposed upon each other. These carious lesions appear in the radiograph as a radiolucent, "half-moon" shape directly under the occlusal enamel and extend into the dentin. As previously stated, mild occlusal caries can very rarely be detected on the radiograph. Therefore, radiographically apparent occlusal caries would be classified as either moderate or severe. Severe occlusal caries would extend more than half way to the pulp of the tooth (Figure 16-36).

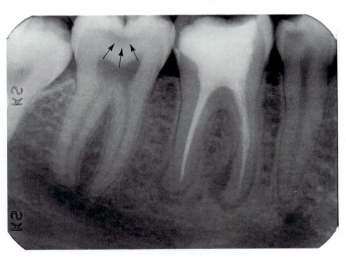

FIGURE 16-36   Occlusal caries

Buccal and Lingual Caries

Buccal and lingual caries may be difficult to detect on radiographs. They appear as radiolucent circular lesions in the middle of the crown. It is difficult to determine from the radiograph if the lesion is present on the lingual or the buccal surface.

Cemental Caries

Root surface caries are present on the cementum of the tooth and also involve the dentin. These lesions appear as scooped out radiolucent areas on the root surface just below the cementoenamel junction. These lesions are often confused with the radiographic artifact known as cervical burnout. Cervical burnout appears as radiolucent areas at the CEJ. This is caused by a decreased density of the tooth structure in that area that results in a lessened absorption of the x-ray beam as it passes through the tooth. This creates wedge-shaped radiolucent areas at the CEJ. Root caries can only be present on root surfaces that are exposed in the oral cavity (where bone loss is present) (Figure 16-37).

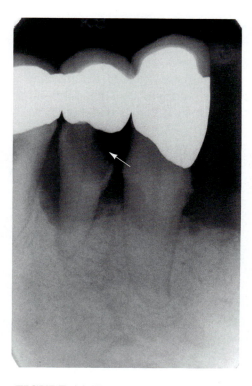

FIGURE 16-37 Cemental caries

Recurrent Caries

Recurrent decay is seen as caries occurring adjacent to existing restorations. These lesions appear as radiolucent areas beneath or below restorations (Figure 16-38).

Lesions that Mimic Caries

Other conditions that appear similar to dental caries in the radiograph include dental attrition and abrasion. Abrasion, which appears as a scooped-out area, is therefore radiolucent on the radiograph. Attrition results in a loss of density of the tooth surface and increased density on the radiograph. Each of these conditions can be ruled out as caries through a clinical examination.

Although dental hygienists cannot legally diagnose radiographic caries, they can use their knowledge about the appearance of carious lesions in calling suspected or "suspicious" areas to the dentist's attention. In addition, identification of carious lesions can aid in treatment planning, the need for oral hygiene instructions, fluoride therapy, and modification of scaling procedures in areas of advanced decay.

RADIOGRAPHIC SIGNS OF LESIONS OF THE PERIODONTIUM

Diseases of the periodontium include gingivitis and periodontitis. Gingivitis is an inflammation of the marginal gingival tissues, not the alveolar bone, and thus does not show any radiographic signs. Periodontitis is also an inflammation, but it involves the supporting tissues

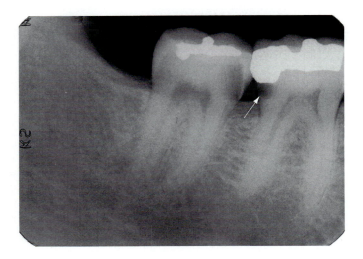

FIGURE 16-38 Recurrent decay

of the tooth, such as the alveolar bone, periodontal ligament fibers, cementum, and gingiva. Changes that occur in the alveolar bone and periodontal ligament space can be seen radiographically. Radiographic signs of periodontal disease are assessed through changes in the crestal bone, periodontal ligament space, lamina dura, and alveolar bone. The appearance of each will be discussed.

Crestal Bone

The crest of the alveolar bone (**crestal bone**) normally appears approximately one to one-and-a-half millimeters below the cementoenamel junction (CEJ). The normal density of the crest is well corticated and, therefore, radiopaque. The appearance should be parallel to a line joining the CEJs of the adjacent teeth in the posterior. In the anterior, the crest will appear pointed. The shape of the crest is a continuous line that forms a sharp angle with the lamina dura (Figure 16-39).

Periodontal Ligament Space

The **periodontal ligament space** appears radiolucent on the radiograph. It is a thin line that follows the contour of the root (see Figure 16-39). In a diseased state, the periodontal ligament space will widen.

Lamina Dura

The **lamina dura** is a radiopaque structure that forms a sharp angle with the crestal bone. It then follows the contour of the root as a continuous line adjacent to the periodontal ligament space (Figure 16-39).

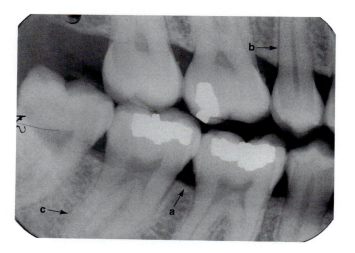

FIGURE 16-39 This radiograph shows the healthy appearance of the periodontium: (a) crestal bone, (b) periodontal ligament space, and (c) lamina dura.

Alveolar Bone

The **alveolar bone** encircles the roots of the teeth. It should appear radiopaque and depict a trabecular pattern (Figure 16-40). When evaluating the periodontal status of a patient, use radiographs that will provide the most accurate information. For the evaluation of periodontal status, both periapicals and vertical bitewings are the radiographs of choice. Periapicals are important because they provide a view of the apical area of the tooth. Bitewings are valuable because of the small vertical angulation used. Bitewings allow for an accurate projection of the crestal bone level and a decrease in the distortion sometimes seen in the periapical radiograph.

Early radiographic signs of periodontal disease involve the crestal bone. There may be a blunting of the crest or a less sharp angle formed by the crestal bone and lamina dura. The cortication of the crestal bone may appear thinner, projecting a more diffuse or irregular border (Figure 16-41).

As the disease progresses, additional changes can be seen in the alveolar bone. These changes include horizontal bone loss, vertical bone loss, and defects between the buccal and lingual cortical plates (interradicular or interdental).

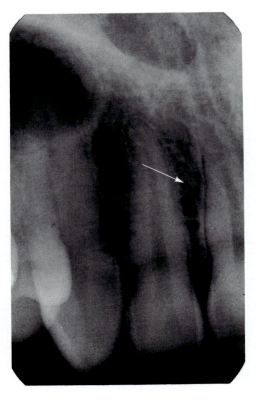

FIGURE 16-40 Healthy alveolar bone will show a trabecular pattern.

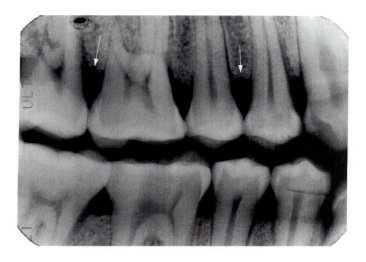

FIGURE 16-41   Diseased alveolar bone will appear with a diffuse irregular border.

Horizontal Bone Loss

Horizontal bone loss involves the level of the crestal bone. The crestal bone resorbs while keeping the same horizontal relationship with the adjacent teeth (Figure 16-42). It includes the loss of both the buccal and lingual cortical plates. This can occur in a localized area or be generalized throughout the mouth.

Vertical Bone Loss

Vertical bone loss occurs when only the mesial or distal surface of the crestal bone resorbs (Figure 16-43). It may also involve the resorption of one of the cortical plates.

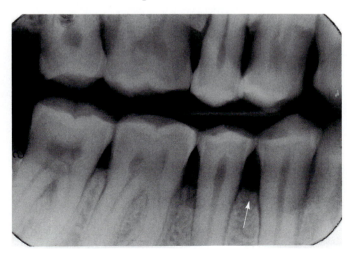

FIGURE 16-42   This is an example of horizontal bone loss.

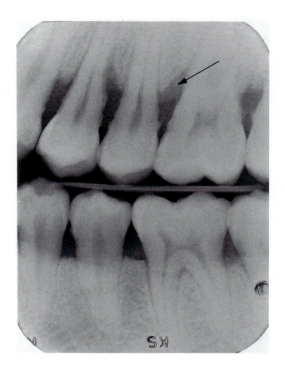

FIGURE 16-43   This is an example of
vertical bone loss.

Interradicular Bone Loss

Advanced stages of periodontal disease will usually involve **inter-radicular bone loss** of multirooted teeth (Figure 16-44). The amount of radiolucency present on the radiograph will be determined by the amount of bone loss in the furcation area.

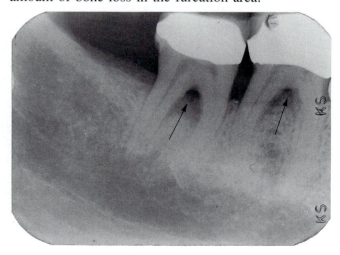

FIGURE 16-44   Severe bone loss occurring in the
furcation area.

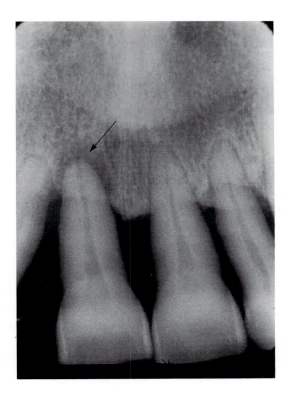

FIGURE 16-45 An abscess present at the apex of the tooth due to periodontal disease.

Periodontal Abscess

The **periodontal abscess** is a lesion that appears around the apex of the tooth. It originates in the bottom of a periodontal pocket where debris or bacteria may be present. Because of the destruction of bone, the lesion may appear radiolucent at the tooth apex (Figure 16-45).

RADIOGRAPHIC SIGNS OF DENTOALVEOLAR TRAUMA

Trauma can occur to the tooth, the surrounding and supporting structures in the oral cavity, or both. Tooth fractures are classified according to location and extent. The following list classifies tooth trauma into four classes:

- Class I   Involves the enamel only
- Class II   Involves the enamel and dentin
- Class III   Involves the enamel, dentin, and pulp
- Class IV   Occurs below the cementoenamel junction

Trauma to the dentition can be identified radiographically as old or recent trauma. Common signs of recent trauma include widening of the periodontal ligament space; fracture lines (appear radiolucent); radiopaque lines that represent overlapping fractured tooth segments; and tooth malaligned or displaced. Old trauma can be identified by an open apex of the tooth and an enlarged or obliterated pulp canal. In addition, periapical radiolucencies may still be present.

Trauma to the maxilla or mandible can display many clinical signs, including pain, tenderness, lacerations, contusions, hemorrhage, edema, and disruption of the occlusion plane. If trauma is suspected after clinical examination, a panoramic radiograph will aid in defining the extent of the trauma. Panoramic radiographs are not as useful in diagnosing maxillary trauma as they are in mandibular trauma. Maxillary trauma can usually be better defined with the use of periapical or occlusal radiographs.

Figure 16-46 illustrates the types of fractures that are most commonly found in the mandible. In the **simple fracture,** there is no communication with the outside environment—no break in the mucosa or skin. In the **compound fracture,** there is communication with the outside environment, as the bone lacerates the skin or mucosa. This is common in the mandible, where teeth are fractured during the trauma. In **comminuted fractures,** the bone is shattered or crushed. In **greenstick fractures,** the bone bends like a twig and fractures only one cortical plate. The bone is thus fractured on one side and bent on the other. This type of fracture is most commonly seen in children.

Compound fractures account for about 74 percent of the mandibular

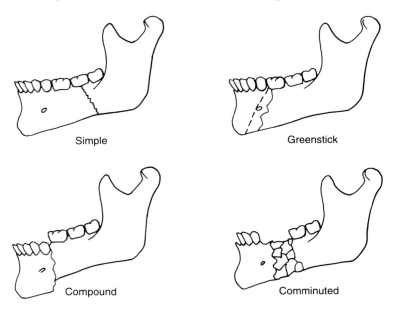

Simple

Greenstick

Compound

Comminuted

FIGURE 16-46 Types of fractures most commonly found in the mandible: (1) simple; (2) compound; (3) comminuted; (4) green-stick.

fractures; simple fractures for 23 percent, and comminuted fractures for the remaining 3 percent.

Mandibular fractures occur in certain anatomic sites more frequently than others. With this knowledge and the knowledge of artifacts in the area, misinterpretation of fracture can be avoided.

BENIGN AND MALIGNANT LESIONS

Dental professionals who are able to recognize the signs of benign and malignant lesions play an important role in the identification, prevention, and management of these lesions. After making an assessment of the area involved, the dentist can then make an appropriate referral. Early detection of benign and malignant lesions is extremely crucial, because treatment is most effective during the early stages of the disease and may result in a less costly and more simple type of treatment.

Benign lesions are new growths containing tissue similar to the tissue from which they originate. They grow slowly and usually do not metastasize (or spread to other parts of the body). Radiographically, they are characterized by well-defined and well-marginated areas with an even and regular shape. The contents of benign lesions may be radiolucent, radiopaque, or mixed. Generally benign lesions cause bone to expand rather than be destroyed. If this occurs in the presence of teeth, they will often cause the dentition to be pushed aside. Figure 16-47 shows an example of a benign lesion found in the mandible.

Malignant lesions grow rapidly and may spread through the vascular

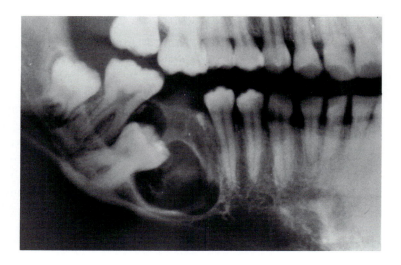

FIGURE 16-47 Panoramic image displaying the presence of a benign lesion. Notice the well defined borders. Courtesy of Dr. Donald A. Tyndall, UNC School of Dentistry.

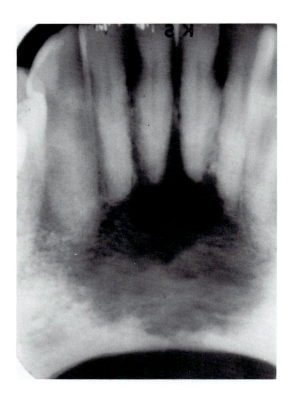

FIGURE 16-48 Intraoral image depicting the presence of a malignant lesion. Notice the irregular borders of the lesion and the invasive inferior expansion. This was diagnosed as metastatic carcinoma. Courtesy of Dr. John B. Ludlow, UNC School of Dentistry.

and lymphatic systems. Many may metastasize and be considered life threatening. Sometimes a variety of projections must be obtained in order to visualize these lesions. In some cases, after patients are referred to specialists, nuclear medicine, ultrasound, computed tomography, magnetic resonance, and/or special procedures may be required to fully assess the lesion. Radiographically, malignant lesions are poorly demarcated because of their rapid and destructive growth. They are irregular in shape, usually radiolucent, and generally cause bone destruction. A definitive diagnosis is made after a biopsy has been performed. Figure 16-48 is an example of a malignant tumor found in the mandible.

SUMMARY

This chapter has discussed the basic principles of radiographic interpretation. These include the terminology, appearance of restorative materials, and the differences between normal and abnormal pathological processes. The radiographic signs of caries, periodontal lesions, developmental abnormalities, trauma, benign, and malignant lesions were also reviewed. With this information, the dental hygienist should be able to increase his/her knowledge and ability to distinguish between normal and pathological processes in the radiograph.

BIBLIOGRAPHY

EASTMAN KODAK COMPANY. *Dental Radiography and Photography: Seminars in Advanced Oral Radiographic Interpretation.* Rochester, NY, 1985, 1–4.

GOAZ PW, WHITE SC. *Oral Radiology Principles and Interpretation,* 3rd ed. St. Louis: CV Mosby, 1994.

HARING JI, LIND LJ. *Radiographic Interpretation for the Dental Hygienist.* Philadelphia: WB Saunders, 1993.

REVIEW QUESTIONS

1. Radiographically, an amalgam restoration appears radiolucent.

   a. True
   b. False

2. What normal radiographic anatomical landmark often mimics a periapical lesion in the area of the apices of the mandibular premolars?

   a. Lingual foramen
   b. Mandibular canal
   c. Mental foramen
   d. Genial tubercles

3. A large radiolucency in the area of an edentulous space in the maxillary molar region may represent

   a. pneumatized sinus.
   b. malar process.
   c. incisive foramen.
   d. hamulus.

4. The most common area(s) for supernumerary teeth is (are)

   a. between the maxillary central incisors.
   b. below the mandibular premolars.

    c. behind the third molars.

    d. All of the above

5. Which teeth are most likely to show signs of microdontia?

    a. Central incisors

    b. Maxillary third molars

    c. Mandibular canines

    d. Maxillary canines

6. Occlusal caries can be seen radiographically before they can be detected clinically.

    a. True

    b. False

7. Cervical burnout is often mistaken radiographically for cemental caries.

    a. True

    b. False

8. Horizontal bone loss involves the mesial or distal level of the crestal bone.

    a. True

    b. False

9. Common signs of recent trauma include

    a. teeth malaligned or displaced.

    b. radiolucent fracture lines.

    c. periapical lesions.

    d. a and b only

10. Radiographically, benign lesions appear well defined and well marginated, with an even, regular shape.

    a. True

    b. False

Radiographic Imaging for the Dental Team,
by Sally Mauriello. J.B. Lippincott Company,
Philadelphia © 1995.

17

Quality Assurance in Dental Radiology

Upon the completion of this chapter, the student should be able to:

1. Define quality assurance.

2. Propose a quality assurance program.

3. Differentiate between quality assurance and quality control.

4. Discuss the American Academy of Oral and Maxillofacial Radiology Quality Assurance Recommendations.

5. Explain the rationale for performing machine tests and checking performance function.

6. Sketch a plan for performing quality assurance in the dental office.

Quality assurance in dental radiology is a comprehensive concept that comprises all of the management practices instituted by the dentist to assure that every imaging procedure is necessary and appropriate to the clinical problem; the images generated contain information critical to the solution of the problem; the recorded information is correctly interpreted; and the examinations result in the lowest possible radiation exposure, cost, and inconvenience to the patient.

Quality assurance represents the highest medical/dental ethical practice and should be every practitioner's goal. An important component of quality assurance is quality control, which is the task/s required to ensure that the equipment being used is working safely and accurately. Quality control minimizes risk, discomfort, cost, and radiation exposure to patients.

The production of high-quality images largely depends on accurate machine calibration and optimum film processing. Dental radiation units must be calibrated, or "tuned up," regularly to ensure their safe operation. In addition, chemical solutions must be monitored on a regular basis, because their stability is also vital to image production. When equipment is properly monitored, the source of faulty images can be more easily isolated, resulting in a safer and more manageable environment.

HISTORY

Several programs have contributed to the improvement of quality assurance in dental radiology. The first was the Surpak program that began in 1961. This program aided in the screening of gross defects in filtration and collimation of large numbers of radiographic installations. After identifying machines lacking sufficient filtration and collimation, the Division of Radiological Health sent corrective devices, such as aluminum disks and lead washers, to dentists to bring their machines into compliance with established standards. The program ended in 1965. The X-ray Exposure Studies (XES) of 1964 and 1970 followed the Surpak program by documenting continuing improvements in collimation and filtration.

In 1972 the Nationwide Evaluation of X-ray Trends (NEXT) program was initiated and coordinated nationally by the Bureau of Radiological Health. Participating state radiation control agencies measured x-ray output using a standardized field survey technique. Data from 1973 to 1976 indicated that the mean skin exposure for posterior bitewing radiographs was 430.00 mR, and the mean exposure for periapical radiographs was 470.00 mR. However exposures ranged from 75 mR to 7000 mR.

In 1972 and 1973, the Bureau of Radiological Health in Nashville, Tennessee, conducted the Nashville Program, which tested the feasibility of using an educational approach for voluntary improvement of dental radiographic practices. Each participating office was visited for three purposes: to obtain data detailing causes of unnecessary exposure, to recommend changes, and to obtain data on the changes.

This successful program was the impetus for the Dental Exposure Normalization Technique (DENT). The DENT was developed to identify dental x-ray facilities where patient exposure fell outside an accepted range. The program consisted of screening, detection, demonstration, and correction phases; it also identified and surveyed new x-ray machines. Data from the first phase of DENT showed that about 40 percent of the dental x-ray units surveyed exceeded the recommended exposure ranges. Much of the overexposure was caused by poor darkroom practices and inadequate equipment. In many cases, film was overexposed to compensate for deficiencies in processing–a practice still seen today. After the correction phase, the exposure was reduced by an average of 200 mR per film.

Quality Assurance Today

All x-ray machines manufactured after 1974 must meet federal government equipment safety specifications. These include minimum filtration, accuracy and reproducibility of milliamperage, timing mechanism, and kilovoltage. In addition, all x-ray equipment, regardless of date of manufacture, is subject to state x-ray equipment regulations. A new program, the 1993 Nationwide Evaluation of X-ray Trends (NEXT), has begun to formally look at areas of dental radiography not previously addressed, such as cephalometric exposures, the number of intraoral, cephalometric and panoramic units in use, step, kVp measurements, and **spatial resolution.** Although a good surveillance mechanism does provide some idea of how equipment functions, it does not offer a real picture of image quality. Recent studies have consistently shown that less than desirable image quality is present in dental radiographs. The literature is replete with studies that consistently point to the same problems. Image quality in dental radiology lags because of a lack of quality control in processing, operator performance, and lack of machine calibration.

RECOMMENDATIONS FOR QUALITY CONTROL

In 1983, at the request of the American Dental Association, the American Academy of Dental Radiology (now the American Academy of Oral and Maxillofacial Radiology) made recommendations for quality assurance in dental radiology. These recommendations called for establishing maintenance and quality assurance monitoring procedures for dental radiology facilities. The recommendations are based on the facilities' size and workload as determined using the point system shown in Table 17-1. Once a facility has been staged, different levels of recommendations apply as listed in the following outlines.

Stage I Dental Practice

It is recommended that facilities qualifying as Stage I use the following program:

1. Reference films

2. Retake log

3. Monthly check of viewboxes

4. Yearly test of the x-ray generator

5. A monthly darkroom assessment

6. Daily visual monitoring of processing

TABLE 17-1
Method to determine the stage of a faculty using the point system

		Points
A. An evaluation of facilities, film processing, and workload		
1. Radiology facilities: equipment and techniques		
Intraoral radiography only (periapical, bitewing)		1
Intraoral and panoramic radiography		3
Intraoral, panoramic, and extraoral skull views		7
2. Film processing method		
Manual (time–temperature development)		1
Automatic development		3
3. Radiographic workload (average number of films per week)		
Under 100 films per week		1
100 to 300 films per week		3
Over 300 films per week		6
B. Recommended monitoring level of quality assurance program (total point value of 1, 2, and 3 above)		
Less than 8 points: Stage 1 dental practice		
8 to 11 points: Stage 2 dental practice		
12 or more points: Stage 3 dental practice		

Adapted from The American Academy of Oral and Maxillofacial Radiology, "Recommendations for Quality Assurance in Dental Radiography."

Stage II Dental Practice

It is recommended that facilities qualifying as Stage II use all Stage I recommendations plus the following:

1. Daily assessment of film development
2. Monthly check of cassettes and intensifying screens

Stage III Dental Practice

It is recommended that facilities qualifying as Stage III use Stage II recommendations in addition to sensitometry and an increased level of effort in administration.

ESTABLISHING A BASELINE FOR QUALITY ASSURANCE

Before a quality assurance program is initiated all systems should be checked and standardized to ensure that they are functioning at the level specified by the manufacturer. In addition, everyone involved should agree that the goal of the quality assurance program is to keep all systems consistently functioning at an optimum level and to intervene before patient services are detrimentally affected. The following systems should be standardized as part of the program:

1. Designate someone to be responsible for overseeing the program.
2. Establish the integrity of the x-ray systems to include the calibration of **kilovoltage,** milliamperage, timer, source to image distance, **half-value layer,** beam diameter and beam alignment, and exposure output.
3. Establish the proper storage and handling of films, screens, and chemicals.
4. Establish processing procedures to include the use of time–temperature development, replenishment, and maintenance schedules.
5. Establish safelighting.
6. Formulate technique charts.
7. Establish a retake log.
8. Establish film standards (reference films) and the maintenance of viewboxes.
9. Create a mechanism for continuing and inservice education.

10. Use recommended selection criteria for the prescription of radiographic exams.

Each of these systems is discussed in detail below.

Assigning Responsibility

Quality assurance in dental radiology reflects concern for patients and is indicative of high-quality care. An individual who has the skills and interest should be assigned the task of monitoring quality assurance in the office. This individual should be able to coordinate all the tasks involved in carrying out the plan and be given the time to complete the duties required to fulfill the program. Assigning responsibility to an individual promotes accountability and creates a contact for resolving problems.

Establishing the Integrity of X-Ray Systems

New x-ray equipment requires calibration upon installation and regular calibration thereafter. Accurate calibration promotes the consistency of equipment performance, and more importantly, reduces radiographic retakes because of equipment malfunctions. X-ray machines should be able to reproduce exposures with a reasonable percentage of accuracy. Properly calibrated units and optimum processing practices should result in exposures falling within the acceptable ranges for operating kilovoltages as recommended by the U.S. Department of Health and Human Services (Figure 17-1). For example, a facility using E speed film and 70 kilovolts should be using exposures between 125 and 165 mR. A figure higher or lower than this range warrants checking the systems for underexposure or overexposure of images. The **National Council on Radiation Protection and Measurements** and the American Academy of Oral and Maxillofacial Radiology recommend the following annual checks for x-ray systems:

1. Kilovoltage (kVp). Peak electrical potential across the x-ray tube affects the radiation intensity reaching the film. A variation of 2 or 3 kVp will measurably affect patient dose and radiographic density. However, to see a change in contrast, a variation of 4 to 5 kVp is necessary. Of the many methods available to evaluate kilovoltage calibration, the simplest is the use of a kilovoltage meter. This method is noninvasive and only requires a few minutes (see Figure 17-2). The test checks for the relationship between the kilovoltage selected on the generator console and the actually obtained kVp.

2. Milliampere-second (mA). Exposure output varies in direct proportion to the milliamperage. Different combinations of mA and exposure times produce the same mAs. For example, 15 mA and 30 im-

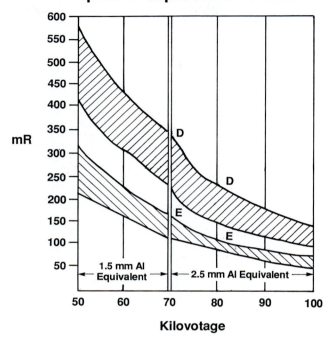

FIGURE 17-1 Recommendations for acceptable exposures (U.S. Department of Health and Human Services).

pulses produces the same mAs as 10 mA and 45 impulses. This is called exposure linearity. Checking exposure linearity allows inspection of the milliamperage. This is an indirect evaluation of the mA values. For units using impulses, the **mAi** (milliamperage impulses) value is kept constant, for example, at 15 mA, 30 impulses and 10 mA, 45 impulses, both of which result in 450 mAi. This test could be performed using an **aluminum step wedge.** The step wedge is imaged using two different mA and time settings, while maintaining the same mAs or mAi. The resulting images are compared. If the corresponding steps in each pattern appear to be of the same density, the mA/s are operating satisfactorily (see Figure 17-3). If the densities of the corresponding steps vary by more than 2 steps, the milliamperages should be adjusted. Machines with a single mA station must be checked invasively and this should be done by a qualified serviceperson.

3. Exposure Control (Timer). Defective timers may cause film **overexposure** or **underexposure.** The simplest way to check for timer accuracy is by using a spinning top, which consists of a disk with a hole

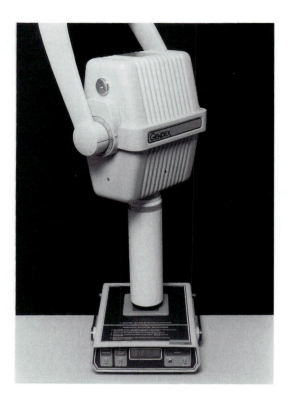

FIGURE 17-2 Setup for testing kilovoltage using kVp meter.

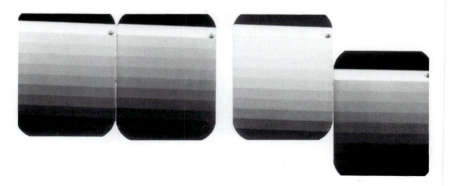

FIGURE 17-3 The set of radiographs on the left were exposed on a unit whose milliamperages were reciprocating. The set on the right demonstrate results from a faulty unit.

in it (Figure 17-4). This test is effective for checking any single-phase radiographic unit. The American Association of Physicists in Medicine recommend the following criteria for the evaluating timers.

- 0 - ¼ sec (0–15 impulses) ±1 density

- ¼ - ½ sec (15–30 impulses) ±2 density

- > ½ sec (>30 impulses) ±5% of set time

Other alternative methods for checking the timer mechanism include the use of a synchronous spinning top and pulse counters.

   4. Establishing the source-to-image distance. The source-to-image distance is determined in part by the length of the cone. The guidelines for machines operated at 50 kVp or less require a 4-inch or longer PID; above 50 kVp, a 7-inch or longer PID.

   5. Half-value layer (HVL). Filtration reduces most low energy x-rays and is perhaps the most important patient protection feature of the x-ray unit. Because measuring filtration directly is not always possible, a measure of the HVL provides a useful index of filtration (Table 17-2). The HVL is the amount of thickness of any material (aluminum is used in radiology) that is required to reduce the exposure to one-half of its original value. The HVL may be measured using aluminum attenuators (filters) of high purity and a **dosimeter.** The HVL is measured at the kilovoltage for which the filtration is being investigated. For example, an exposure is made using a combination of kVp, mA, and time that produces a reading of 300 mR. Repeated exposures are then made placing aluminum attenuating sheets in front of the beam. Each time a sheet of aluminum is added, a dosimeter reading is taken, until the output of the x-ray intensity has been reduced to half its original value—in this case, 150 mR. The amount of aluminum used is the HVL.

   6. Beam diameter and beam alignment determination. This test is important because a great deal of radiation can be delivered to the patient if the field size is too large or the system is misaligned. If the source to skin distance (SSD) is 18 centimeters (6 inches) or more, the x-ray field at the SSD shall be containable in a circle having a diameter of no more than 7 centimeters (2.75 inches). As shown in Figure 17-5, this can be verified by imaging either four no. 2 dental films in the form of a cross or by using a film large enough to cover the radiation field. If the exposed area is greater than 2.75 inches in diameter, the collimator opening is too large and should be replaced. If the circumference or shape of the exposed area is different than the shape of the collimator, then the collimator or a component of the tube head may be misaligned.

   7. Exposure output and exposure reproducibility. Exposure factors

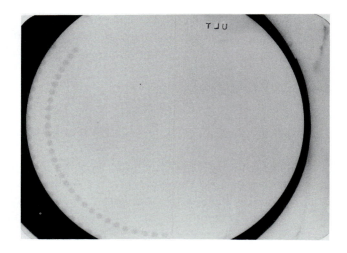

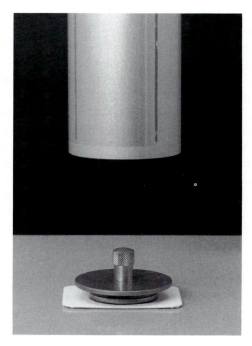

FIGURE 17-4 Setup for checking the timer using a spinning top and results from testing the 30 impulse setting.

on a per film basis should fall within acceptable dose ranges and should be reproducible if all or any of the factors are changed and then returned to the previous value. A radiation dosimeter is required to check exposure output and reproducibility. One method is to make a series of 5 exposures at the same technique while moving the technique controls

TABLE 17-2
Minimum half-value layer values

kVp	Minimum HVL (Millimeters of Aluminum)
50–70	1.5
80	2.3
90	2.5

between exposures and resetting them to the same technique. The average of the readings is indicative of the output and if the readings are within ±10 percent of each other, the exposure is considered reproducible.

Establishing Storage Conditions and Handling of Films and Screens

Unexposed and unprocessed film should be kept in a cool, dry place. High temperatures are known to increase the sensitization of the film emulsion, causing the production of **fog** and the loss of contrast. Ideally, film should be stored at temperatures between 50 and 70°F at 30 to 50 percent relative humidity. Extraoral film boxes should be stored on edge to prevent creating pressure artifacts. All film should be used before the expiration date. The film with the nearest expiration date should be used first. Chemicals should also be stored in a cool dry place at between 40 and 80°F. When the manufacturer's recommendations for storage are followed, chemicals should maintain their proper activity and a shelf life of two years. Film should be handled by the edges, and always with clean hands. Avoid touching the emulsion surface of films, because this may induce unwanted artifacts. The same applies to screens—avoid touching or bending them. A fingernail mark will permanently damage the screen. Screens should be cleaned and inspected at least once a month, following the recommendations of the manufacturer. There are commercially available cleaning agents, but a mild soap and water solution is highly effective. After cleaning allow the screen to dry and apply an antistatic solution to the surface of the screen. This can be done by spraying the antistatic solution on to gauze and then applying it to the screen.

Processing Monitoring

Monitoring film processing is one of the most important aspects of quality assurance. The need to adhere to the manufacturer's specifications and guidelines for processor operation cannot be overemphasized.

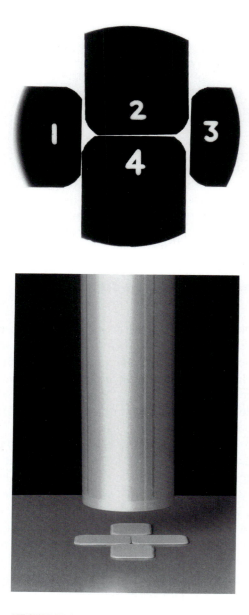

FIGURE 17-5 Setup for performing image diameter test using 4 films and the results of the test.

Tables 17-3 and 17-4 depict the appropriate combinations of time and temperature which, when used as indicated, contribute to the production of high-quality images. A film that is properly processed exhibits high quality and maintains archival properties. Archival quality is important because it allows the practitioner to compare radiographic im-

TABLE 17-3
Time–temperature recommendations for manual processing

Develop		Rinse	Fix	Wash
68°F (20°C)	5 min			
70°F (21°C)	4½ min	30 sec	2–4	10 min
72°F (22°C)	4 min	agitate	min	
76°F (24.5°C)	3 min	continuously		
80°F (26.5°C)	2½ min			

ages exposed at different times. Although the practice of sight development still exists, this practice should be discontinued, because it does not make a positive contribution to consistency in image production nor to the archival quality of the film. All processors should have a maintenance schedule. Included in the schedule should be cleaning, **replenishing,** changing of solutions, start up and shut down procedures, and frequency for testing solutions. The following guidelines are recommended for processor maintenance:

■ Clean processor and replace solutions at regular intervals. Average time periods are every 10 working days for manual processors and every 20 working days for automatic processors. The recommendations only apply if the proper amount of replenishment is done. Replenishment aids in maintaining the chemical activity of the solutions; lack of replenishment results in the loss of concentration of the chemical activity of solutions. This translates into films of inconsistent quality, density, and contrast. The recommended replenishment values for automatic and manual processing are 8 ounces each of developer and fixer daily. Replenishment should be performed even when films are not processed. When a large volume of films is processed, consult the manufacturer's recommendation for the proper amount of replenishment.

TABLE 17-4
Time-temperature recommendations for automatic processing

Cycle for Developing, Fixing, Rinsing, and Drying	
4 Min	85°F (29.5°C)
4½ Min	83°F (28.5°C)
5½ Min	82°F (28°C)

- Tanks should be thoroughly cleaned at each solution change. Cleaning the tanks removes chemical deposits and any contaminants that may exist. Rinse everything thoroughly to remove any traces of soap or cleaner.

- On automatic processors, inspect rollers, gears, belts, chains, and the turning mechanism for signs of wear. Fix if appropriate.

- Always change developer and fixer solutions at the same time. To prevent contamination of the developer, fill the fixer tank first.

- Set the correct temperature and processing time. For optimum processing in automatic processing and other temperature and time combinations, consult your owner's manual.

Aeration and Daily Clean Up

At the end of each day, remove the main cover and the developer and fixer covers from the automatic processor to allow them to aerate. For manual processors this is not necessary. At start-up time in the morning, replenish solutions and run a "clean-up" film, such as the 8 x 10 Kodak Roller Transport "Clean-Up" Film, to remove any residual gelatin or dirt from the rollers.

Monitoring Methods

Sensitometry measures the response of film to exposure and development and is the preferred method for monitoring the activity of the processor. It requires the use of a sensitometer, a device that produces a simulated exposure and a densitometer, a device that measures the density of a film. The data obtained from the sensitometric film objectively allows the determination of malfunctions before they affect patient films. Sensitometry is used in hospitals, large medical offices, some dental schools, and some large practices. However, monitoring chemical activity of dental processors can be accomplished by the use of simpler tools and methods, such as the Dental Radiographic Normalizing and Monitoring Device, the dental quality control test tool, the Spectroline, and the film monitoring strip. The first three methods require exposure of a step wedge or filter that is used for comparison with standards that are provided with the tools. Based on the appearance of the test film, the operator either intervenes or establishes the proper operation of the processor. The last method, utilizing the film monitoring strip, requires preexposure of the number of films that are going to be used for monitoring purposes. The following method is recommended to prepare the required number of strips.

Expose about 20 number 2 periapical films individually, with a step wedge on top, using identical exposure conditions and the bitewing technique. Once the processor has been cleaned and new solutions put in place, turn the processor on and allow it to warm up. Process one of the preexposed strips and save the remaining 19 films in a cool, dry place. Inspect the processed film and select a density approximately in the middle of the film that should be used as the standard for monitoring purposes (Figure 17-6). On the second day, after replenishment has taken place, warm up the processor and process another prepared strip. Compare this film with the standard and verify that it does not differ from it by more than two steps (Figure 17-7). This procedure should be repeated daily, early in the morning. When the strip shows a deviation of more than two steps, check for malfunctions in the temperature regulation system, water temperature, replenishment rate (if automatic), variations in development time, contaminated solutions, frequency of solution changes, and even safelighting. If a problem is identified, correct the problem and run an additional strip to determine the results of the corrective action.

The Dental Aluminum Step Wedge

Step wedges may be made from aluminum foil or purchased directly from manufacturers. The dental aluminum step wedge may contain up to nine consecutive steps of increasing thickness. It is big enough to fit on a number 2 film and it serves multiple purposes. A radiograph of the wedge produces an image made up of multiple densities, with each density representing a different thickness of aluminum. The thickest step results in the most **radiopaque** image; the thinnest step results in the most **radiolucent** image, with several graded densities in between. Comparing the densities of the wedge on test films is very effective because one can detect density changes before they affect patient films. For example, the radiographs in Figure 17-7 differ from each other by two steps. The difference is determined by placing the image of radiograph 1 next to the image of radiograph 2 and aligning the densities until they match. To properly use the step wedge, assign a number to each step beginning with the lightest density and progressing to the

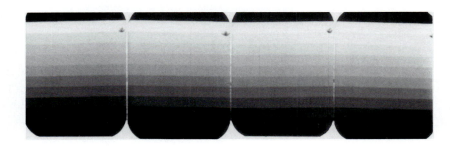

FIGURE 17-6 The strips next to each other demonstrate successful monitoring by matching densities with the chosen standard.

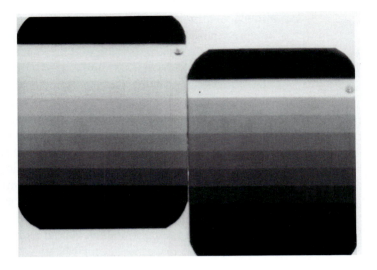

FIGURE 17-7 Two images of strips that differ from each other by two steps.

darkest. Number one would be the lightest density and number nine the darkest density. In Figure 17-8 the images match at steps five and seven. As such, images 1 and 2 differ from each other by 2 steps $(7 - 5 = 2)$.

Safelighting

Film processing should take place under safelighting conditions. Improper, or unsafe, lighting causes film fog and is detrimental to image

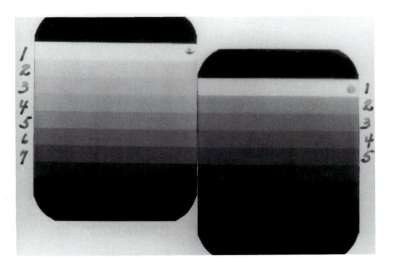

FIGURE 17-8 Images matching at steps 5 and 7.

quality. Elimination of light leaks and the selection of the correct type of **safelight** filter are important because not all films can be processed under the same lighting conditions. The use of a universal red filter, such as the Kodak GBX-2, provides safelighting conditions for both intraoral and extraoral films. Regardless of the filter used, safelighting conditions should be assessed every six months. The following method is recommended for this purpose. Expose a number 2 film to a very small amount of radiation, such as 10 mA, 2 impulses, 70 kVp. This is done because film is always more sensitive after it has been exposed, and one would only develop exposed films. Turn off all of the lights in the darkroom or insert your hands and the film in the daylight loader. Open up the film and place a coin on it and wait for two minutes. After the two minutes have elapsed, process the film and then examine it. An image of the coin on the film is indicative of unsafe safelighting conditions (Figure 17-9). If this occurs, check for faded filters and higher than recommended wattage lightbulbs. Wattage should not exceed 15. Safelights do fade with age and should be replaced every few years. As a rule of thumb, if a safelight is on for 12 hours a day, the filter should be replaced every 2 years.

Formulate Technique Charts

Technique charts should be posted above all x-ray controls. The chart should include the projection, the kilovoltage, the milliamperage, the exposure time, film speed, and the patient's size. Figure 17-10 depicts a technique chart that was formulated to consistently provide the same

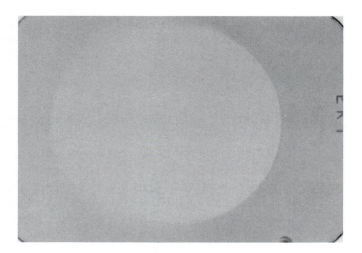

FIGURE 17-9 Safelight test demonstrating the poor condition of the filter. Notice image of coin.

TECHNICS CHART: GENDEX (GE) 1000

PROJECTION	mA	kVp	TIME in SECONDS	FILM TYPE
ANTERIOR	15	70	21/60	E
PREMOLAR	15	70	24/60	E
MOLAR	15	75	24/60	E
BITEWING	15	75	30/60	D
OCCLUSAL	15	75	30/60	D

For **Large** Patients Add 5 Killovolts (kVP)
For Small Patients Reduce 5 Killovolts (kVP)

FIGURE 17-10   Technique chart.

contrast and density ranges in a facility. Even with technique charts, special conditions may require that the radiographer adapt the technique to a given situation. Situations that require changes in technical factors may be dictated by the patient's condition—for example, a patient unable to hold still, or a pathological condition that causes bone density to increase. Guidelines should be provided for changing technical factors in special conditions. This will not only help the technologist, but insure that patients are receiving the best care available. If possible, produce a series of phantom test images and select the best image of the group. Perform a clinical trial examination, and, if acceptable, implement the technique. Establish an on-going, fine-tuning system. Whenever the technique chart produces unacceptable images and the cause is not obvious, perform quality control tests to isolate the problem. To minimize radiation exposure to patients, consider using E speed film, rectangular collimation, kilovoltages no lower than 60, and rare earth screens for panoramic and extraoral radiography.

Retake Log

One of the goals of a quality assurance program is to reduce the number of retakes on patients. A retake log will serve to monitor not only the number of retakes but the reason(s) for the retakes. By looking at a history of retakes, individuals in charge of quality assurance can more easily identify areas that may require improvement or corrective action. For example, if a retake log consistently reveals that most film retakes are the result of poor processing conditions, then more attention needs to be given to processing quality control. If, on the other hand, many retakes result from operator error, then inservice or continuing education may be necessary. Figure 17-11 shows a sample log, which is really a short inventory list of the most common imaging errors. A

UNC-SCHOOL OF DENTISTRY SECTION OF ORAL RADIOLOGY
RETAKE LOG

MONTH_____YEAR_____

Date					
	Mon	**Tues**	**Wed**	**Thurs**	**Fri**
Pt. Positioning					
Movement					
Dark Film					
Light film					
Double exposure					
Fogged film					
Processing error					
Mechanical					
Packet placement					
Exposed backwards					
Horizontal angulation					
Vertical angulation					
Cone cut (cc)/ Precision cut (pc)					
Artifact					
Miscellaneous					
Total					

FIGURE 17-11 Sample of retake log for keeping track of types and number of errors.

careful analysis of the number of retakes can result in a significant reduction in exposure dose, radiographer's time, effort, and supply costs.

Establishing Film Standards

The American Academy of Maxillofacial Radiology recommends the use of reference films, which are radiographs of diagnostic quality chosen by the person interpreting the images. Reference films represent the desired radiographic quality, including the positioning, density, and contrast. These radiographs serve as a standard and should be used as a reminder of the diagnostic quality expected.

Inservice Education

Inservice education should be a component of quality assurance. The retake log is a good source for obtaining ideas for review. If, for example, a pattern of retakes is the result of head malposition in panoramic radiographs, then an inservice on proper head positioning, anatomical landmarks, and patient instructions is appropriate. Blind film reviews, which consist of random examinations of radiographic studies, should also be performed on a regular basis. Technical merit, diagnostic quality, and appropriateness of the exam should be checked. This type of activity presents many opportunities for learning and improving technical proficiency. A resource library with references, videotapes, slides, and professional literature will also provide a means for enhancing skills. Employees should be encouraged to attend professional meetings, seminars, subscribe to professional journals, and even attend classes to further their knowledge.

Use of Selection Criteria

The use of selection criteria is a sound, rational method for prescribing radiographs on patients. By no means should radiographic examinations be performed either on a routine basis or for administrative purposes. Radiographic examinations should be determined following a thorough clinical exam and using the Food and Drug Administration Guidelines for prescribing dental radiographs.

STATE INSPECTIONS

Many states have adopted their own regulations for the use and operation of ionizing producing equipment. To find out about these regulations, contact the Department of Health and Human Resources in your state. Regulations may range from requiring yearly inspections to a simple annual registration. If practitioners fail to comply with state regulatory guidelines, they may face stiff penalties. In certain cases, they may not be allowed to use the equipment until it is brought into compliance. It is the responsibility of the dentist to properly register all x-ray equipment and to meet any state and federal installation guidelines.

RECORDS

All facilities operating x-ray equipment should maintain records of machine purchases, registrations, inspections, maintenance, and quality control procedures. Records help identify the frequency of machine

UNC-School of Dentistry Section of Oral Radiology
Processor Quality Control Chart

Processor									Location								Month/year							
Date																									
Day of wk	M	T	W	Th	F	M	T	W	Th	F	M	T	W	Th	F	M	T	W	Th	F	M	T	W	Th	F
Major clean up																									
New chemistry																									
Replenishment																									
Dev Temp																									
86																									
85																									
84.5																									
84																									
83																									
82																									
Density (step#)																									
7																									
6																									
5																									
4																									
3																									
2																									
1																									

FIGURE 17-12 Sample form used for documenting quality control tests on processors.

breakdowns, the level of machine functioning, the quality of care imparted at a facility, and evidence that care is being taken to ensure that a facility is operating according to agreed standards. Figure 17-12 displays a sample of a record that may be utilized to document procedures performed for quality control purposes. Records should also show that operators are properly credentialed in the use and operation of radiographic equipment.

SUMMARY

Quality assurance, quality control, and quality improvement result in higher quality service. Monitoring the activities associated with the operation and delivery of radiology services benefits not only the patient but also those involved in providing care. Significant improvements can result from careful monitoring of x-ray systems, processing, exposures, and operator performance. With today's technical advances and the new information generated in maxillofacial radiology, continuing education is extremely important. Dental radiographers must be able to answer patients' questions about radiation concerns. Table 17-5 summarizes the recommended tests and their frequency of performance. To further your knowledge, contact the manufacturer of your x-ray film or equipment. These companies often offer literature and/or

TABLE 17-5
Summary of quality control recommendations

General	Reference films
	Retake log
	Use thyroid shields and lead aprons
	Use technique charts
	Use rectangular collimation
	Use the fastest film speed and screens available
Daily	Clean darkroom
	Perform processor quality control
Monthly	Clean screens and cassettes
	Check viewing conditions and viewboxes
	Perform safelight test
Yearly	Check stability of tube head
	kVp accuracy
	mA accuracy
	Timer accuracy
	Half value layer
	Beam alignment and field size diameter
	Representative skin exposure

Adapted from The American Academy of Oral and Maxillofacial Radiology, "Recommendations for Quality Assurance in Dental Radiology."

technical assistance to help the consumer establish a quality control program. Professionals who concentrate in maxillofacial radiology in dental schools and dental auxiliary programs in universities, community colleges, and technical schools are also good resources.

BIBLIOGRAPHY

BUSHONG SC. *Radiologic Science for the Technologists,* 5th ed. St. Louis: CV Mosby, 1993.

GRAY JE, WINKLER NT, STEARS J, FRANK ED. *Quality Control in Diagnostic Imaging.* Baltimore: University Park Press, 1983.

NATIONAL COUNCIL ON RADIATION PROTECTION AND MEASUREMENTS, *Quality Assurance for Diagnostic Imaging Equipment.* Report No. 99, Bethesda, MD, 1988.

PLATIN E, MATTESON SR. *Quality Assurance for Dental Imaging.* Rochester, NY: Eastman Kodak, 1992.

REVIEW QUESTIONS

1. According to the recommendations of the Department of Health and Human Services, a facility using D speed film and 75 kilovolts should be using exposures in the range of

   a. 120–170 mR.
   b. 100–140 mR.
   c. 240–350 mR.
   d. 170–260 mR.

2. An x-ray machine operated at 70 kilovolts requires a PID of at least

   a. 4 inches.
   b. 7 inches.
   c. 12 inches.
   d. 16 inches.

3. Which x-ray field diameter is acceptable if the source to skin distance is 12 inches?

   a. 2.60
   b. 2.75 inches
   c. 2.50 inches
   d. Only two of the above
   e. All of the above

4. Replenishment of developer and fixer are recommended daily because replenishment
   I.   helps maintain the concentration of solutions.
   II. results in consistent quality.
   III. prevents the loss of contrast resulting from "bad" solutions.
   IV. accelerates film development.

   a. I, II, and III
   b. I, II, and IV only
   c. II, III, and IV only
   d. I, II, III, and IV

5. Which parameters should be inspected if a film monitoring strip differs by more than two steps from the standard?
   I.   Temperature regulating system
   II. Rate of replenishment
   III. Exposure conditions
   IV. Integrity of solutions

   a. I, II, and III only
   b. I, II, and IV only
   c. II, III, and IV only
   d. I, II, III, and IV

6. Which of the following is *not* considered an advantage of keeping a retake log?

   a. Provides clues for the source of most retakes
   b. Serves as a guide for continuing education topics
   c. Provides some measure of the operators competence
   d. Reduces the amount of paperwork

7. Design a quality assurance program for your facility using the American Academy of Maxillofacial Radiology guidelines.

Radiographic Imaging for the Dental Team,
by Sally Mauriello. J.B. Lippincott Company,
Philadelphia © 1995.

18

Pitfalls in
Dental Imaging

Upon the completion of this chapter, the student should be able to:

1. Understand the basic pitfalls in dental imaging.

2. Differentiate between exposure, processing, handling, and storage pitfalls.

3. Detect causes responsible for basic imaging pitfalls.

4. Solve basic imaging pitfalls.

The quality of a radiograph depends on multiple variables that must work together to make a positive contribution to the final image. Figure 18-1 illustrates most of the factors that are involved in this process. Quality improvement in dental imaging is partially dependent on the ability of the radiographer to solve problems that arise from poor image production. When one of the variables fails to perform at an optimum level, the results are usually detrimental and are reflected in the final image.

Chapter 17 established that a quality assurance program can drastically reduce the chances of creating conditions that result in image degradation. This is accomplished by the periodic assessment of equipment function and a series of checks performed on a regular basis. The decision tree in Figure 18-2 suggests a method for identifying problems that may occur during image production.

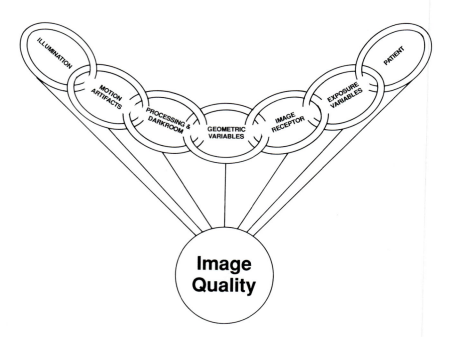

FIGURE 18-1 Variables involved in image production. Notice how failure of only one system weakens the entire system.

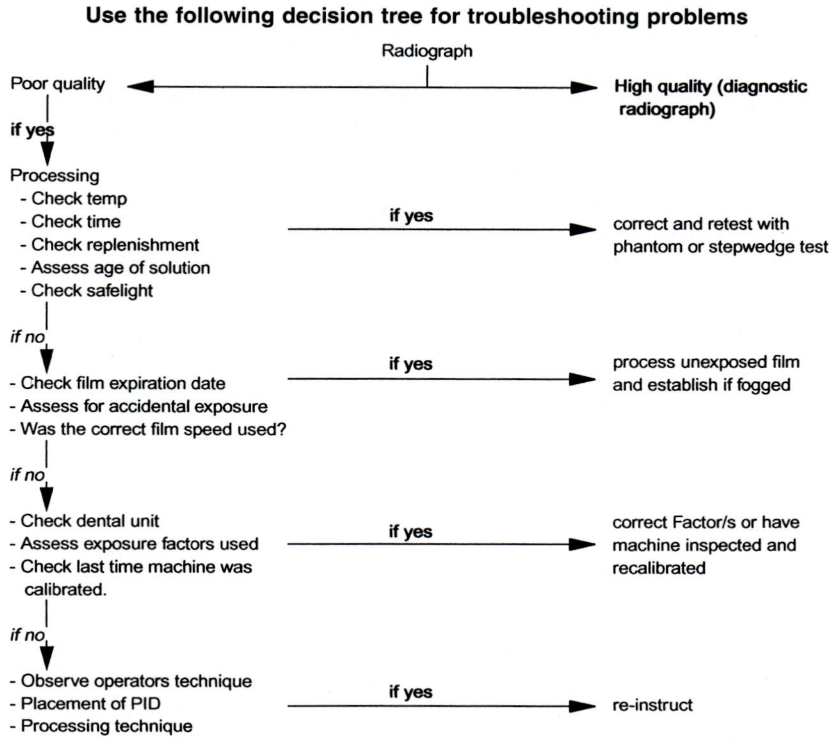

Use the following decision tree for troubleshooting problems

Radiograph

Poor quality ◄────────────────────────► High quality (diagnostic radiograph)

if yes

▼

Processing
  - Check temp
  - Check time ──────── *if yes* ────────► correct and retest with phantom or stepwedge test
  - Check replenishment
  - Assess age of solution
  - Check safelight

if no

▼

  - Check film expiration date ──────── *if yes* ────────► process unexposed film and establish if fogged
  - Assess for accidental exposure
  - Was the correct film speed used?

if no

▼

  - Check dental unit
  - Assess exposure factors used ──────── *if yes* ────────► correct Factor/s or have machine inspected and recalibrated
  - Check last time machine was calibrated.

if no

▼

  - Observe operators technique
  - Placement of PID ──────── *if yes* ────────► re-instruct
  - Processing technique

FIGURE 18-2 The decision tree represents the progression suggested when identifying problems that occur during image production.

RADIOGRAPHIC PITFALLS

Radiographic pitfalls are those events that result in images of poor diagnostic quality. They may be divided into exposure pitfalls, processing pitfalls, handling pitfalls, storage pitfalls, and other pitfalls.

Exposure Pitfalls

These are generally related to improper exposure techniques. Figures 18-3 through 18-7 are representative of exposure pitfalls. To the right of each image are the probable cause(s) and recommended variables to check.

FIGURE 18-3 Blank film with no image resulting from having a faulty exposure switch.

PROBLEM: NO IMAGE

Probable Causes: Faulty generator, faulty exposure switch, switch not on, placement of film between teeth and cheek.

Action: Check machine, review proper film placement.

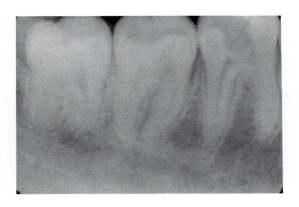

FIGURE 18-4 Light image resulting from incomplete exposure. The operator failed to keep exposure switch fully depressed, thereby delivering only a fraction of the radiation needed for the exam.

PROBLEM: LIGHT IMAGE

Probable Causes: Incomplete exposure (failure to depress the exposure switch for the entire time), faulty generator, not enough exposure (mA, kVp, time), too much distance, incorrect film speed, film exposed backwards.

Action: Check proper switch operation, check exposure factors and increase if necessary, check film speed.

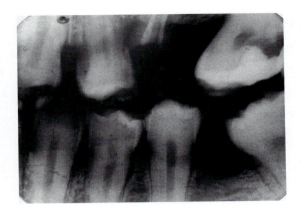

FIGURE 18-5 Dark image resulting from using incorrect film speed. The operator inadvertently used E speed film instead of D speed film.

PROBLEM: DARK IMAGE

Probable Causes: Faulty generator, too much exposure (mA, kVp, time), not enough distance, incorrect film speed.

Action: Check exposure factors and decrease if necessary, check film speed.

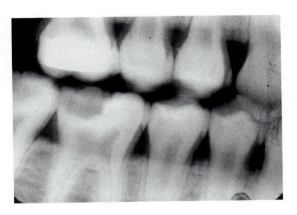

FIGURE 18-6 Radiograph of a right premolar bitewing in which the patient moved during the exposure.

PROBLEM: BLURRED IMAGE

Probable Causes: Patient motion, film motion.

Action: Give patient proper instructions not to move.

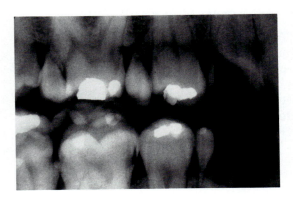

FIGURE 18-7 Radiograph of a film used twice—once to expose a premolar bitewing and once to expose a molar bitewing. Notice the multiple cusps in the molar area.

PROBLEM: DOUBLE IMAGE

Probable Causes: Double exposure, film movement during exposure.

Action: Organize workspace and after each exposure place film in paper cup to avoid mixing exposed and unexposed films.

Processing Pitfalls

Processing pitfalls usually occur from the use of improper development time and development temperature, from inadequate chemical activity, processor condition, and sloppy darkroom practices. Figures 18-8 through 18-13 illustrate common processing errors. To the right of the image are listed the probable causes and recommended functions to check.

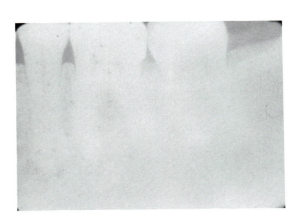

FIGURE 18-8 Light image resulting from film processed at low temperature. The developer temperature was 10 degrees lower than expected.

PROBLEM: LIGHT IMAGE

Probable Causes: Lack of mixing solutions to prevent stratification, temperature too low, development time too short, inactive solutions (too old), under- or no replenishment.

Action: Check thermostat, heating pad, development time, and replenishment frequency.

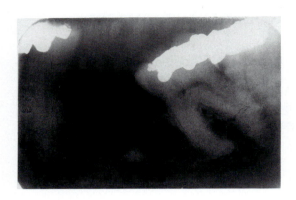

FIGURE 18-9 Dark image resulting from film processed in a unit whose thermostat had failed. The temperature was recorded 15 degrees higher than the normal setting.

PROBLEM: DARK IMAGE

Probable Causes: Temperature too high, development time too long, overreplenishment.

Action: Check thermostat, heating pad, development time, and replenishment frequency.

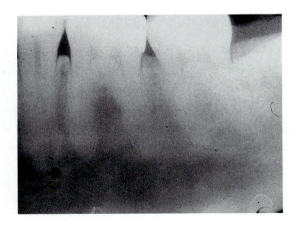

FIGURE 18-10 Brown-orange image resulting from a film that was not properly fixed or washed.

PROBLEM: BROWN IMAGE

Probable Causes: Oxidized developer, old developer, film not in fixer and wash long enough.

Action: Replenish or replace chemicals, check processing procedure.

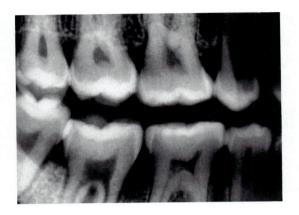

FIGURE 18-11 Although hard to appreciate, this radiograph was wet to the touch when it emerged from the processor. Inspection of the unit revealed that the dryer was malfunctioning.

PROBLEM: WET IMAGE

Probable Causes: Dryer not working, old fixer or lack of replenishment.

Action: Check dryer temperature, last time fixer was changed and change or replenish if necessary.

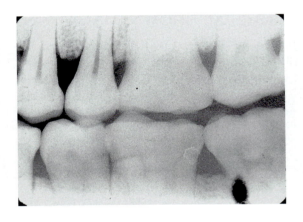

FIGURE 18-12 This image appears gray, washed out, and low in contrast. Close inspection of the processor revealed that the replenishment lines were clogged and the solutions had not been replenished for a few days.

PROBLEM: GRAY IMAGE

Probable Causes: Contaminated solutions, old solutions, lack of replenishment, improper washing after exposure to chemicals.

Action: Check replenishment frequency, last time solutions were replaced and change if necessary. Pour fixer first and then developer. When replenishing use caution not to contaminate developer with fixer.

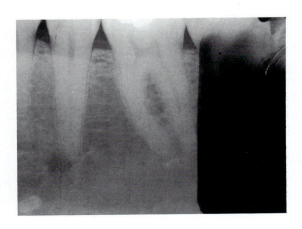

FIGURE 18-13 Radiograph demonstrating line of overlap that resulted when films were processed too close together. The first film was not given enough time to travel before the second film was fed through the machine.

PROBLEM: OVERLAPPING LINES

Probable Causes: Films were processed too close together, dirty rollers.

Action: Check processing technique.

Handling Pitfalls

These generally result from poor or rough handling of films. Figures 18-14 through 18-18 depict examples of artifacts produced by poor handling.

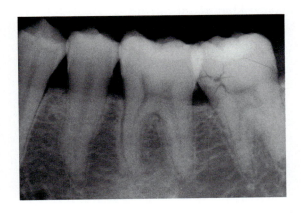

FIGURE 18-14 Radiograph demonstrating evidence of static electricity in the mesial of a mandibular molar.

PROBLEM: TREE-LIKE ARTIFACT

Probable Causes: Static electricity, static from clothing or carpet.

Action: Use antistatic solution in intensifying screens, install humidifier in processing room if necessary, stand on antistatic pad while processing, and open cassette slowly.

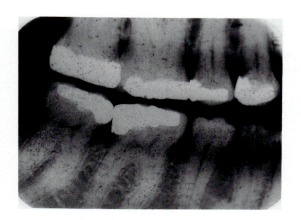

FIGURE 18-15 What appears to be dirt on this film actually turned out to be smudge static electricity. We were able to duplicate the artifact in the clinic during the winter while wearing a clinic gown and rubber gloves.

PROBLEM: SMUDGE STATIC

Probable Causes: Same as above. Impermeable materials used in new clinic attire have been known to be responsible for this type of artifact. It may be related to the high content of polyester in the clothes.

Action: Use antistatic fabric softener when drying clothes.

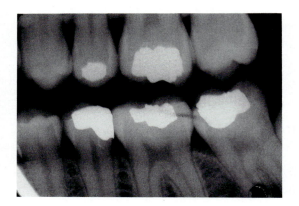

FIGURE 18-16 Radiograph displaying fingernail artifact on the distal and mesial of mandibular molars.

PROBLEM: CRESCENT OR HALF MOONS

Probable Causes: Rough handling of film, fingernail pressure, bending or creasing.

Action: Handle film gently.

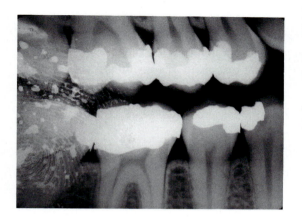

FIGURE 18-17 Radiograph displaying fingerprints resulting from handling the film with a moist hand containing fluoride.

PROBLEM: FINGERPRINT PATTERN

Probable Causes: Moist hands, touching film before processing.

Action: Wash and dry hands before processing films.

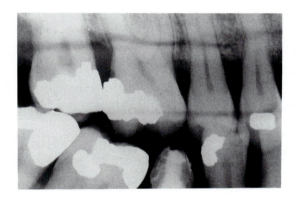

FIGURE 18-18 Bitewing radiograph showing black lines representative of sites where the film was severely bent.

PROBLEM: BLACK LINES

Probable Causes: Black horizontal lines across film.

Action: Do not bend film before or after exposure. Film should be handled gently without creasing it; if necessary roll film rather than bend to help fit the contour of the oral cavity.

Storage Pitfalls

Storage pitfalls result from improper storage of film—that is, storing film in a hot place with poor air circulation, lack of rotating film stock, and so on. Figure 18-19 depicts an image that resulted from poor film storage.

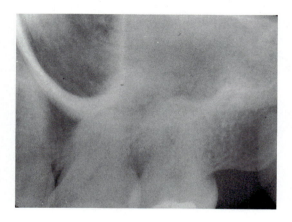

FIGURE 18-19 Low-contrast radiograph resulting in low-contrast film that was used eight months past the expiration date.

PROBLEM: LOW-CONTRAST IMAGE

Probable Causes: Storage temperature too high, high humidity, expired film.

Action: Store film in cool, dry place away from radiation sources. Use film before expiration date.

Other Pitfalls

Pitfalls that do not normally fall under any of the categories described above will be listed here. Figures 18-20 through 18-25 display a series of errors commonly found in periapical radiography.

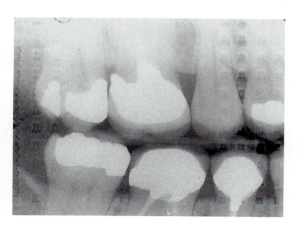

FIGURE 18-20 This bitewing radiograph shows the embossing pattern found in the foil. Notice that the film is also very light because the foil absorbed a high percentage of the primary x-rays.

PROBLEM: EMBOSSING PATTERN

Probable Cause: Film exposed backwards.

Action: This can be avoided by concentrating on the task and always making sure that the white portion of the film packet faces the x-ray source.

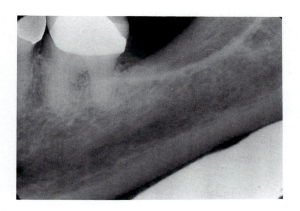

FIGURE 18-21   Molar periapical demonstrating radiopaque area at the inferior border of the mandible. This resulted from the thyroid shield being too loose around the neck and the vertical angulation too steep.

PROBLEM: RADIOPAQUE AREA

Probable Cause: Apron cut.

Action: Apron cuts occur when the thyroid shield is loose and intercepts the path of the beam. They are prevented by properly securing the shield around the patient's neck.

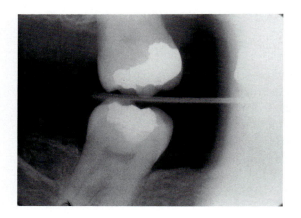

FIGURE 18-22   Bitewing radiograph showing radiopaque area with a circular border that resulted from improper beam centering.

PROBLEM: HALF-MOON SHAPED RADIOPAQUE AREA

Probable Cause: Cone cut.

Action: Properly center the x-ray beam to film.

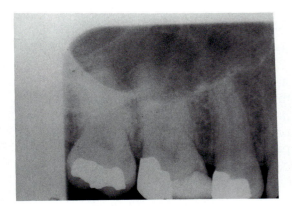

FIGURE 18-23 This maxillary periapical radiograph displays a rectangular radiopaque region on the distal and superior portions of the film. This resulted from not having the central ray perpendicular to the collimator face of the precision instrument.

PROBLEM: RECTANGULAR CLEAR AREA

Probable Cause: Collimator cuts.

Action: These are due to improper centering of beam when using precision instruments, XCP instruments with rectangular collimators, or rectangular PIDs. Cuts are horizontal, vertical, or both. They result when the beam is not properly aligned with the film or when XCP is improperly assembled.

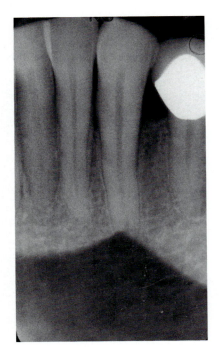

FIGURE 18-24 Black area on the inferior border of this lateral canine projection resulted from partial opening of the film packet in the presence of white light.

PROBLEM: BLACK AREA

Probable Cause: Film exposed to light.

Action: Blackened areas on films may occur from exposure to light. To prevent this from happening, only open film packets under safelight conditions. When processing with daylight loader, avoid exposure through sleeve.

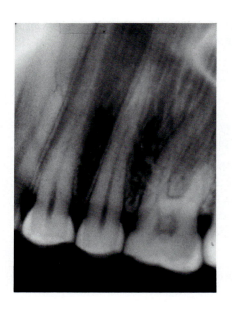

PROBLEM: DISTORTED ROOTS

Probable Cause: Bent film. This occurs when the film is bent during the exam.

Action: Avoid film bending by making sure there is enough clearance when patient occludes, or the film does not shift position when occlusion takes place. Use cotton rolls to stabilize bite block if necessary. However, the cotton roll should not be placed between the occlusal surface of the teeth of interest and the bite block, but rather between the bite block and the opposing teeth.

FIGURE 18-25   Periapical film showing severe distortion of the roots of the maxillary teeth due to film bending.

SUMMARY

Film errors can be reduced by establishing a quality assurance program and by carefully monitoring image production. Unusual artifacts and film problems should be documented; if possible, the films should be saved. They will serve as a guide for solving problems at a later time. In addition, discussion of radiographic pitfalls should be a part of inservice education. When problems persist, consult the technical sales representative, vendor, or call a university or community college that offers dental or dental auxiliary programs. Members of the faculty are often excellent resources.

BIBLIOGRAPHY

EASTMAN KODAK CO. *Successful Intraoral Radiography*. Rochester, NY, 1990.

MATTESON SR, WHALEY C, AND CRANDELL CE. *Dental Radiology (Dental Assisting Manual V)*. Chapel Hill; University of North Carolina Press, 1988.

PLATIN E, MATTESON SR. *Quality Control for Dental Imaging*. Rochester, NY: Eastman Kodak, 1992.

REVIEW QUESTIONS

1. Which of the following variables may be responsible for the production of light radiographs?

   I.   Kilovoltage too low
   II. Milliamperage too high
   III. Exposure time too long
   IV. Development time too short
   V.   Source to image distance too long

   a. I, II, and V only
   b. II, IV, and V only
   c. I, IV, and V only
   d. I, III, IV, and V

2. Which of the following methods is the most effective way to decrease the chances of static electricity production?

   a. Wearing clinic gowns made from polyester materials
   b. Increasing the level of humidification
   c. Installing a polyester rug under the processor feeding area
   d. Removing films quickly from cassettes

3. The use of outdated films may result in images that are

   a. gray.
   b. low in contrast.
   c. orange in color.
   d. a and b
   e. a, b, and c

4. Radiographic films that are not properly fixed

   I.   may turn orange-brown in color.
   II. emerge wet from the processor.
   III. lose archival quality.
   IV. show an increase in contrast.

   a. I, II, and III only
   b. I, II, and IV only
   c. II, III, and IV only
   d. I, II, III, and IV

5. Discuss the impact of a quality assurance program in the reduction of errors in dental radiography.

Radiographic Imaging for the Dental Team,
by Sally Mauriello. J.B. Lippincott Company,
Philadelphia © 1995.

19

Radiographic Administration

Upon the completion of this chapter, the student should be able to:

1. Describe the appropriate procedures for keeping accurate radiographic records.

2. Discuss legal issues that surround the exposure and use of radiographs.

3. Discuss the components necessary for developing policies on radiation use and infection control.

4. Understand the importance of continuing education.

In addition to being a competent radiographer, the clinician must be adept at developing, maintaining, and monitoring accurate records and policies pertaining to radiographic procedures. This would include accurate record-keeping, legal considerations, policies governing radiation use and infection control, and keeping abreast of current radiographic practice through continuing education. Well-kept dental records enhance communication between the patient and dental professional, defend against malpractice litigation, and document treatment rendered.

RECORD-KEEPING

Patient Record

Patient records are considered legal documents in a court of law and should be kept up-to-date with accurate information. Documentation is of the utmost importance. Records that clearly reflect the treatment rendered can also serve as a basis for communication among the patient, dental professionals, and third-party payors. Good record-keeping for radiologic purposes should include the following critical information.

All radiographic records should include the patient's name, social security number, and date of exposure. Entries should be made in ink and signed by the operator. The patient history should include both medical information and radiation therapy exposures. The purpose for exposing radiographs should also be stated, such as the detection of interproximal caries. A record of informed consent (patient's agreement for treatment) or refusal is a necessary component of risk management. The patient must be thoroughly informed or educated as to the need for dental radiographs, the benefits, the risks of exposure to ionizing radiation, and the consequences of not receiving dental treatment. The patient should have ample opportunity to ask questions or receive clarification on the information presented. Finally, the patient must clearly indicate acceptance or refusal of the treatment suggested. The conversation and patient response should be clearly documented in the permanent record and be signed by the patient. Treatment of minors requires signed approval for treatment from a parent or guardian. An area in the chart should also be allocated for the exposure history. This would include exposure dates, the number and type of films exposed (including retakes), and exposure amount (that is, mR).

Film Mounting

Film mounting is an essential component of accurate record-keeping. Obviously, an incorrectly mounted radiograph could result in extraction of the wrong tooth, thereby leaving the operator vulnerable to malpractice litigation. Therefore, the following steps should be used to prevent improper film mounting of a full series.

1. Place all films on the **viewbox** with the bump facing up (convex). Films mounted with this orientation will be viewed as though you are looking into the patient's mouth (Figure 19-1).

2. Separate the films based on projection type, that is, bitewing and periapicals (Figure 19-2).

3. Mount bitewings. The premolars should be located closest to the middle of the mount. If mounted correctly, a smile should be apparent due to the Curve of Spee (Figure 19-3).

4. Separate periapical projections based on anterior and posterior positions. These can be further separated based on maxillary and mandibular projections. Clues that may help to achieve this are the presence of sinuses and three-rooted teeth (Figure 19-4).

5. Begin to mount the periapicals using the bitewings as a guide. Restorations, bridges, and other landmarks can be used to make sure films are correctly positioned in the mount (Figure 19-5).

LEGAL ISSUES

The need to transfer radiographs may occur at some point in time; this raises the question of ownership. Although at one time radiographs

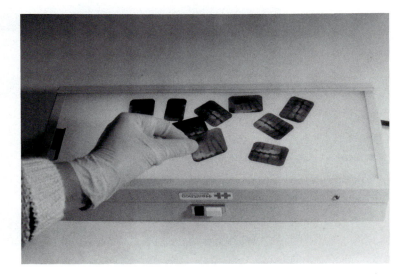

FIGURE 19-1 Radiographs are shown placed on the viewbox with the bump up (convex).

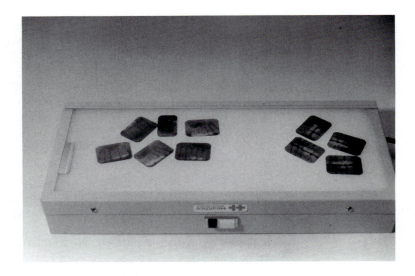

FIGURE 19-2 Radiographs are being sorted based on a bitewing or periapical projection.

were considered the property of the dentist, this is no longer an absolute condition. Because people move, patients must be allowed access to charts and radiographs. Copies of radiographs can be achieved by the use of double-packet film or by duplicating radiographs. Either is acceptable and the ability of the office to provide a copy for a small clerical fee is becoming a necessary service. Transferral of radiographs

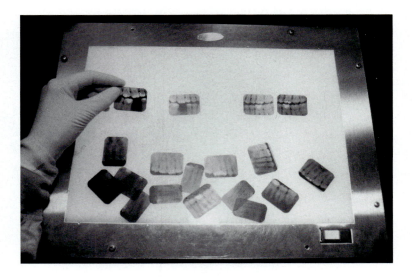

FIGURE 19-3 A set of bitewings demonstrating the Curve of Spee.

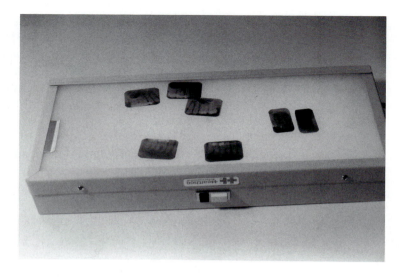

FIGURE 19-4 Radiographs are further sorted by anterior/posterior positions and maxillary/mandibular projections.

should be documented in the chart. Due to confidentiality, the patient must provide a written request for transfer of radiographs. This authorization is also necessary when supplying information to an insurance company. In the event that the dental practice is sold, the patient must still give permission for the transfer of records to a new dentist. Origi-

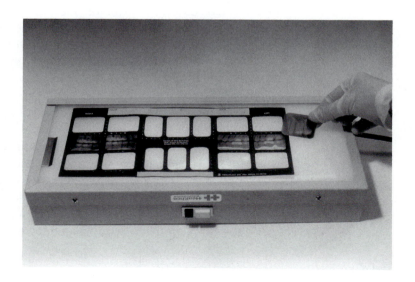

FIGURE 19-5 Use restorations in the bitewings to match periapical projections. Include date of exposure.

nal radiographs should remain in the patient chart and copies made for transfer. All records should be kept for at least ten years.

Negligence is the most common form of malpractice that patients wage against their dentist. Radiographically, this could result from the failure to take the needed projection or not referring to a radiograph that is available. Therefore, all films should be interpreted and used during dental treatment.

Radiographs are also used as evidence. In forensics, dental radiographs can be used for identification of a body. The radiographs are useful in identifying domestic violence (including child/elder abuse), documenting malpractice, and personal injury.

USE OF AN IONIZING RADIATION POLICY

Each dental office should develop a policy on the use of ionizing radiation that provides a guideline for both new and experienced office personnel. The policy should address equipment, processing, radiographic technique (including a retake policy), interpretation of the radiographic image, quality assurance, and protection of dental personnel.

Equipment

The film of choice should be the fastest speed available. Double-packet film is a good mechanism for providing duplicate information if a film copier is unavailable. In extraoral radiography, intensifying screens provide an excellent means for reducing the radiation dose to the patient. A long focal spot to film distance will enhance image clarity. Collimation of the beam to the size of the film will also enhance the image and reduce exposure to the patient. Various filter materials (that is, rare earth filters) can be used to improve the quality of the film and reduce patient dose. Lead aprons and thyroid collars should be worn for patient protection.

Federal and state agencies also monitor equipment to some degree. The Center for Devices and Radiological Health of the Food and Drug Administration requires that manufacturers of x-ray equipment include several safety features. State agencies inspect dental x-ray machines on a regular basis. The date of purchase of each piece of equipment should be kept in a log with dates that the equipment is inspected.

Intraoral Procedure

The radiographic technique of choice should use the paralleling principles, collimate the beam to the size of the film, and align the beam to the film with a position-indicating device and film holder. A kVp that will produce a good range of densities for dental structures should be employed. This is usually in the range from 70 to 90 for intraoral radiography. The exposure time should be short to help decrease the possibility of movement on the film. Processing should follow the appropriate time/temperature method. Under no circumstance should films be overexposed so that films can be underdeveloped and thus, decrease the processing time.

Interpretation of Image

The best radiographic technique will not reveal all of the diagnostic information if the films are not viewed properly. Care should be taken to use conditions that will maximize the display of information. Primarily, radiographs should never be held up to a light or window for interpretation.

Retake Policy

A statement should address the retake policy of the office. This should be determined by the dentist through discussion with office personnel. The retake policy should address the number of films that can be reexposed on a patient. In addition, a log of technique errors should be kept to help identify such problems. Once identified, assistance can be provided to correct them.

Protection of Personnel

The physical barriers used for protection should be regularly monitored based on room use. An increase in the workload may alter the protection level. Operators should also monitor their radiation exposure by wearing a **radiation monitoring badge.** Professional companies can provide this service.

QUALITY ASSURANCE POLICY

As discussed in Chapter 17, a quality assurance program should be established for each office, with one person assigned to monitor the program and make sure the appropriate tests are implemented. This would include developing, implementing, and monitoring quality assurance logs for the radiology operatory, darkroom, and interpretation of films. As mentioned earlier, operator errors would also be included.

INFECTION CONTROL POLICY

Each office should have an established, written policy that describes the infection control procedures to be employed. This will serve as a good reference for new employees. Infection control in the radiology area should be consistent with that used in other areas of the office. Procedures should also be in compliance with those stated by the American Dental Association, OSHA, and local state and regional agencies. All patients should be treated as though they are infectious. A protocol should be designed that would prevent the transmission of disease from patient to patient, operator to patient, and patient to operator. One person in the office should be designated as the infection control coordinator. The responsibilities of this person would include establishing, implementing, and monitoring policies and procedures governing infection control. New personnel should receive training in proper infection control techniques and information should be updated and training documented.

CONTINUING EDUCATION

The continued education of dental professionals in current radiologic practice cannot be overstressed. This can be accomplished by reading journals, attending meetings, and participating in continuing education programs. Up-to-date knowledge will help to provide the best care possible to your patient.

SUMMARY

This chapter discussed various components of the dental office that should be monitored and evaluated on a regular basis to ensure the rendering of good dental care to patients. To obtain desired results, these responsibilities should be assigned to specific personnel. Good record-keeping is a must in withstanding today's legal challenges. Established written policies describing the use of ionizing radiation and infection control procedures are necessary to improve communication between dental personnel and with patients and to aid in the provision of good dental care. Finally, dental professionals should recognize the need for lifelong learning in order to remain current in providing acceptable care.

BIBLIOGRAPHY

BURRINGTON B. Selling Your Practice: Legal Considerations When Transferring Patient Records. *Wisconsin Dent Assoc J*. 1987; 63:575.

COMMITTEE ON INFECTION CONTROL GUIDELINES. American Academy of Oral and Maxillofacial Radiology Infection Control Guidelines for Dental Radiographic Procedures. *Oral Surg Oral Med Oral Pathol*. 1992; 73:248–249.

CURTIS JW, ZARKOWSKI P, FERINGA SD. Risk Management: Protecting against Litigation in Dentistry. *J Mich Dent Assoc*. 1987; 69:497–502.

DILLON MT. Records: Your Most Reliable Witness. *Wisconsin Dent Assoc J*. 1986; 62:252–253, 255.

GOSSELIN CE. The Use and Transfer of Patient Records. *J Dentaire Du Québec* 1989; 26:472–473.

KERSTETTER CA. Informed Consent: A Professional Obligation. *Ohio Dent J*. 1988; 62:34–36.

MILES DA, LOVAS JGL, LOYENS S. Radiographs and the Responsible Dentist. *Gen Dent*. 1989; 5:201–206.

NORA RL. Dental Malpractice: Its Causes and Cures. *Quintessence International* 1986; 17:121–126.

RAUCHER F, SCHWARTZ H, RUBIN A. The Biodontics of Informed Consent. *NY State Dent J*. 1981; 47:533.

VOLD M. Good Recordkeeping Vital in Dental Risk Management. *CDS Review* 1986; 79:30–31.

VOLD M. More on Dental Recordkeeping. *CDS Review* 1987; 80:43–45.

WEBER RD. Dental Records: Ownership and Access. *J Mich Dent Assoc*. 1987; 69:623.

REVIEW QUESTIONS

1. For legal purposes, all radiographic records should

    a. be written in pencil or erasable pen.
    b. include the patient's social security number only.
    c. include date of exposure.
    d. All of the above
    e. None of the above

2. Informed consent is a necessary component of risk management.

   a. True
   b. False

3. Films should be mounted with the bump —————.

   a. Convex
   b. Concave

4. The transfer of radiographs should include

   a. chart documentation.
   b. verbal request from patient.
   c. original radiographs.
   d. All of the above
   e. None of the above

5. A policy on the use of ionizing radiation should include all *except*

   a. retake policy.
   b. interpretation of the radiographic image.
   c. quality assurance.
   d. equipment.
   e. All of the above

Answers
to Review Questions

Chapter 1

1. a. Exhibits differential
      attenuation
   b. Causes a screen to
      fluoresce
   c. Made of pure energy
      (has no mass)
   d. Travels in straight lines
   e. Has no charge
2. b
3. a
4. b
5. a

Chapter 2

1. d
2. e

3. a
4. b
5. Environmental Protection
   Agency (EPA) and
   American Dental
   Association (ADA)

Chapter 3

1. a
2. c
3. b
4. a. Mitotic delay
   b. Cell death
   c. Genetic damage
5. a
6. a. Skin
   b. Thyroid gland
   c. Lens of the eye

d. Bone marrow
e. Reproductive organs
f. Fetus/embryo

7. (N-18) × 5 rem
8. a. Time
   b. Distance
   c. Shielding

Chapter 4

1. b
2. c
3. c
4. a
5. d
6. b

Chapter 5

1. a
2. a
3. d
4. d
5. b
6. b
7. b

Chapter 6

1. a. Silver bromide
   b. Silver iodide
2. a. Developing
   b. Fixing
   c. Washing
   d. Drying
3. c
4. Water
5. Fixer
6. The radiograph will eventually fade and discolor.
7. b
8. a

Chapter 7

1. a. X-rays should be emitted from the smallest source of radiation possible.
   b. The focal spot to target distance should be as long as possible.
   c. The object to film distance should be as short as possible.
   d. The film and long axis of the object should be parallel.
   e. The x-ray beam should be perpendicular to the film.
2. e
3. e
4. b
5. a

Chapter 8

1. a. Periapical
   b. Bitewing
2. a. Film placement, vertical alignment, horizontal alignment, cone centering
   b. Film placement, horizontal alignment, cone centering, vertical alignment
   c. Film placement, horizontal alignment, vertical alignment, cone centering
   d. Film placement, cone centering, horizontal alignment, vertical alignment
3. d
4. a

5. b
6. c
7. Vertical
8. a

Chapter 9

1. b
2. d
3. d
4. b
5. a.

Chapter 10
1. a. To locate pathology
   b. With patients with limited opening
   c. To locate fractures
   d. To locate supernumerary or impacted teeth
   e. To locate foreign bodies
   f. On small children
2. b
3. a
4. a. Buccal object rule
   b. Tube shift technique
5. b

Chapter 11

1. b
2. d
3. a
4. e
5. d

Chapter 12

1. c
2. d
3. c

4. b
5. a
6. a

Chapter 13

1. c
2. d
3. a
4. b
5. b
6. c

Chapter 14
1. c
2. d
3. d
4. d
5. c
6. a

Chapter 15

1. b
2. a
3. d
4. a
5. b
6. a

Chapter 16

1. b
2. c
3. a
4. d
5. b
6. b
7. a
8. b
9. d
10. a

Chapter 17

1. d
2. b
3. e
4. a
5. b
6. d

Chapter 18

1. c
2. b

3. d
4. a

Chapter 19

1. c
2. a
3. a
4. a
5. e

Glossary

Aberrations   Deviations from standard.

Absorbed dose   The amount of energy imparted by ionizing radiation to a unit mass of irradiated material at a place of interest. The unit of absorbed dose in the traditional (cgs) system is the rad (100 ergs/gram). The currently accepted unit of absorbed dose is the gray (Gy). (Gy = 1 Joule/kilogram)

Accelerators   This chemical serves to swell the film emulsion and provides an alkaline medium during processing.

Activator   This gives the solution the proper ph and neutralizes any remaining developer on the film. It also acts to aid the other processing chemicals in their activity.

Actual focal spot   That area of the target (tungsten) that is always larger than the effective focal size. It is the area of the anode upon which the electrons strike.

Acute effects   Effects that are usually the result of high doses of radiation (usually over the whole body). The symptoms of these "acute" effects

Some definitions were taken and/or adapted from (by permission) Schiff, TS. Glossary of Maxillofacial Radiology. 3d ed. American Academy of Oral and Maxillofacial Radiology, 1990.

may include nausea, vomiting, hemorrhage, diarrhea, fever, loss of hair, and death.

ALARA Principle This principle emphasizes that the dose to the patient should be kept as low as reasonably achievable under the given set of circumstances. It should be employed in all radiographic procedures.

Alternating current A flow of electrons in one direction followed by a flow of electrons in the opposite direction.

Aluminum filter Any of various thicknesses of aluminum used as filtration in an x-ray beam to absorb the longer wavelength, less-penetrating x-radiation.

Aluminum step wedge A device consisting of increments of different thicknesses of an absorber (aluminum, plastic, etc.) through which a radiographic exposure is made on film. A radiograph of the step wedge produces an image of multiple densities with each density representing a different thickness and a different amount of radiation reaching the film. From such data, conclusions may be drawn as to the initial intensity and penetrative power of the radiation, the effect of processing on density, and the quantitative assessment of machine parameters.

Alveolar bone The part of the maxilla and mandible in which the sockets for the teeth are situated.

Ampere The unit of intensity of an electric current produce by 1 volt acting through a resistance of 1 ohm.

Angulation The direction of the primary beam of radiation in relation to object and film.

Anode The positive terminal of an x-ray tube; a tungsten block embedded in a copper stem and set at an angel to the cathode. The anode emits x-rays from the point of impact of the electron stream from the cathode.

Anomaly A marked deviation from the normal or a departure from the regular order of things.

Anterior nasal spine This structure appears as a radiopaque area at the base of the nasal septum. It represents a bony protuberance to which the nasal cartilage is attached.

Anterior wall of the maxillary sinus A radiopaque line separating the nasal fossa and the maxillary sinus that appears around the maxillary canine region.

Arthrography Radiographic evaluation of a joint after injection of radiopaque contrast material.

Atom The smallest particle of an element that has the characteristic properties of that element.

Atomic number The number of protons in the nucleus.

Attenuation The process by which a beam of radiation is reduced in intensity when passing through some material. It is the combination of absorption and scattering processes that leads to a decrease in flux density of the beam when projected through matter.

Autotransformer A special single-coil transformer that provides the voltage selected by the kVp dial.

Base layer The thin, transparent sheet of cellulose acetate or similar material that carries the radiation- and light-sensitive emulsion of x-ray films.

Beam An emission of electromagnetic radiation or particles.

Benign lesions New growths containing tissue similar to the tissue from where they originate. They grow slowly and usually do not metastasize (or spread to other parts of the body).

Binding energy The energy needed to eject an electron from a particular shell in the atom.

Bisecting angle technique A technique for the radiographic exposure of intraoral films whereby the central axis or central ray of the x-ray beam is directed at right angles to a plane determined by bisecting the angle formed by (1) the long axis of the tooth or teeth being radiographed and (2) the plane in which the film is positioned behind the teeth.

Bite block In intraoral radiography, a film holder that the patient bites on to provide stable retention of the film packet or orientation of tooth position. In panoramic radiography, a tooth positioned to obtain correct orientation of the dentition within the image layer of the panoramic machine.

Bitewing The x-ray shadow images of crown, necks, and coronal third of the roots of both upper and lower teeth and dental arches.

Bitewing tab A cardboard tab or "wing" in the center of the film packet that the patient bites upon when exposing the projection that images the crowns of the maxillary and mandibular teeth.

Bremsstrahlung radiation (white radiation) A spectral distribution of x-rays ranging from very low energy photons to those produced by the peak kilovoltage applied across an x-ray tube. Bremsstrahlung or "braking radiation," refers to the sudden deceleration of electrons (cathode rays) as they interact with highly positively charged (high atomic number) nuclei such as tungsten.

Buccal object rule This rule states that a buccal (or facial) object will move in the same direction as the beam is directed. For example, as the beam is directed mesially, the buccal object appears to shift mesially.

Bureau of Mines and Mining Safety and Health Administration This bureau is responsible for occupational radiation protection regulation for uranium mines.

Bureau of Radiological Health (BRH) (now the National Center for Devices and Radiological Health) This organization regulates the manufacturing of radiation producing equipment such as x-ray machines and microwaves.

Cancellous bone Bone having a reticular, spongy, or lattice-like structure and corresponding medullary radiographic appearance.

Canine fossa This fossa may be seen in the canine region because of an indentation in the surface of the maxilla in that area (this is also known as the lateral fossa).

Caries A radiolucent lesion that appears in the crown or root of the tooth. Also known as tooth decay.

Cassette A light-tight container in which x-ray films are placed for exposure to x-radiation.

Cathode A negative electrode from which electrons are emitted. In x-ray tubes, the cathode usually consists of a spiral tungsten filament housed in a molybdenum focusing cup to focus the electron emission toward the target of the anode.

Cathode rays A stream of electrons passing from the hot filament of the cathode to the target or anode in an x-ray tube; the speed will be approximately one-third the speed of light, depending on the impressed potential.

Central ray The theoretical center of the x-ray beam. The term is employed to designate the direction of the x-rays in a given projection; may be considered to extend from the focal spot of the x-ray film.

Cephalostat A head holder used in cephalometric radiography. An instrument that makes it possible to reposition the patient's head for reproductibility purpose.

Cervical burnout This appears as radiolucent areas at the CEJ. It is caused by a decreased density of the tooth structure in that area and thus a lessened absorption of the x-ray beam as it passes through the tooth. This creates wedge-shaped radiolucent areas at the CEJ. Cervical burnout mimics the appearance of caries.

Characteristic curve The relationship between the blackness or density on a film and the amount of x-ray exposure the film has encountered can be measured and plotted on a graph

Characteristic (discrete) radiation Electromagnetic radiation produced by electron transitions from higher energy orbitals to replace ejected electrons of inner electron orbitals. The energy of the electromagnetic radiation emitted is unique or "characteristic" of the emitting atom (element). The wavelength of the emitted radiation is specific for the element used.

Chronic effects (because of radiation exposure) These effects, which are usually shown as a decrease in the tissue to resist trauma and infection, are usually produced over a long period of time.

Clarke's rule This rule states that a buccal (or facial) object will move in the same direction as the beam is directed. For example, as the beam is directed mesially, the buccal object appears to shift mesially.

Clearing agents These chemicals change the unexposed silver halide crystals to soluble compounds that can be washed away. This helps to produce the gray and clear areas on the fully processed film.

Collimation/collimator A device used for the elimination of the peripheral, divergent, portion of the useful x-ray beam, by means of metal tubes, "cones," or diaphragms interposed in the path of the beam. Rectangular technique to limit the primary beam to approximate the size of intraoral radiographic film.

Comminuted fracture A fracture in which the bone is shattered or crushed.

Compound fracture A fracture in which there is communication with the outside environment. The bone lacerates the skin or mucosa. This is common in the mandible where teeth are fractured during the trauma.

Compton scatter radiation (scatter radiation) The incident radiation has sufficient energy to dislodge a bound electron, but attacks a loosely bound electron. The remaining radiation energy proceeds in a different direction as scatter radiation.

Computed tomography (CT) The technique by which multidirectional x-ray transmission data through a body is mathematically reconstructed by a computer to form a cross-sectional representation (slice) of a patient's anatomy. CT is used as an acronym to designate any technical field associated with these techniques.

Cone A device on a dental x-ray machine designed to indicate the direction of the central ray and to serve as a guide in establishing a desired source to film distance. Such may be rectangular or cylindrical. Provision for beam collimation and/or added filtration is often incorporated in the construction of the cone.

Cone cut Failure to cover or expose the entire area of a radiograph with the useful beam, thereby only partially exposing the film.

Contrast The difference in densities appearing on a radiograph, representing the various degrees of beam attenuation.

Contrast media A radiopaque material introduced into organs so that the outline of structures can be discerned.

Coronoid process The superior, anterior process of the ramus of the mandible, to which the temporal muscle is attached. The notch of the superior ramus directly posterior to the coronoid process.

Cortical bone A dense, lamellar structure, the layers of which are a three-dimensional system. Cortical or compact bone comprises the hard surface of all bones, but varies in thickness in different bones.

Coulomb per kilogram (C/kg) The unit of electrical charge equal to 3×10^9 esu, and equal to the total charge of 6.25×10^{18} electrons.

Crestal bone   That portion of the alveolar bone that extends from tooth to tooth. It appears radiopaque

Critical organs   Those which either react most unfavorably to radiation or, by their nature, attract and absorb specific radiochemicals.

Cross-sectional occlusal   A view of the mandible that allows dental practitioners to study the floor of the mouth. This view is similar to looking at the mandible from below.

Daylight loader   Method of loading, unloading, and feeding films into the processor in normal room light. This system entails the use of special equipment; there is no need for a darkroom.

Dead-man switch   A switch or control that can maintain function only by continuous pressure by the operator.

Density   The degree of darkening of exposed and processed photographic or x-ray film.

Detail   A visual quality that depends on sharpness. Factors that influence detail include: (1) the size of the tube focal spot, (2) the source to film distance, (3) the distance of the object from the film, (4) motion of the object or x-ray source, (5) type of intensifying screens, and (6) image contrast.

Developer   A chemical solution with active ingredients designed to change the silver halide crystals to metallic silver, and thus change the latent image to a visible image.

Direct effect   This occurs when a molecule is in the direct path of the radiation and is altered in its function. Subsequently, it can lead to cellular changes.

Direct exposure film   Film that has high sensitivity to the direct action of x-rays, but has low sensitivity to screen fluorescence.

Distal   Remote; farther from any point of reference; e.g., midline

Disto-oblique radiograph   An image useful for viewing the most posterior areas of the mouth, such as impacted third molars.

Distortion   An inaccuracy in the size or shape of an object as it is displayed in the radiograph. Distortion is brought about by misalignment of the cone relative to the object or by excessive film-object distance.

Dose equivalent   The product of absorbed dose and modifying factors, namely the quality factor, distribution factor, and any other necessary factors. The traditional unit of dose equivalence is the rem (rads $\times$ qualifying factors). The SI (mks) unit of dose equivalence is the Sievert (Grays $\times$ qualifying factors).

Dose rate   The dose, in rads, absorbed per unit time, in rads/sec.

Dose response curve   Shows the relationship between the radiation dose given and the biological response that is exhibited.

Dosimeter (radiation meter)   An instrument used to detect and measure an accumulated dosage of radiation.

Double exposure   Two superimposed exposures on the same radiographic or photographic film.

Edge gradient   The area that surrounds the umbra and has a shady or hazy appearance.

Effective focal spot   The apparent size and shape of the focal spot when viewed from a position in the useful beam. With the use of a suitably inclined anode face, it is smaller than the actual focal spot size.

Electromagnetic radiation   Forms of energy propagated by wave motion as photons or discrete quanta. The radiations have no matter associated with them. They differ widely in wavelength, frequency, and photon energy and have strikingly different properties. Covering an enormous range of wavelengths (from 10^{17} to 10^{-6} Angstroms) they include radio waves, infrared waves, visible light, ultraviolet radiation, x-rays, gamma rays, and cosmic radiation.

Electron   A negatively charged elementary particle with a mass of 0.000549 amu, or 9.1×10^{-28} grams.

Elongation   A form of radiographic distortion in which the image is longer than the object radiographed.

Emulsion layer   This contains the actual material with which the x-rays interact in order to record the radiographic image. The emulsion is composed of a mixture of gelatin and silver halide crystals.

Energy   The ability to do work.

Environmental Protection Agency (EPA)   The agency responsible for setting acceptable environmental radiation standards.

Exposure   A measure of the ionization produced in air by x- (or gamma) radiation. It is the sum of the electrical charges on all of the ions of one sign produced in air when all electrons liberated by photons in a volume element of air are completely stopped in air, divided by the mass of the air in the volume element. The traditional unit of exposure is the roentgen (R). No specific unit of exposure is designated in the accepted SI (mks) system, although the coulomb/kilogram would be conceptually equivalent.

External oblique ridge   A ridge originating from the anterior border of the ramus of the mandible extending to the lateral body of the mandible in the molar region.

Extraoral   An examination of the teeth and bones made by placing the film or cassette against the side of the head or face and projecting the x-rays from a position opposite to the side of the head or face.

Extraoral radiography   Examination in which the film is placed outside of the mouth.

Faceplate   That portion of the film-holding device that aligns the cone.

Filament   A coiled tungsten wire, which when heated to incandescence, emits electrons.

Film-holding devices   Devices that not only decrease the retake errors made on radiographs, but can decrease the amount of tissue irradiated by blocking the portion of the beam that does not reach the film.

Film mount   A holder designed to organize radiographs so that they can be displayed for diagnosing films.

Film packet   A light-proof, moisture-resistant, sealed paper or plastic envelope containing x-ray film used in the making of radiographs.

Film speed   The amount of exposure to light or x-rays (the latter in roentgens) required to produce a given image density. It is expressed as the reciprocal of the exposure in roentgens necessary to produce a density of 1.0 above base and fog; films are classified on this basis in six speed groups, from A through F.

Filter   Material (usually aluminum) placed in the path of the useful beam to absorb preferentially the less energetic (less penetrating) x-rays.

Filtration   The use of absorbers or filters for the preferential attenuation of radiation of certain wavelengths from a useful primary beam of x-radiation.

Fixer   The solution in which the manifest image is fixed and hardened, removing the silver halide crystals from the exposed film that has been unexposed to or unaffected by the action of the x-radiation.

Floor of the nasal cavity   The floor of the nasal cavity is a thin line of bone that forms the lower boundaries of the nasal fossae. This structure appears as a curved, radiopaque line.

Floor of the nasal fossa   This thin, radiopaque line is often seen over the maxillary premolar area and represents the floor of the nasal fossa.

Fluorescence   Light emitted promptly within 10^{-8} seconds after absorption of an x-ray photon by photoelectric or compton interaction. The emission occurs essentially only during the period of irradiation.

Fluorescent layer   The active part of the screen. This layer contains the phosphors that convert the x-ray photons into visible light.

Focal spot   That part of the target anode of an x-ray tube that is bombarded by the focused electron stream when the tube is energized.

Focusing cup   Along with the filament, the focusing cup determines the size and shape of the target (focal) spot. The cup is constructed of molybdenum.

Fog (fogging)   A darkening of the whole or part of a radiograph by sources other than the radiation of the primary beam to which the film was exposed.

Foramen An opening through the skull that allows for the passage of nerves.

Foreshortening A form of distortion in which the image is shorter than the object radiographed. In the angle bisecting technique, it is caused by misdirecting the x-ray beam perpendicular to the plane of the film instead of the plane of the bisector (i.e., the vertical angulation is too steep).

Fractions Intervals between exposures.

Frankfort horizontal plane A plane made from the inferior border of the orbit through the superior border of the external auditory meatus.

Full mouth examination A series of projections that provide a radiographic view of the maxilla and mandible. It generally consists of 18 films with periapicals and bitewing projections.

Gag reflex An involuntary reaction when an object is placed or thought to be placed too far down the throat.

Gamma radiation Short wavelength electromagnetic radiation of nuclear origin, within a range of wavelengths from about 10^{-8} to 10^{-11} cm.

Genetic effect Changes produced in the genes and chromosomes of all nucleated body cells. In customary usage, the term relates to the effect produced in the reproductive cells.

Genial tubercles Bony prominence on the posterior surface of the mandible on either side of the symphysis.

Gray (Gy) A new unit of radiation measurement established in 1974 by the International Commission on Radiation Units and Measurements to be phased into general use by 1985. One gray (Gy) = 1 joule/kg = 100 rads. The gray is a unit of absorbed dose and will replace the rad.

Green-stick fracture The bone bends like a twig and fractures only one cortical plate.

Grid A device used to prevent scattered radiation from reaching the film. It consists essentially of a series of narrow lead strips closely spaced, and separated by spacers of low-density material.

Grid ratio The ratio of the height of the lead strips to the width of the interspacing, the height being conventionally stated first, and considerably exceeding the interspace width.

H and D curve A characteristic curve of a photographic emulsion obtained by plotting film density against the logarithm of the exposure. Also called the Hurter and Driffield curve, after the British scientists who developed it.

Half-life (physical half-life) The time required for a radioactive substance to lose 50 percent of its activity by decay. Each radionuclide has a unique half-life, a characteristic often used in the identification of radionuclides.

Half-value layer (HVL) The thickness of a layer of a specified material that reduces the beam intensity to one-half its original value.

Hamulus   This bony projection appears radiopaque and extends downward from the medial pterygoid plate. It is located behind the maxillary tuberosity region.

Hardener   Hardeners help to toughen and shrink the gelatin in the film emulsion. This also helps to reduce the drying time needed at the completion of the processing.

Heel effect   A variation of intensity over the cross-section of a useful x-ray beam that occurs as a result of the angle at which the x-rays emerge from beneath the surface of the focal spot. This causes a differential attenuation of photons comprising the useful beam.

Horizontal angulation   The position of the cone/position-indicating device, with movement occurring in a right-to-left direction (horizontal).

Horizontal bone loss   Bone loss that occurs evenly between two adjacent teeth.

Hydroquinone   This is responsible for blackening the exposed silver halide crystal and for bringing out the contrast.

ICRP   Abbreviation for International Commission on Radiologic Protection

ICRU   Abbreviation for International Commission on Radiation Units and Measurements

Image contrast   The result of two factors: film contrast and subject contrast.

Image receptor   This receives the x-ray image after the x-ray photons have interacted and passed through the patient. Dental x-ray film is one such image receptor. Other types of image receptors used in everyday life include the television monitor and photographic film.

Incisive foramen   This structure is an opening through which the nasopalatine nerves and artery pass. This area appears as a radiolucent, oval-shaped structure between the central incisors.

Indirect effect   This occurs when the impaired cell or molecule induces disruptions in the structure or function of regulatory molecules.

Indirect exposure film   This is used in combination with a cassette film holder and screen.

Inferior border of the mandible   If a mandibular radiograph is exposed using an extreme negative angulation, the inferior border of the mandible can be seen as a radiopaque ridge below the anterior teeth.

Intensifying screen   A devise used to convert x-ray energy to light energy. It consists of a card or plastic sheet coated with fluorescent material, positioned singly or in pairs in a cassette to contact the film. When the cassette is exposed to x-radiation, the light emitted from the fluorescent screen exposes the film and produces the latent image.

Internal oblique ridge (mylohyoid ridge)   This ridge is a bony prominence that provides an attachment site for the mylohyoid muscle to the internal surface of the mandible. It is seen as a wide, curved, radiopaque line extending downward and anteriorly in the molar region. It is often superimposed over the roots of the molar teeth.

Interpretation   The study of a radiograph, the analysis of what is seen, and the integration of the findings with the case history and laboratory and clinical examination to arrive at a diagnosis. The dentist does not diagnose the radiograph; rather he/she studies and interprets its image.

Interproximal   The mesial and distal surfaces of the tooth crown where the adjacent tooth touches.

Interradicular bone loss   Bone loss that occurs between the roots.

Intraoral radiograph   Radiograph produced on a film placed intraorally and lingually, or palatally, to the teeth.

Inverse Square Law   A law that states that in either vacuum or matter, radiation intensity decreases with distance from the source. In the case of a true point source, the reduction is inversely proportional to the square of the distance from the source. In the case of sources of finite size, the decrease of intensity is less rapid, particularly in the vicinity of the source.

Ionization   The process or the result of a process by which a neutral atom or molecule acquires either a positive or a negative charge.

Ionizing radiation   Electromagnetic radiation (e.g., x-rays or gamma rays) or particulate radiation (e.g., electrons, neutrons, protons), capable of ionizing air directly or indirectly.

Ion pair   Two particles of opposite charge, usually referring to the electron and the positive atomic residue resulting after the interaction of an ionizing radiation photon with an orbital electron of an atom. The average energy required to produce an ion pair is approximately 33 eV for air.

Kilovoltage (in x-ray machines)   The potential difference between the anode and cathode of an x-ray tube.

Lamina dura   The thin plate of dense or compact bone that lines the tooth sockets. It appears on a radiograph as a fine radiopaque line passing around the tooth.

Latent image   The invisible change produced in an x-ray or photographic film emulsion by the action of x-radiation or light, from which the visible image is subsequently developed and fixed chemically.

Latent period   The period between the time of exposure of tissue to an injurious agent (e.g., radiation) and the clinical manifestation of a particular response.

Lateral fossa   This fossa appears as a radiolucent area between the lateral incisor and the canine. This structure represent a depression in the surface of the maxilla in that area.

Lateral jaw projection (lateral oblique of the mandible)   An examination in which the film is placed adjacent to the ramus or the body of the mandible. The rays are directed obliquely upward from the opposite side and the central beam is directed at the point of interest. The vertical angulation is such as to cast the image of the near mandible superior and/or anterior to the area of interest.

Lateral skull projection   An examination in which the film is placed parallel to the sagittal plane of the head with the rays directed at right angles to the plane of the film. The entire skull is shown.

Linear energy transfer (LET)   The linear rate of loss of energy by an ionizing particle traversing a medium.

Line-focus principle   A principle employed in the design of x-ray tubes, by which the effective focal spot is sharply reduced relative to the actual focal spot, which is made larger, to compensate for the heat generated.

Lingual foramen   This structure appears as a tiny, radiopaque hole below the roots of the mandibular central incisors. This foramen provides an opening through which a small blood vessel can pass.

Lip line   Often the soft tissue of the lip can be seen as a radiopaque, curved line below the crowns of the mandibular teeth.

Localization   The making of a radiograph for the purpose of identifying a site in relation to surrounding tissues.

Mach band effect   A simulated appearance of caries due to the optical illusion presented from a light and dark object placed next to one another.

Magnetic resonance imaging (MRI)   Use of magnetic resonance to create images of the body. Currently it primarily involves imaging the distribution of mobile hydrogen nuclei (protons) in the body.

Magnification distortion   The enlargement or distortion of a radiographic image recorded on film emulsion. It can be minimized by reducing the object-film distance and increasing the focus-film distance.

Malar process (Typical "U" or "J" shape)   This radiopaque shape appears superimposed over the maxillary molars and represents the bony structure which joins the maxilla, frontal, and temporal bones.

Malignant lesions   These grow rapidly and may spread through the vascular and lymphatic systems. Many may metastasize and be considered life threatening.

Mandibular canal   This canal extends the length of the mandible and provides a passageway for blood vessels and nerves. It appears as a radiolucent band following the roots of the mandibular posterior teeth.

Mandibular tori   Tori are bony protuberances often seen as small, rounded, radiopaque areas superimposed on the roots of the teeth in the canine and premolar regions of the mandible.

Maxillary sinus   This is an air-filled space above the maxillary premolars and molars that appears radiolucent.

Maxillary tuberosity   This bony structure appears as a bulge distal to the maxillary molars and at the end of the maxillary alveolar ridges.

Maximum permissible dose (MPD)   For radiation workers, 5 rad per year is permissible. The MPD formula is: MPD = 5(N-18) rads or rems. Five represents the permitted yearly dose. N represents the individual's present age. Eighteen represents the 18 years of the individual's life when he/she was not exposed to radiation.

Mental foramen   This structure provides a means for the blood vessels and nerves to supply the lower lip. It appears as a radiolucent, round or oval-shaped area located near the apices of the mandibular premolars. This structure is often misinterpreted as some type of periapical lesion.

Mental ridge   The mental ridge is a bony prominence on the external portion of the mandible, which extends in a sloping fashion from the premolar area to the central incisors. It appears as a radiopaque, curved ridge below the mandibular anterior teeth.

Mesial   The proximal surface of the tooth toward the center of the dental arch.

Midpalatine suture   This structure appears as a thin, radiolucent line between the central incisors. This line represents the area where the bony plates come together to form the palate.

Milliampere-impulses (mIs)   The product of the x-ray tube operating amperage and exposure time, in impulses.

Milliampere-seconds (mAs)   The product of the x-ray tube operating amperage and exposure time, in seconds.

Molecule   The smallest quantity of matter that can exist by itself and retain its chemical properties. It is composed of one or more atoms.

Multilocular   Term used to describe the inner portion of a radiolucent lesion that exhibits more than one compartment.

Nasal fossa   This is the air-filled radiolucent area inside the nasal cavity.

Nasal septum   This is the thin line of bone that separates the right and left nasal cavities. In the radiograph, the nasal septum appears as a radiopaque line.

National Council on Radiation Protection and Measurements (NCRP)   A nonprofit agency that makes recommendations on occupational radiation exposure.

National Evaluation of X-ray Trends (NEXT)   A program carried out jointly by the state and federal governments in order to compile nationwide data on radiation exposure in dental offices.

Neutron   An elementary particle having a rest mass of 1.00894 atomic mass units of no electrical charge.

Nonstochastic effects   These have threshold doses. It is believed that below these threshold doses, the effects do not occur. In addition, the severity of the effect is increased as the dose is increased. An example of this is erythema of the skin.

Nuclear medicine   The branch of medicine concerned with the diagnostic and therapeutic use of radionuclei.

Nuclear Regulatory Commission (NRC)   An organization that establishes radiation protection regulations

Nucleus, atomic   The small central part of an atom containing the protons and neutrons and in which most of the mass is concentrated.

Nutrient canals   These canals provide a means for the blood vessels and nerves to reach the teeth. Nutrient canals can be seen as radiolucent lines extending downward from the mandibular anterior teeth.

Occlusal radiographs   A radiograph made with a film designed for placement between the occlusal surfaces of the teeth, with the x-ray beam directed caudad or cephalad.

Occupational Safety and Health Administration (OSHA)   The agency responsible for occupational radiation protection regulation.

Osteoradionecrosis   Damage and death of normal bone that may result from a curative dose of radiation used in the treatment of malignant or nonmalignant disease.

Overlapping   The projection of one tooth surface onto another (superimposition). It results from incorrect horizontal angulation.

Palate   The roof of the mouth.

Paralleling technique   An intraoral radiographic technique that requires the film to be stabilized in a film holder and positioned so that the film and long axis of the teeth are parallel.

Parallel objects   Two objects equidistant from all other points

Pathogens   Microorganisms that can cause disease.

Penumbra   The secondary shadow that surrounds the periphery of the primary shadow. The term pertains to the shadow proper. A penumbra is the ill-defined margin or shadow produced by light. In radiography, it is the blurred margin of an image detail also called geometric unsharpness.

Periapical projection   A radiograph made by intraoral placement of film for recording shadow images of the outline and the position and mesiodistal extent of the teeth and surrounding tissue. It is the best means available for redisclosing the apices of the teeth and their contiguous tissues.

Periodontal abscess   A radiolucent lesion that develops in the base of a periodontal pocket.

Periodontal ligament space   A radiolucent space that exists between the root of the tooth and bone.

Perpendicular lines   Two lines that intersect at right angles (90 degrees).

Phenidone   This chemical works quickly to develop the lighter areas of the film, thereby creating the gray areas in the processed radiographs.

Photoelectric effect   The ejection of bound electrons by an incident photon such that the whole energy of the photon is absorbed and transitional or characteristic x-ray emissions are produced.

PID   Film-holding device that allows technicians to align the film and the beam in the proper manner to produce a good quality radiograph.

Pneumatization   Formation of pneumatic cells or cavities in tissue.

Position indicating device   A device that aligns the cone/collimator to the film holding device.

Preservatives   Chemicals that inhibit oxidation of the reducing agents by air. Sodium sulfite is the chemical usually employed. See also under Developer and Fixer.

Primary radiation beam   All radiation coming directly from the target of the anode of an x-ray tube.

Processing, film   Chemical transformation of the latent image into a stable image. The usual procedure is basically a selective reduction of affected silver halide salts to metallic silver grains (development), followed by the selective removal of unaffected silver halide (fixation), washing to remove the processing chemicals, and drying.

Processor   The equipment that houses the processing chemicals needed to develop exposed radiographic film. This may be an automatic machine or manual tanks.

Projection   A term for the position of a part of the patient with relation to the x-ray film and the x-ray beam.

Protective layer   A layer placed on the screen to make it more resistant to such damages as scratches and abrasions. In addition, this layer reduces the chance of static electricity production.

Proton   An elementary nuclear particle with a positive electric charge equal to 1.007594 mass units.

Pulp   The anatomical portion of the tooth that contains the nerve and blood supply for the tooth. The radiographic appearance is radiolucent.

Quality assurance   Refers to the mechanisms used to assure the continuous optimal functioning of both technical and operational aspects of radiology.

Quality factor (QF)   The linear-energy-transfer-dependent factor by which absorbed doses are multiplied to obtain (for radiation protection purposes) a quantity that expresses the effect of the absorbed dose on a common scale for all ionizing radiations.

Radiation absorbed dose (rad)   A unit of measurement for the absorbed dose of any type of ionizing radiation in any medium. One rad is the energy absorption of 100 ergs per gram.

Radiation caries   Caries caused by changes in the saliva due to radiation therapy. The decreased flow, increased acidity, and shift in oral flora all contribute to increased caries action. Usually the caries occur at the gingival margin. The patient's risk for increased caries remains high throughout his/her lifetime.

Radiation monitoring badge   A device that monitors the amount of exposure a person receives to ionizing radiation through occupational exposure. This is usually monitored for a specified time period (i.e., monthly).

Radioactive tracer (radioisotope)   The isotope of an element used for diagnostic observations. The observations may be made by measurement of radioactivity or isotopic abundance.

Radiograph   A visible image on a radiation-sensitive film emulsion produced by chemical processing after exposure of the film emulsion to ionizing radiation that has passed through an area, region, or substance of interest.

Radiographic mottle   This is often compared to "snow" on a television picture or static on radio. Radiographic mottle is any undesirable variation in density caused by have too few photons creating the image.

Radiography   The process of making radiographs.

Radiolucency   The appearance of dark images on film because of the greater amount of radiation that penetrates the structures and reaches the film.

Radiolucent   This permits the passage of radiant energy with relatively little attenuation by absorption.

Radiolysis of water   The water molecule represents about 75 percent of the body's total number of molecules. As such, it is involved in the greatest number of interactions when the body is exposed to x-ray photons.

Radiopacity   The appearance of light images on film because of the lesser amount of radiation that penetrates the structures and reaches the film.

Radiopaque   A structure that strongly inhibits the passage of radiant energy.

Radioprotectors   Chemical agents that inhibit the indirect effects of radiation by taking up the free radicals and thus arresting the production of hydrogen peroxide.

Radiosensitizers   Chemicals that can increase the radiation effects.

Rectification   Conversion of alternating current to direct current.

Reducing agents   Chemicals that "reduce" (or change) the exposed silver halide crystal to black metallic silver.

Reflective coat (on screens)   This is placed next to the base and serves to redirect light from the fluorescent layer back to the film. This helps to increase the number of light photons reaching the film.

Relative biological effectiveness (RBE)   The relative biologic potency of a given kind of ionizing radiation. Quantitatively, this is the number of rads of 250 kV x-rays required to produce a given biologic end point, divided by the number of rads of the given type of radiation needed to produce the same effect, for identical timing, dosage distribution, and other relevant exposure factors. Used primarily in radiobiologic research and radiotherapy; the more approximate quality factor (QF) is used in radiation protection work.

Replenishment   The addition of solution to the original developer and fixer. In order to maintain the activity of the solutions, as well as the level (or volume) of the solutions (some evaporates and some is carried out on the films into the water), replenishment is necessary.

Resolution   A term that relates to the ability of a film to record an in-focus or true image. This is often seen as the ability of the radiographic image to discern the boundaries between two objects that are close together.

Restrainers (antifogging agents)   The restrainers act to block the action of the reducing agent on unexposed crystals. Without this chemical, the processed radiographic film would be totally black.

Right angle technique   This technique is accomplished by taking a standard periapical radiograph of the area of interest and then exposing an occlusal radiograph of that arch.

Roentgen (R)   An international unit of exposure based on the ability of radiation to ionize air; an exposure to x- or gamma radiation such that the associated corpuscular emission per 0.0001293 gram of air produces, in air, ions carrying 1 electrostatic unit of quantity of electricity of either sign (2.083 billion ion pairs).

Roentgen-Equivalent-Man (rem)   A unit of dose of any radiation to body tissue in terms of its estimated biological effects relative to an exposure of 1 R of x- or gamma radiation.

Safelight   Special lighting used in the darkroom. It permits film to be transferred from cassette to processor without fogging.

Scatter radiation   Radiation that, during passage through a substance, has been deviated in direction. It may also have been modified by an increase in wavelengths. It is one form of secondary radiation.

Secondary radiation   Particles or photons produced by the interaction of primary radiation with matter.

Self-rectification   Suppression of one-half the sine wave of the alternating current across an x-ray tube. This result from the absence of electrons at the anode side when the polarity is reversed.

Sensitivity speck   This is produced by adding sulfur-containing compounds to the emulsion. These compounds react with the silver halide to form silver sulfide. This area is located on the surface of the crystal and referred to as a sensitivity speck.

Shadow of the nose   The nose can be seen as a soft tissue shadow, usually radiopaque, along the roots of the maxillary incisors.

Sialograph   A radiograph made using contrast media to determine the presence of disease or calcareous deposits in a salivary gland or its ducts.

Sievert (Sv)   The SI unit associated with rem. One rem equals 100 Sv.

Silver halide   Silver compounds, usually silver bromide and silver iodide, embedded in the photographic emulsion of film.

Simple fracture   A fracture in which there is no communication with the outside environment.

Sinus   An air space that appears radiolucent.

Sinus septum   These thin, radiopaque lines appear within the sinuses and represent the bony walls that form the compartments of the sinuses.

Solvent   As with developer, water is the solvent used as the vehicle for mixing the chemicals in the fixer.

Somatic effect   Damage that is manifested in the individual who is exposed to radiation.

Spatial resolution   The smallest distance between two points in the object that can be distinguished as separate details in the image. Generally indicated as a number of black and white line-pairs per millimeter.

Static electricity   A stationary charge of electricity produces tree-like artifacts in film.

Stochastic effects   Those effects effects in which the risk of getting the effects is dependant upon the dose of radiation received. There is no known threshold below which the effects do not occur. An example of a stochastic effect is cancer.

Subject contrast   The difference in image density appearing on a radiograph, representing various degrees of beam attenuation.

Submandibular fossa   A depressed area on the lingual side of the mandible. It appears radiographically as a radiolucent area below the internal oblique ridge.

Submento-vertex projection (base film)   A skull projection with the central ray entering under the chin at right angles to the canthomeatal line.

Subtraction radiography   A photographic or digital method of eliminating background anatomical structures from the final image to bring out the differences between the images being subtracted.

Supplemental radiographs   These include occlusal radiographs, disto-oblique radiographs, localization techniques, edentulous and partially edentulous surveys, endodontic and pediatric projections. Some of these projections require specific types of film as well as unique packet placement and adjustment of technique factors (machine settings).

Target   The area on the anode subject to electron bombardment, usually consisting of a tungsten insert on the end face of a solid copper anode.

Thermoluminescent dosimeter A determination of the amount of radiation to which a thermoluminescent material has been exposed. This is accomplished by heating the material in a specially designed instrument that relates the amount of luminescence emitted to the amount of radiation exposure.

Time–temperature method This method is the most accurate for obtaining a good quality finished radiograph. The film is immersed in the developer for a specific time, according to the temperature of the solution. The film is then washed for approximately 30 seconds and immersed in the fixer for twice the clearing time (the time required for the visible image to appear on the film, not the total developing time), usually 2 to 4 minutes. Finally, the films are placed in the water tank for a 10-minute wash.

Tomography A general term for a technique that provides a fairly distinct image of any selected plane through the body. Tomography is sometimes referred to as "body-section radiography."

Topographical occlusal A radiograph that demonstrates the anterior area of the arch. This view can be taken on either the maxilla or mandible.

Torus A rounded bony growth that has a radiopaque appearance.

Towne projection A skull projection with the central ray entering the frontal bone at 30 degrees to the canthomeatal line.

Transformer An electrical device in which the alternating current in the primary windings induces an alternating voltage in the secondary windings.

Transillumination Transmitting light through the tooth surface to illuminate the interior portion of the tooth.

Trismus Radiation of the mastication muscles or the temporomandibular joint can result in fibrosis of these areas. This can limit the patient's ability to open his/her mouth.

Tubehead The metal housing that contains the anode, cathode, glass envelope, and insulating oil. It is attached to the extension arm mounted on the wall.

Tube shift technique This technique is based on the concept that images will shift in position as the projection angle changes.

Typical Inverted "Y" formation (Y of Ennis) This is a "Y"-shaped, radiopaque line that represents the intersection of the nasal cavity and the maxillary sinus.

Ultrasound Sound waves that are above 20,000 cycles per second or 20,000 Hertz (Hz)—that is, beyond the range of human hearing.

Umbra A complete shadow produced by light, with sharply demarcated margins. In radiography, a sharply delineated image detail.

Unilocular A term used to describe the inner portion of a radiolucent lesion that exhibits only one compartment.

Unit of exposure   The traditional unit of exposure is called the Roentgen (R). This unit is defined as the measurement of exposure of air.

Universal precaution policy   A policy developed for use with all patients, regardless of their medical history, to prevent the transmission of infection and disease.

Vertical angulation   The movement of the cone or position-indicating device in an up and down direction. Improper alignment of the vertical angulation will result in elongation or foreshortening of the radiographic image.

Vertical bone loss   Bone loss that occurs along the root of one tooth at a rate unequal to the adjacent tooth.

Viewbox   A uniform light source on which radiographs are viewed.

Waters projections   A skull radiograph with the central ray projected through the chin 37 degrees below the canthomeatal line. Used primarily for an anterior–posterior view of the maxillary sinuses.

Wavelength   The distance between the peaks of waves in any waveform, such as light, x-rays, and other electromotive forms. In electromagnetic radiation, the wavelength is equal to the velocity of light divided by the frequency of the wave. The distance from any point on a wave to the identical point on an adjacent wave.

Xerostomia   Dry mouth.

X-ray (roentgenrays)   A type of electromagnetic radiation characterized by wavelengths of 100 Angstroms or less.

X-ray tube   An electronic tube in which x-rays are generated.

Index

The letter *f* following a page number indicates a figure; the letter *t* following a page number indicates a table.